MAN OF THE EASTERN SHORE:

The World War II Letters of James Bordley, Jr.

MAN OF THE EASTERN SHORE:

The World War II Letters of James Bordley, Jr.

Charles A. Webb, Jr.

PALMETTO
PUBLISHING
Charleston, SC
www.PalmettoPublishing.com

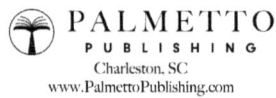

Man of the Eastern Shore: The World War II Letters of James Bordley, Jr.
Copyright © 2023 by Charles A. Webb, Jr.

First Edition

Hardcover ISBN: 979-8-8229-2823-7

CONTENTS

PART TWO
WAR LETTERS

DEDICATION

This is written for the descendants of James Bordley, Jr. who did not have the opportunity to know him. Here is his story and many letters in his own voice. He is an ancestor that you can be proud to have. He saw opportunities that his times provided and was sharp enough to take advantage of them—may you be able to do the same.

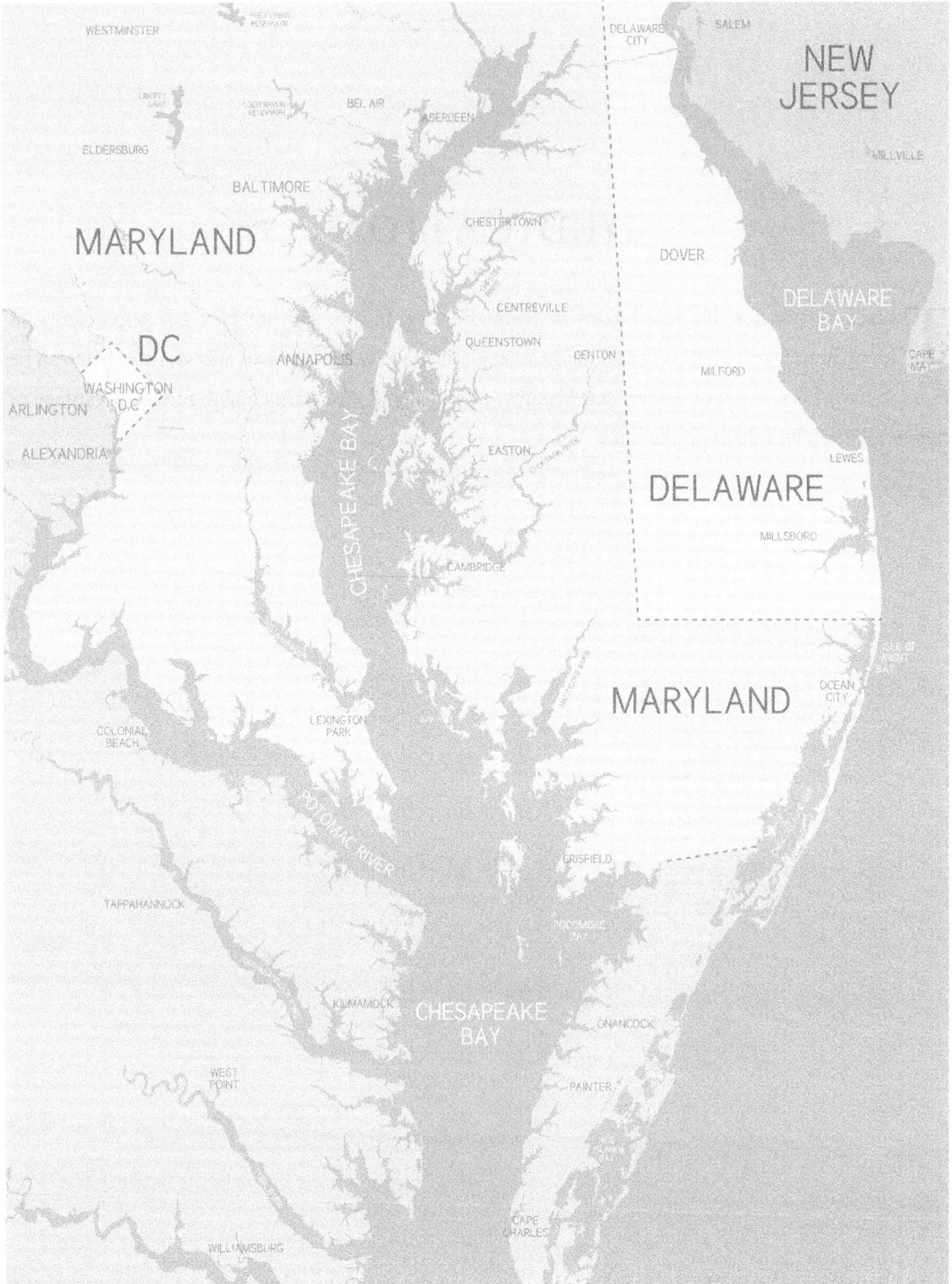

FOREWORD

In June 1942 the two sons of James Bordley, Jr. shipped out to the Pacific. They were both physicians with the 118th General Hospital, a unit formed by the Johns Hopkins Hospital at the start of World War II.

Dr. Bordley started typing letters to them. During the war, he sent over two hundred letters and kept a carbon copy of each letter. These carbons have been in a manila file folder in a cardboard box for at least fifty-five years—first under his son John's bed, then later forgotten in the top of the author's closet.

The question now is what to do with them; I decided to try to have them printed so that his heirs could see them. But this led to the need of trying to explain to his descendants, who never knew him, who Dr. James Bordley, Jr. was.

What started out as a brief biography for a background to the letters turned into a longer-than-intended piece of work. As we started researching and writing, the story of an incredibly vigorous and dynamic man emerged. It is the story of a man of rather impressive accomplishments, whom we had only known as a friendly, warm grandfather we took for granted.

So, the book is in two sections: First is the biography and then come the letters. Either can be read independently, but they complement each other. We doubt that many readers will really want to read all the letters, but we hope that the descendants will want to at least read something of their interesting ancestor and the extraordinary times that shaped his life.

This era, 1870 to 1970, is so well summarized in a March 27, 2016, article by George W. Will, a writer and political commentator for the *Washington Post*, that we will start by quoting several sections. George was reviewing a book by Robert J. Gordon, *The Rise and Fall of American Growth*. It is a pessimistic view on the potential occurrence of another century to follow one of such explosive change. It starts with a nice review of those hundred years, and it is exactly the period of Dr. Bordley's life. George writes,

In many ways, the world of 1870 was more medieval than modern. Three necessities, food, clothing, and shelter absorbed almost all consumer spending. No household was wired for electricity. Flickering light came from candles and whale oil, manufacturing power from steam engines, water wheels and horses. Urban horses, alive and dead, complicated urban sanitation. Window screens were rare, so insects commuted to and fro between animal and human waste, and the dinner table. A typical North Carolina housewife in the 1880s carried water into her home 8–10 times daily walking 148 miles a year to tote 36 tons of it. Few children were in school after age 12.

But on Oct. 10, 1879 Thomas Edison found a cotton filament for the incandescent light bulb. Less than 12 weeks later in Germany, Karl Benz demonstrated the first workable internal combustion engine. In the 1880s refrigerated rail cars began to banish "spring sickness," a result of winters without vegetables. Adult stature increased as mechanical refrigeration and Clarence Birdseye's frozen foods improved nutrition. By 1940, households were networked—electrified, with clean water flowing in and waste flowing out, radio flowing in and telephonic communication flowing both ways. Today's dwellings, Gordon says, are much more like those of 1940 than the 1940 dwellings were like those of 1900. No more lack of privacy for people living and bathing in the kitchen, the only room that was warm year-round. Since 1940, however, only air-conditioning, television and the Internet have dramatically changed everyday life, and these combined have not remotely matched the impact of pre-1940 changes.

He goes on,

Nineteenth century medicine mostly made patients as comfortable as possible until nature healed or killed them. In 1878, yellow fever killed 10% of the Memphis population. But 20th century medicine moved quickly from the conquest of infectious diseases (the cause of 38 percent of deaths in 1900; 2 percent in 2009) to the management of chronic ailments of the elderly. There were 8,000 registered automobiles in 1900 but 26.8 million in1930. Ford's Model T. introduced in 1908 at $950, sold in 1923 for $269." "Gordon says two calamities – the Depression and World War II – fueled the post war boom. The Depression by speeding unionization (hence rising real wages and declining work hours), the war by high pressure "productivity-enhancing learning" that, for example, manufactured a bomber an hour at Michigan's Willow Run plant.

Finally, he discusses "the classic modernization trek from rural conditions into sanitized urban life and the entry of women into the workforce" as vast advances.

And so, as an unintended consequence of studying Dr. Bordley's life, we will see how these factors spinning the world into a modern society affected him and those around him.

Charles A. Webb Jr., MD

PART ONE

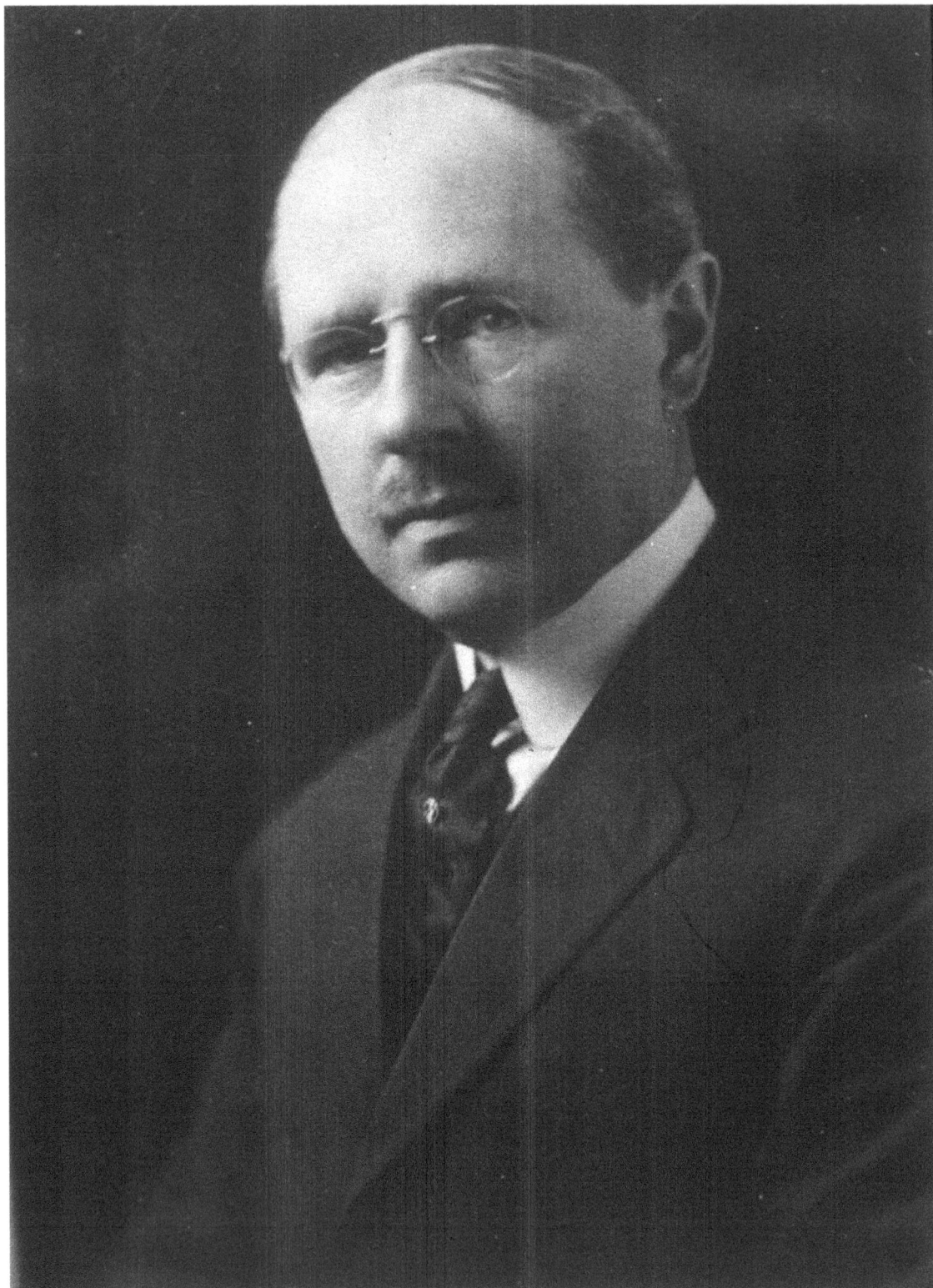

James Bordley, Jr., MD
Photo from the National Library of Medicine

JAMES BORDLEY, JR.

The coffin was surprisingly heavy—I was eighteen and had never carried one before. Eight of us lifted the long box by the polished brass bars; we carried it down the hill from the hearse to the open grave at Green Mount Cemetery in Baltimore. The weight seemed to be due mostly to the rich mahogany wood. It was a raw, gray winter day. The grass was wet. I worried that some of the other pallbearers who were elderly would have trouble with their load. We placed the coffin on straps over the open grave—the view downward into that hole provided what was probably my first serious contemplation of mortality; looking around at the group of family and friends was reassuring. I was one of the youngest there and realized that with a bit of luck, I would outlast most of them. So, I have and can record the history of my grandfather, James Bordley, Jr., who we buried on that sad day: January 7, 1956.

The mourners knew him variously as Dr. Bordley, Dr. Jim, Uncle Doc, Jim, Pop, or Poppy. After the minister said soothing words, the coffin made its descent. We each threw a handful of dirt after it. There were hugs all around and we went off to a brief family get-together.

His wife—Margaretta Carroll Hollyday, Minnie, Cousin Minnie, or Ma—would be placed in the adjacent plot ten years later October 7, 1966. Her death came at an awkward time for the family. We all had tickets to the World Series the day of the funeral. The underdog team of the Orioles were taking on Sandy Koufax and the world champion Dodgers. Brooks and Frank Robinson, Jim Palmer, Milt Pappas, and company were blowing the Dodgers away in a four-game sweep, to the delirium of Baltimore. The funeral had to be timed for the morning so we could get Ma laid to rest and make the opening pitch—such an indiscretion was justified by the fact that in her later years, she had become a baseball fan through the miracle of television. We *knew* she wouldn't want us to miss the game.

CENTREVILLE, 1874–1900

Jim Bordley was born on February 20, 1874, in Centreville, Queen
Anne's County. This was on the Eastern Shore of Maryland's Chesapeake Bay. He was born ten years
after the end of the Civil War. It was the year George Armstrong Custer led an escort party of the Seventh
Cavalry to protect the Black Hills Expedition. There were rumors of gold in the Black Hills. This was
legally Sioux territory. Army protection was needed for yet another act of our aggressive trespassing into
Indian lands. Two years later, in 1876, Sitting Bull annihilated Custer at the Battle of Little Big Horn.
That year, 1876, was also America's centennial year. The country was avidly celebrating its founding. As
Jim grew up, he must have been engulfed in this enthusiasm, and it probably accounts for his lifelong
interest in colonial history, architecture, and decorative arts.

The celebration in 1876 included a great Centennial Exposition in Philadelphia with three miles
of fence encircled red buildings. Ulysses S. Grant, who was in his final year as president, delivered the
opening address. The exhibitions centerpiece was a giant Corliss steam engine. New products that were
introduced included Heinz Ketchup, Hires Root Beer, and the Remington typographic machine, later
known as the typewriter. Alexander Graham Bell displayed his telephone.[1]

A post–Civil War economic boom was developing that would transform the country over the
next fifty years. As Brutus said to Cassius, "There is a tide in the affairs of men which, taken at the flood,
leads on to fortune."[2] So Jim was born at a rising tide in the affairs of this country—and he was able to
ride it to a remarkable life.

Centreville was on a hill at the head of the Corsica River, a branch of the Chester River, which
led into the Chesapeake Bay. The town had been established by an act of the state legislature in 1782 to
replace Queenstown as the county seat. It was a central location in an expanding county. The spelling
was in honor of the French, whose help had been so critical in the War of Independence. The town was

built on part of the Chesterfield farm near Chester Mill, on what passed for a road between Queenstown and Church Hill. The first construction got underway after 1789, and the courthouse, which is still in use today, was completed in 1795.

In 1800, an assessment list showed the Hackett family owning the lots that eventually became the Brown-Bordley residence. By 1816 there were seventy-seven lots sold. The first public water pump was on the courthouse green. In 1835 there were four public pumps.[3]

By the time that James Bordley, Jr. was born, the town was a thriving small port and seat of a county serving eighteen thousand people. It had steamboat service to Baltimore and slow, bumpy stage-coach service to Philadelphia. There was a newspaper, the *Centreville Times*, but no telegraph service until the mid-1880s. Houses did not have electricity, running water, or central heating—all they had were oil lamps, privies, and fireplaces.

Mail came from Baltimore by steamboat. The boat was really the main source of communication with the rest of the world. The Queen Anne's and Kent Railroad arrived in Centreville about the time Jim was born, but it communicated mostly with Philadelphia, a city in another state and with which relatively little commerce occurred. It was faster and easier to take the steamer to Baltimore than the train up the peninsula. The rail trip required riding nearly to Wilmington, changing trains, and then going back down to Baltimore.

The *B. S. Ford* was a typical steamboat at the height of the era. It was an iron-hulled side-wheeler built just after Jim was born. It carried passengers and freight on the Chester River run. Except when winter ice made the rivers impassable, she would leave Baltimore at seven a.m. and make stops at Rock Hall, Kent Island, Queenstown, Centreville, Spaniard's Point, Quaker Neck, Bookers Wharf, and Rolph's Wharf before arriving at Chestertown in the afternoon.[i] From there, one could transfer to a smaller steamer, the *Corsica*, and go on upriver as far as Crumpton. Freight coming from Baltimore consisted of the city's manufactured goods; on the return run she carried seafood and local produce. Peaches were a major Eastern Shore crop until a blight in the early twentieth century. When they were in season, it was not uncommon for baskets to be piled all the way to the overhead on the steamer's freight deck. She would spend the night in Chestertown and start the return run at seven a.m. the next day.[4]

---

i   Jim's future in-laws, the Hollydays, had their plantation, Readbourne, almost directly across the Chester River from Quaker Neck Landing. On the Hollydays' side is Ashland Landing, three-quarters of a mile down river (apparently not on the *Ford*'s run). Bookers Wharf is a mile upstream also on the same side.

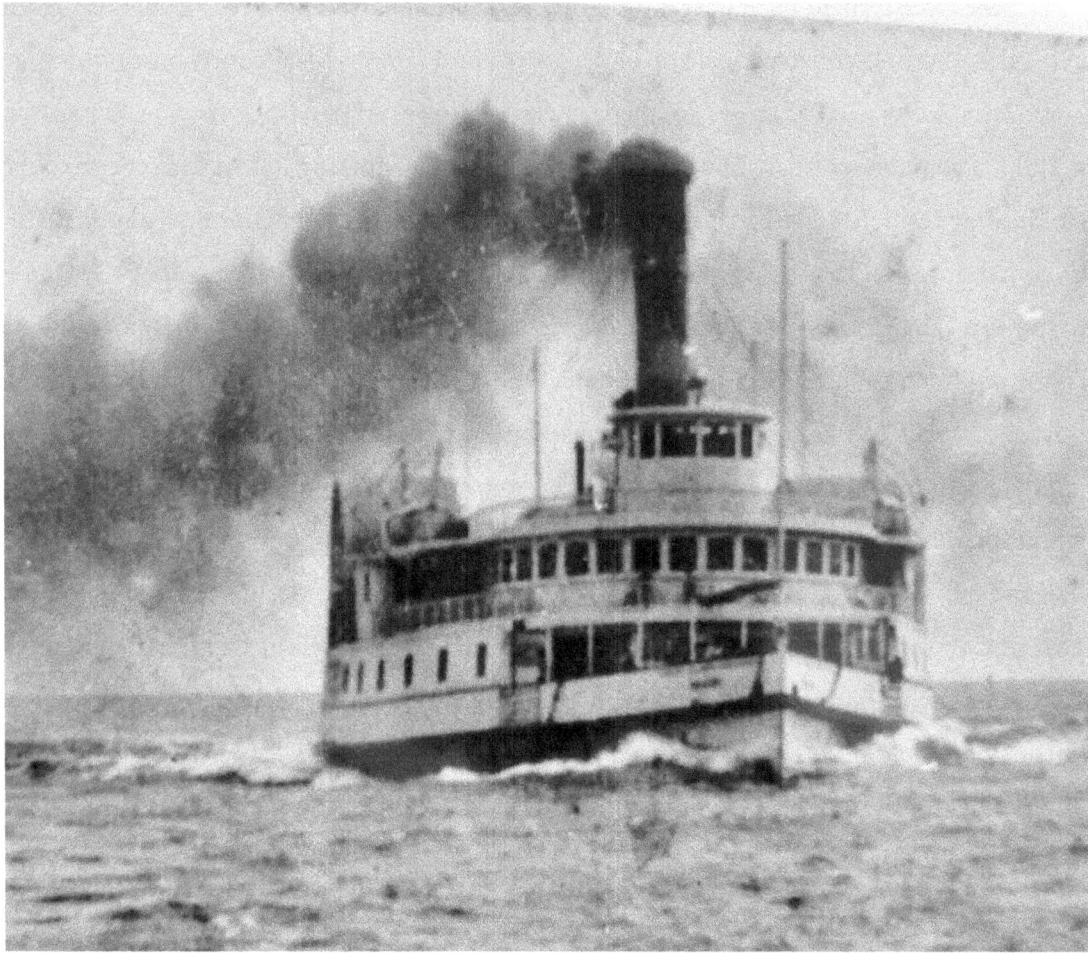

B. S. Ford, courtesy of the Chesapeake Bay Maritime Museum

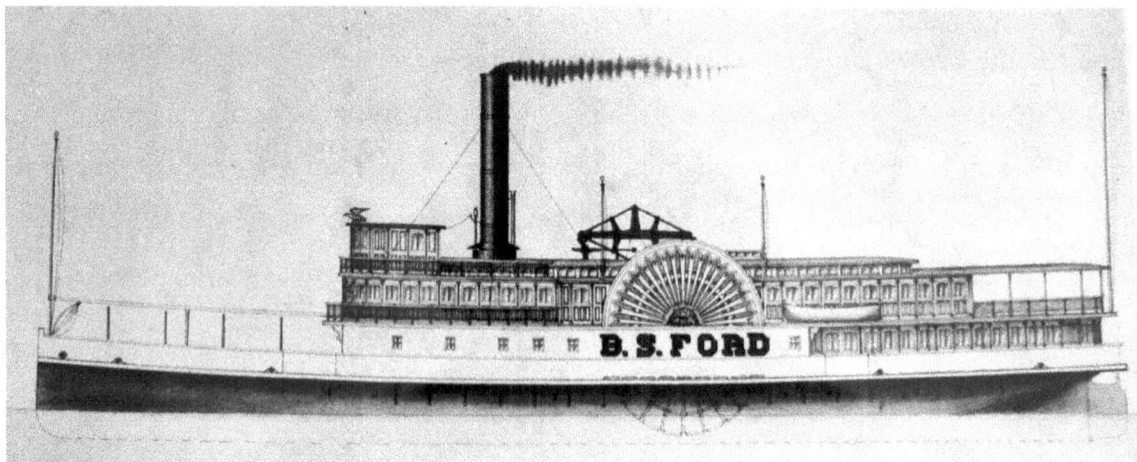

Courtesy of the Chesapeake Bay Maritime Museum

Roads were not paved until well into the next century, and there were few main roads. Most roads ran through someone's farm, so there were gates at property lines to contain livestock. There were many delays in opening and closing these barriers when traveling locally. The farm owner was expected to maintain the road section on his property. The legislature finally passed an act prohibiting these gates in 1870, but it took a while for them to disappear. Automobiles did not come on the Eastern Shore scene in any numbers until after 1910. They were only used in good weather. The horse and buggy remained the mainstay of travel for some time because when it rained, the horseless carriage bogged down quickly in the muddy country roads. My mother could recall as a young girl in about 1916 coming by steamer from Baltimore to visit her Centreville grandparents. She was later taken to Easton to visit other family members. They went in the horse and buggy, and it took much of the day to get there—it is a thirty-minute trip by car today.

Our subject could trace his ancestry back six generations to the Reverend Stephen Bordley, a newly ordained Anglican minister who emigrated from England to Annapolis in 1697 with his younger brother Thomas. Thomas stayed in Annapolis and became a prominent attorney. Stephen was assigned St. Paul's Parish across the bay in what was then Kent County. The county subsequently was split, leaving St. Paul's in the new Queen Anne's County. Stephen's descendants were mostly well educated, being clergymen, lawyers, and doctors. Most had farms as well as professional careers. A quick peek at the family tree reveals an almost unending supply of James Bordleys in Stephen's branch. The first was born in 1763. Except for the first, who was a judge, most were physicians. The current one graduated from medical school in 2010, almost two-hundred and fifty years later. He is named as the fifth JB, but from the top he is really the seventh. And for the first time there is a female Dr. Bordley: his sister, Jessica. The newest, JB IV, was born in 2018.

James Bordley Sr.—really the third JB, (1846–1904), our subject's father—was a physician. He was trained at the University of Maryland, getting his MD in 1868. He practiced in Centreville all his life. In 1890 he was a principal figure in getting a medical licensure bill passed in the Legislature.[5] He was elected second president of the Maryland Board of Medical Examiners in 1893 but resigned in 1896 because of the problem of having to travel frequently to Baltimore to fulfill his obligations. He served as county health officer. He was also second president of the Centreville National Bank[6]—and he was the president of the Centreville Opera Company—which creates an image of wonderment for such a small town.[ii] Besides a

---

ii   There was a theater in Centreville known as the Opera. Eventually it became the movie house. Also, there was a barge that was fitted out as a theater. It went from town to town on the river giving shows. In an era without electricity, such productions must have been very important.

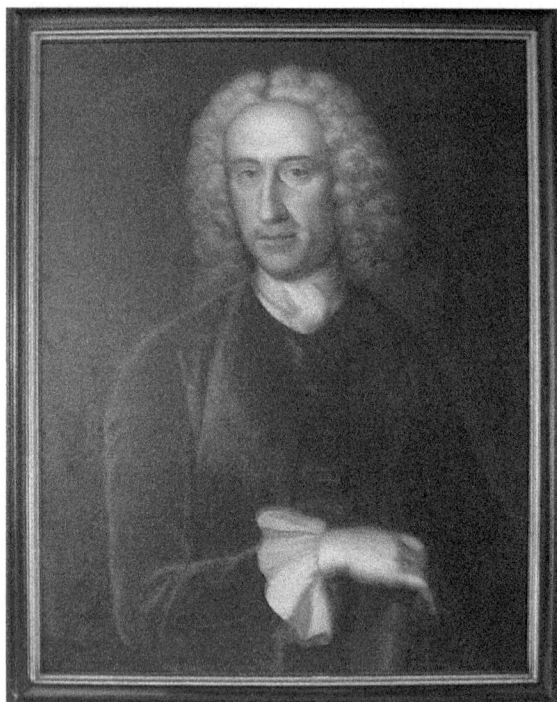

Thos. Bordley, Esq. 1677–1726
G. Hesselius, given to the Paca House by James Bordley III

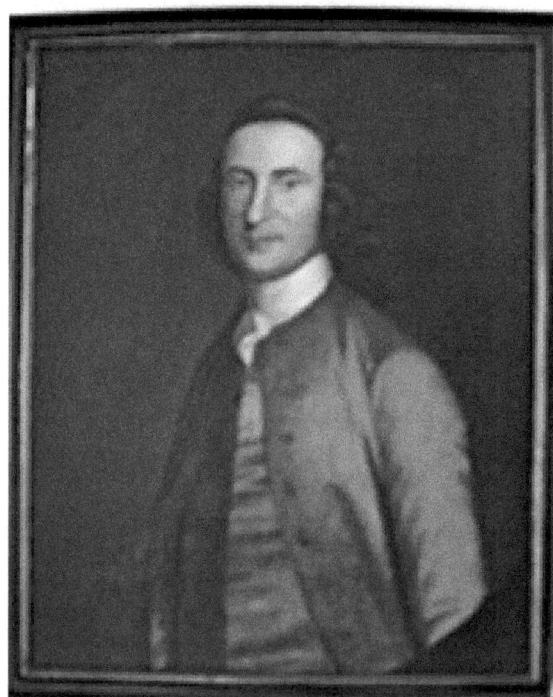

Rev. Stephen Bordley 1674–1709
Wollaston, given to the Paca House by James Bordley III

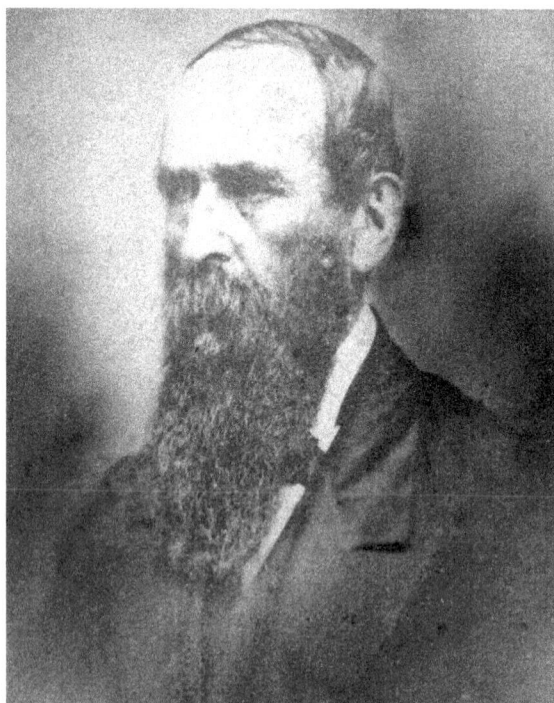

Grandfather
James Bordley, MD, 1808–1872

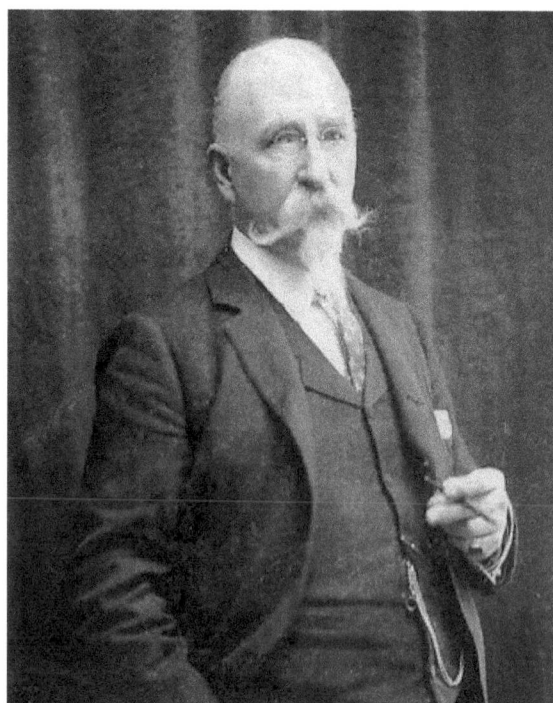

Father
James Bordley, MD, 1846–1904

house in town, he had a farm outside of town. Dr. Bordley's office was on Lawyers Row across from the courthouse.[iii] It contained an impressive library of the classics, some in Greek and Latin. There were medical books and genealogical records, but it was all lost in the Centreville fire of 1905.

So, James Jr. was born into a locally prominent family. He grew up at 202 South Liberty Street—it is a brick home on a large lot about three blocks from the courthouse.[iv] William Hackett built it in 1805. In an interesting exchange, Hackett's heirs swapped the house with Richard Tilghman Earle for Pascall's Chance on September 23, 2014, a 279-acre farm on the Corsica River. Earle's daughter, Mary Earle Davidson, inherited it. Mary's heirs rented the house to Madison Brown. Later, in 1860, he bought it from the Davidson estate. Madison's daughter, Ella Fassitt Brown, inherited it and was the owner until her death. She married James Bordley Sr. and they lived in the house—this is where her son, our subject, was raised.

In his manuscript *Bordleys of the Eastern Shore*, Jim says that he was born in a house on Front Street. His parents must have started their marriage there. Ella inherited the Liberty Street house upon her father's death in 1871. Her mother surely stayed on in the house until her death in 1885. We do not know when Ella's family moved back in.

The house was one of the finest homes in Centreville, and today it is considered a good example of the early Federal period. The front hall extends the length of the house. The living room is on the south side of the hall, and the dining room is further down the hall on the same side. There are no rooms on the north side of the hall.[v] Large doors allowed the living room and dining rooms to be closed in winter to retain what heat could be had from their fireplaces. In summer, the doors were left open for air to circulate. The house had six fireplaces: One was in the basement for the kitchen; the living room and dining room each had one; two second floor bedrooms had one; and there was one on the third floor.

---

iii   From Judge John Sause, who is knowledgeable about Centreville history and who now owns the Brown/Bordley house at 202 S. Liberty St.

iv   This is really lots 202 and 204 of the original Centreville layouts, plus some more land in the rear purchased by James Bordley Sr.

v   Orlando V. Ridout, *Md. Historic Trust Inventory of Historic Properties*, describes the layout of the first floor as "a side passage with double parlor plan. The overall width of the passage is ten feet wide but a double stair extends three feet seven inches into that space along much of the north wall. This stair is one of the most unusual in the county. It rises from both ends of the passage to a landing in the center of the hall. These straight runs then join, turn 90 degrees and rise an additional six steps to the second-floor passage. This transverse section of stair is positioned above an elliptical arch that, combined with the stair, creates a highly ornamental effect."

Originally there were four bedrooms on both the second and third floors, but no bathrooms. With the twentieth-century addition of plumbing, the number of bedrooms is now reduced. In 1955, Jim commented in a letter about that winter's weather. He said that he had not been so cold since he was a boy—surely, he was referring to those unheated bedrooms where he grew up.

Although the house was in town, the town had only two primary streets, Liberty Street and Commerce Street, parallel to each to other, running north and south. There was open land behind the house and a stable. Dr. Bordley Sr. bought the lot behind to add space to the property.[vi] Almost surely, they had some domestic help. Slaves had recently been freed and labor was cheap. There was probably a man in the stable to look after horses and hitch up the wagon. It was also likely there was help to do cooking, housekeeping, laundry, and probably childcare. They raised their own chickens—we know this from Madison Bordley Jr., who related that when he stayed in the house as a boy, he was given the job of crawling under the porch to remove dead chickens. He said it was so nasty a task that he was never able to eat chicken again. The Bordleys had two gardens, one for "eating" and one for "cutting" flowers. In the backyard there is a sinkhole that must be filled in periodically—this is presumed to be the site of the well. The location of the privy is unknown.

During the time Jim grew up, the house went through several changes. Marble coal-burning fireplace inserts were added. A gas generator was buried in the backyard to supply gas lights inside. Gas lights replaced the candles and oil lamps that had been the only source of illumination at night. Finally, perhaps after he had left for medical school, there came electricity, running water, toilets, central steam heat, and the telephone. At some point cement floors replaced the hard packed dirt in the basement and the kitchen was moved up to an addition in the back on the northwest corner of the house.

It was in 1905, after Jim had grown up, that his parents "modernized" the house in Victorian style. They added the wide front porch—that young Madison had to crawl under—lengthened the living room windows to floor level and put in parquet flooring in the main rooms. We know the date because the current owner, Judge Sause, found a 1905 newspaper clipping under the parquet when it and the Victorian marble fireplaces were removed to restore the original character of the house.

So that is the background of the times when Jim grew up. The Civil War was over, and the country was switching from an agricultural to an urban society. The industrial revolution was gearing up, and one modern convenience after another arrived to help make life better. Some of the most remarkable changes of all were just beginning to happen in medicine as he was completing his medical training—

---

vi   Ella was the owner of the house, but her husband owned the lot behind it.

ether anesthesia was making it reasonable to do surgery and the risk of surgical infections was vastly reduced as germ theory was coming to be understood. At Hopkins, Dr. Halstead was developing modern surgical procedures. In Germany, William Roentgen had just discovered the X-ray.

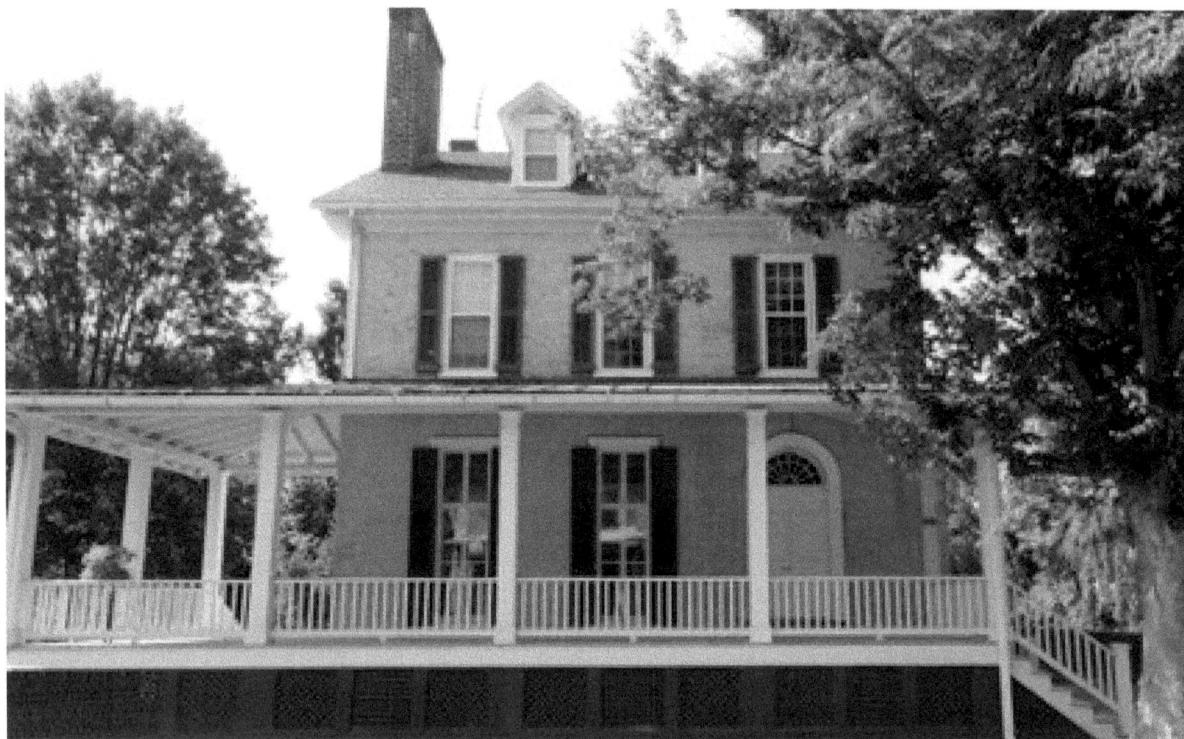

202 South Liberty St., Centreville, MD

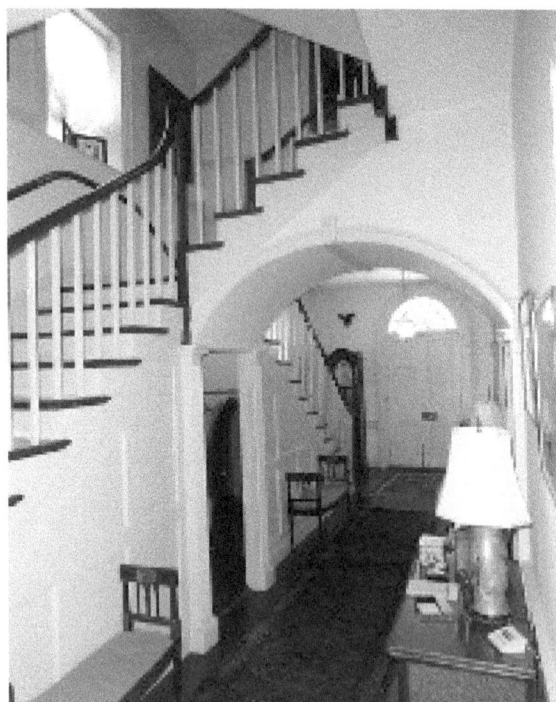

Front Hall, 202 S. Liberty St.

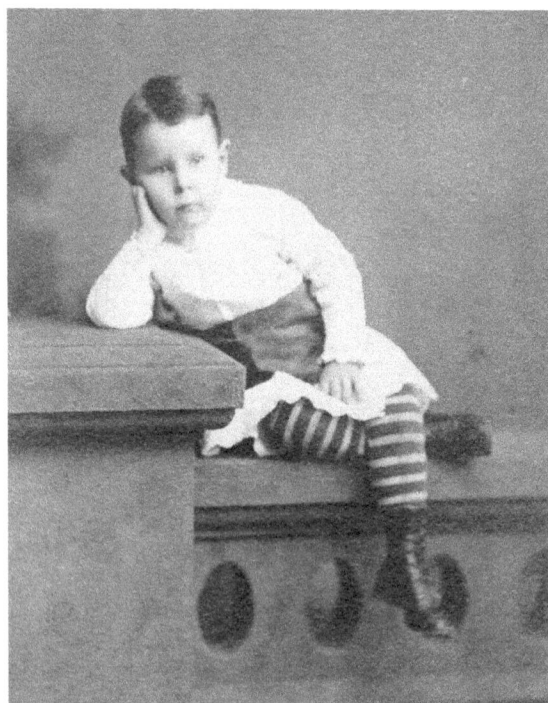

JB Jr., 1878 or 1879

EDUCATION AND WEDDING, 1890–1900

James Bordley, Jr.—really the fourth—was the middle of three sons. His older brother, Madison, became a lawyer, married, and initially continued living on Liberty Street. Eventually he moved to Ripley near Church Hill.[vii] Younger brother Worthington moved to Baltimore, got married, had a family, and worked for Bendix. Jim probably attended the Centreville Academy, where his older brother had gone. Then he went to the Davis Military College in Winston-Salem, North Carolina, graduating in 1893. He went to the University of Maryland School of Medicine, finishing the three-year curriculum in 1896. He did an internship at the University of Maryland and Baltimore City Hospital.[viii] Of his early training, he wrote: "My first operation was forty-three years ago…when I went out to help Ridge Trimble remove a large fatty tumor from a man's back. Griff (Davis) gave the anesthetic. It was in the days when most operations were performed at home. Ever since Griff has given anesthetics for me, first chloroform and then ether."[ix]

He returned to Centreville to practice with his father for about a year but did not like it. So, he went back to Baltimore and became associated with Dr. Samuel Theobold, clinical professor of ophthal-

---

vii   "Ripley" was another Brown house. Madison married his first cousin Helen Brown, granddaughter of Madison and Ella Brown, daughter of James Brown.

viii   Balto. City Hospital was also known at various times as the Baltimore Infirmary or the Bayview Asylum. In 1845 Dr. John Charles Earle, grandfather of Jim's wife, was the first resident physician of the institution then called the Baltimore Infirmary. Today the complex is known as Bay View Hospital and is part of Johns Hopkins Hospital.

ix   James Bordley, Jr., April 27, 1943, letter to sons Jim and John. His recollection of the date may be off a bit as he was past his training in 1900. More likely it was about 1897.

mology and otolaryngology at Johns Hopkins. He got a position on the visiting staff of the Franklin Street Eye and Ear Hospital. In March of 1899, he opened a private office for the practice of eye, ear, nose, and throat surgery.[7]

He also found time to do research. His early investigative work, dealing with experimentally induced choked optic disc and decompressive cranial operations, was done in conjunction with Dr. Harvey Cushing. He became a frequent contributor to the medical literature.[x] Many of his papers dealt with ocular manifestations of diseases of the paranasal sinuses.[8]

On November 29, 1899, with his practice established in Baltimore, he married Margaretta Carroll Hollyday at St. Paul's Church in Centreville.[9] We have no information about their courtship. He was a year and a half older than she was and they had grown up in moderate proximity of each other. The Hollydays were from Readbourne, a plantation a few miles up the Chester River from Centreville. He was from the town, she from the farm. But there was a social difference—the Hollydays were members of the old "landed aristocracy." Plantation owners were a cut above the folks in town.

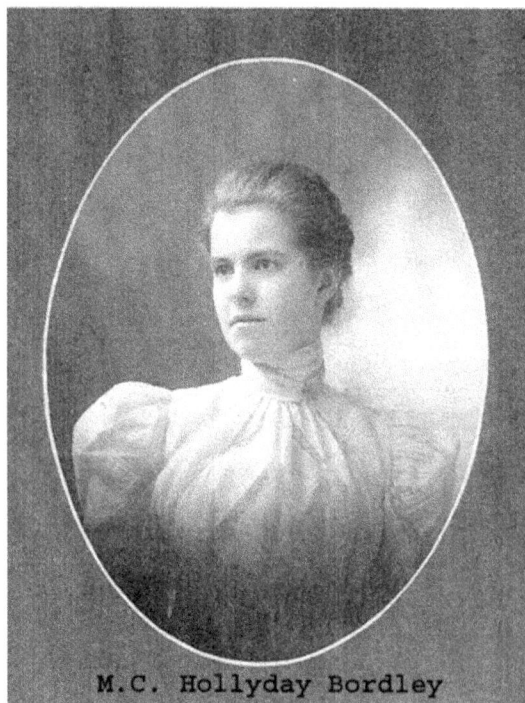

M.C. Hollyday Bordley

Minnie about age 20

The story of Readbourne began with James Hollyday. He married Sarah Covington Lloyd at Wye plantation in 1720 or 1721. She was a Quaker and the widow of Edward Lloyd II (1680–1718) and

---

x   See Appendix for a bibliography of his medical papers.

thus became one of the richest women in Maryland. James Hollyday was an Annapolis attorney. He had come to Wye to help settle the estate after the forty-eight-year-old Edward Lloyd died. He lived at Wye for three years working with Sarah. Although Hollyday was a good bit younger than she was (twenty-six and thirty-four respectively), Sarah married him. They lived at Wye until her oldest son, Edward Lloyd III, grew to maturity and could manage the vast Lloyd fortune, farms, and shipping interests. While still at Wye, she had three more children by James Hollyday; two survived. In 1733, James purchased Readbourne. It was a tract of over one thousand acres on the Chester River. It eventually was enlarged to over two thousand acres. The land had only a small house, and we know that it took until about 1740 to complete the construction of the manor house. When Sarah left Wye, she came with her two sons, James and Henry Hollyday, plus her youngest three Lloyd children, James, Rebecca, and Richard. There was also domestic help—they brought or acquired the men with skills necessary to make bricks, gather lumber, and do the building. Where they lived while Sarah oversaw the construction of the house is unknown. Her husband went to England, perhaps for health reasons, perhaps to establish buyers for his tobacco.[10] He also made purchases for the house.[11]

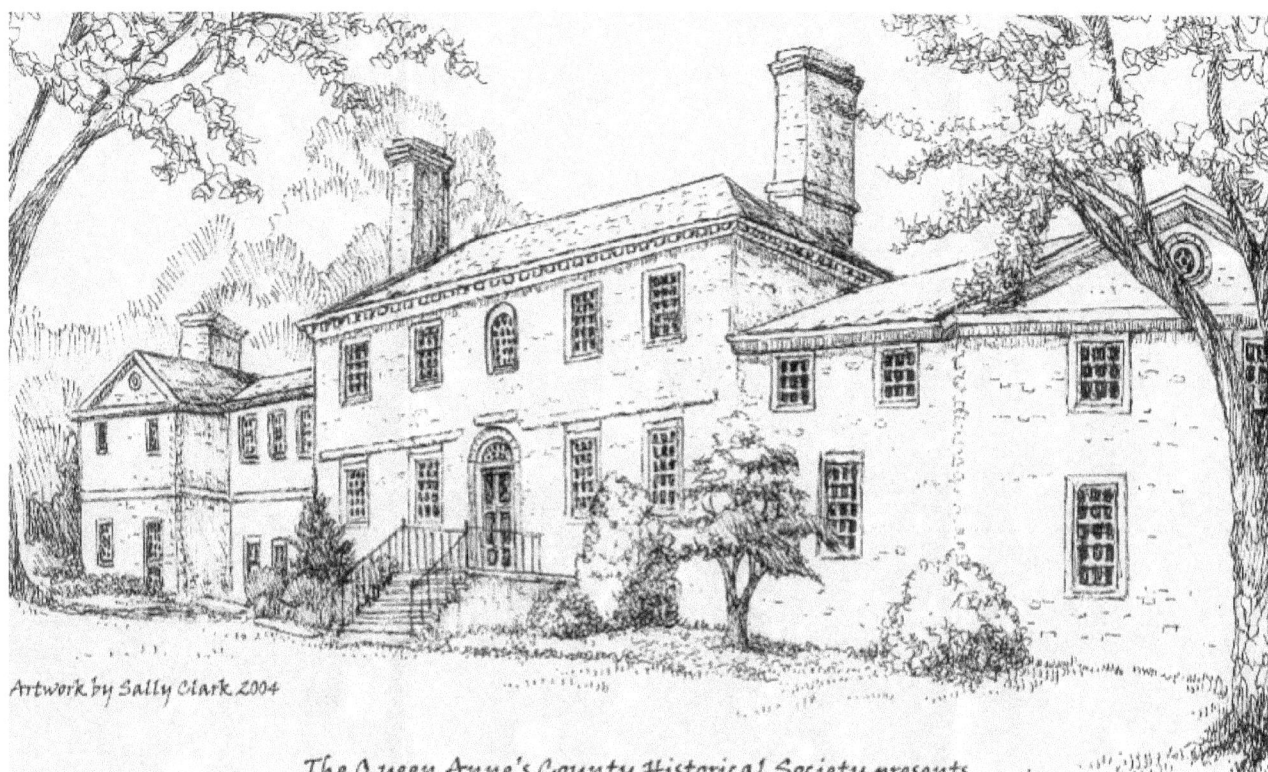

Artwork by Sally Clark 2004

The Queen Anne's County Historical Society presents
An Afternoon at Readbourne

In 1740, Readbourne consisted of the central building and a separate kitchen on the right.
The kitchen burned, was rebuilt, and later was joined to the main building by the hyphen.
The wing to the left is a twentieth-century addition.

In any event, the Hollydays were members of a tight colonial society who tended to marry among themselves. In part this was because of their financial distinction, but also because they were educated, in contrast to most of the local population in the eighteenth century, who were not. However, by the nineteenth century, the War of Independence had reduced trade with English markets. Then the Civil War had destroyed the remaining affluence of the plantations. Although the Hollydays still had land and social status, they were short on cash by the end of the nineteenth century. So when Minnie Hollyday decided to marry Jim Bordley, it was a good match. She got an up-and-coming city physician and he benefited from her social standing. Why they were married in Centreville and not at Readbourne is not known to us. Notices in the *Baltimore Sun* reported that six hundred invitations were sent out! Surely that many did not come. Still, St. Paul's Church in Centreville was filled with relatives and friends. It had been decorated for the Thanksgiving service. The bride wore a brown broadcloth traveling dress and carried a bouquet of American Beauty roses. Madison, Jim's older brother, was best man. After the ceremony there was a reception and luncheon at the residence of Dr. James Bordley Sr., which was walking distance up the street from St. Paul's. At two-thirty p.m., the bride and groom left for a wedding trip, probably by steamboat or perhaps train—we do not know. Of note is the fact that twenty-eight years earlier, November 30, 1871, Jim's parents were married in the same church, at the same hour. It had also been Thanksgiving Day.

BALTIMORE, 1900–1920

Jim and Minnie established a home at 10 East Mount Royal Avenue in Baltimore.[12] Children came promptly. Minnie returned to Readbourne to deliver her first child, James Bordley III, on December 9, 1900. But in 1902 she stayed in Baltimore to deliver John Earle Bordley. There is family lore that Minnie came down with diphtheria during this pregnancy, recovered, and was advised to have an abortion because of the risk of complications, presumably myocarditis. She refused. John was born at Johns Hopkins Hospital—an interesting coincidence as John eventually made his career at Hopkins as professor of otolaryngology. There followed a pause in childbearing. Ellen Ffassitt, their last child, did not arrive until December 31, 1909.[xi]

The medical practice did well. His initial office was at 520 North Charles Street.[13] Dr. Bordley acquired hospital appointments as clinical assistant, University of Maryland; assistant resident physician, Bayview; and clinical assistant in ophthalmology and otology at the Johns Hopkins Hospital Dispensary. He was appointed professor of diseases of eye and ear at the Woman's Medical College in 1902, and he was on the staff at Church Home and Infirmary. On October 2, 1901, the *Baltimore Sun* reported: "The South Baltimore Free Eye and Ear Hospital, which was established last May at 1017 Light Street, has proved to be a great boon to the citizens of that section of the city. Between 600 and 700 patients have been treated. Drs. H.E. Peterman and James Bordley, Jr., the founders, are the attending physicians, and Mrs. C. D. Grafton is the nurse. There are four rooms for the accommodation of patients compelled to remain for treatment. On the first floor are two examination rooms. It is the intention of the founders to have the institution incorporated in the near future."

---

xi   Ffassitt was from a Welsh ancestor. The double *F* is usually dropped in contemporary spelling.

Over the next nineteen years, there were many articles in the press documenting the remarkable growth of this little hospital. It expanded to a much larger facility at 1211 Light Street in 1905. The building was "thoroughly renovated and converted to a modern hospital for the treatment of diseases of the eye, ear, nose and throat with a capacity of 20 beds. Among the improvements are a new and well-equipped operating room, steam heating plant and sanitary plumbing."[14] That also tells us what was not in the original hospital. By 1909 the hospital reported there were 10,456 patients seen in the dispensary for the year, and 1,230 inpatient days of care. About one-fifth of this was paid in full or in part, and they were beginning to get the support of state funds. The social section of the *Sun* throughout these years recorded many charitable events to help raise money for the hospital and Minnie served on the women's committee.

In 1913, funds were raised for another expansion on the adjacent lot and a three-story building was erected. Then with growth of manufacturing at Locust Point and Curtis Bay, the need for a hospital to treat industrial accident cases was strong, and the board voted to expand and become a general hospital renamed the South Baltimore General Hospital. Jim remained active and on the board until 1918, when he joined in the army and became director of the effort to rehabilitate blinded soldiers, known as the Evergreen project. South Baltimore General Hospital moved in 1960 from Light Street to Hanover Street. It was renamed Harbor Hospital; today it serves the Cherry Hill district.

On May 30, 1903, he went to Europe. He traveled with Dr. H. E. Peterman and Dr. Charles Hollyday, Minnie's brother. They sailed out of New York for London on the Atlantic Transport liner *Minnetonka*—it was one of the new modern ships under full steam power and carried no sails. They were to be away until the last of August to visit London, Paris, Berlin, and Vienna. Late in life he wrote, "I remember when I got back to the U.S. after four months in Europe in 1903. What a glorious feeling it was to be home again. I have never wanted to repeat the experience."[15]

In 1904 Jim was elected to membership in the American Ophthalmological Society. He joined the American Medical Association, was a member of the American Academy of Ophthalmology and Otolaryngology, the Baltimore Medical Society, and the Medical and Chirurgical Faculty of Maryland.

Dr. Bordley developed a national reputation; his position in the AMA has been mentioned. As we shall see, he held a high position on the surgeon general's staff during World War I. He had patients coming to see him from out of state. The *Sun* noted that in 1916 Mr. Samuel S. Dunlap of Macon, Georgia, was "successfully operated on by Dr. James Bordley at South Baltimore Eye, Ear, Nose and Throat Hospital." (So, it was not entirely a charity hospital.) He was convalescing at the Belvedere Hotel with his two sisters. They did not have much in the way of inpatient care in those days, at least that the affluent were willing to tolerate. In 1922 the Princess Miguel de Braganza, Duchess de Viseu and wife to the Portuguese pretender to the throne, came for "a slight throat problem." She stayed at the Stafford Hotel with a maid and declined to stay in a hospital.

He joined the Maryland Club, which was the gathering spot for Baltimore gentlemen and where he could play squash. The excellent dining room served terrapin stew—it became one of his favorite dishes. Minnie made it or arranged for it to be sent to the house for his birthday dinners for years.

He had a lifelong love of golf and joined the Elkridge Club for that purpose. His tee shots were never the longest, perhaps because he was not a tall man. In fact, he was not more than five feet six or seven inches, so he did not have great leverage in his swing. But with very accurate chipping and putting, he was able to pick up strokes. We can remember him in his senior years during the long summer evenings at Rye Beach. The Farragut Hotel where he stayed was next to one of the holes on the local golf course. He loved working on his chipping skills, and often did so after dinner until it was so dark he could barely be seen on the green.

The years 1904 and 1905 were a bad period for urban fires. We have mentioned the fire in Centreville of 1905 that destroyed his father's library. In 1904 there had been a devastating fire in Baltimore—it burned out much of the business district around the harbor. In the rebuilding enthusiasm that followed, it was realized that Baltimore needed a fine arts museum. In 1911 a Founding Committee was established, and it served until 1914. It included a group of very distinguished Baltimoreans, and James Bordley, Jr. was on the committee. The minutes of the museum show he was an active participant. Although not placed on the original board of trustees, he subsequently served on it from 1924 to 1955.[xii] In 1944 he was asked to be head of the board, but as we shall see, he declined.

When the museum first opened in 1923, it was temporarily housed in Mrs. Thomas Carey's mansion at the corner of Cathedral and Monument Streets, the western end of Mount Vernon Square.[xiii] In the meantime, Johns Hopkins University donated six acres on the southern edge of its campus for a new museum building. John Russell Pope was hired as the architect— later he designed the National Gallery in Washington. The Maryland legislature authorized one million dollars in bonds to raise money for construction. The corner stone was laid in 1927. The museum opened on April 18, 1929. It was the roaring twenties and the opening just beat the October stock market crash. There is a floor-to-ceiling marble plaque beside the front door that names and honors the Founding Committee, including Dr. Bordley.

[xii]   Emily Rafferty, a museum librarian, noted that he was active initially, but in the later years his name was not listed in attendance at Board meetings too frequently. We were not allowed to study those minutes.

[xiii]   This residence has been taken down.

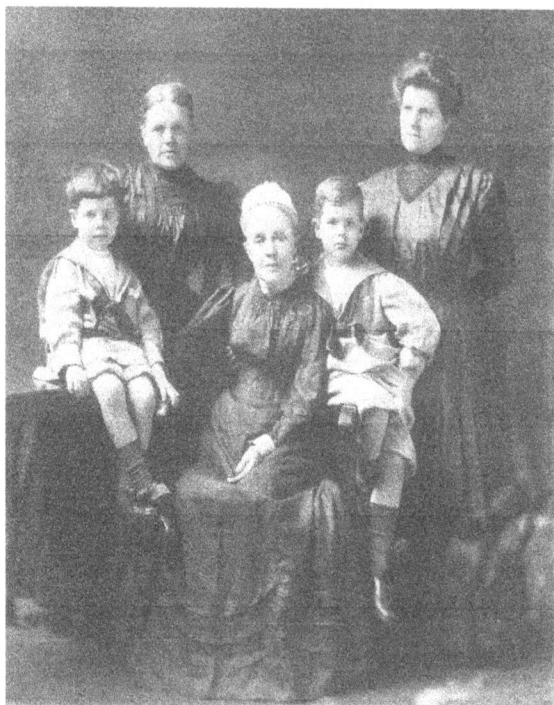

Four Generations
Top left: Elizabeth Tilghman Earle (Mrs. R.
Hollyday) Top right: Minnie (Mrs. JB Jr.)
Bottom: John Bordley, Clara Goldsborough
(Mrs. John Earle), Jim Bordley III

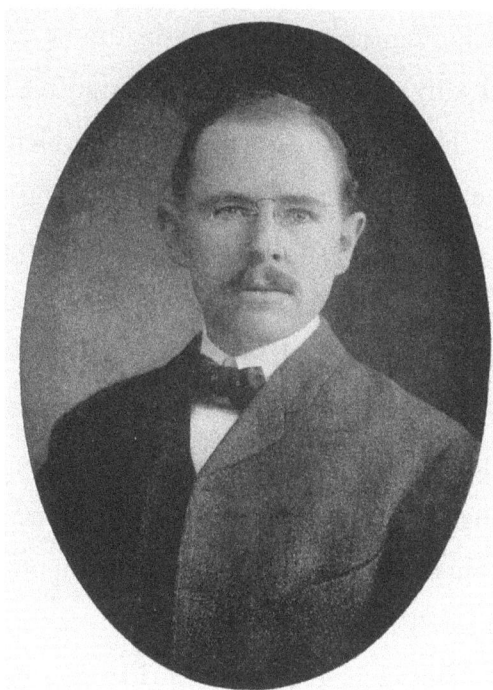

JB Jr.

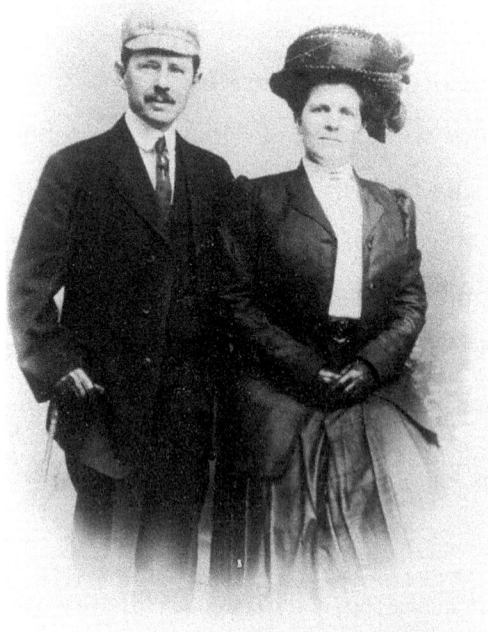

Jim and Minnie in Atlantic City

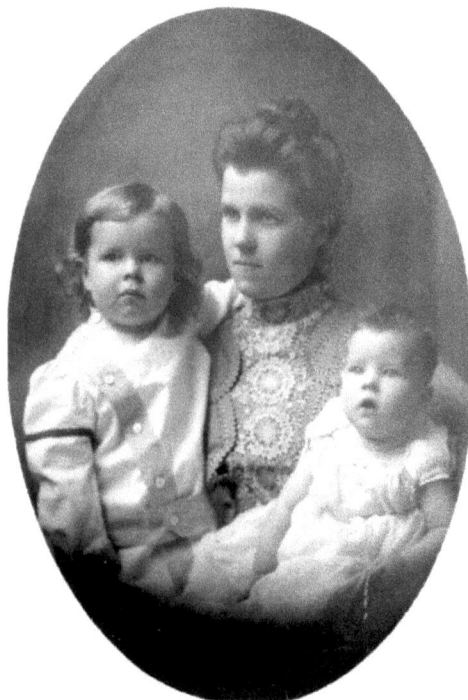

Jim III, Minnie, and John, 1903

ART MUSEUM
BUILDING COMMISSION
1926
BLANCHARD RANDALL, PRESIDENT
LEMUEL T. APPOLD, SECRETARY
THE MAYOR
THE COMPTROLLER
THE PRESIDENT OF THE CITY COUNCIL
HENRY ADAMS, DR. JAMES BORDLEY JR.
VAN LEAR BLACK,   HENRY F. BROENING
THOMAS C. CORNER, DR. A. R. L. DOHME
JACOB EPSTEIN,   ROBERT GARRETT
MRS. JOHN W. GARRETT,   E. H. GOTTLIEB
DR. HENRY BARTON JACOBS, JULIUS LEVY
J. HEMSLEY JOHNSON, EDGAR G. MILLER
C. MORGAN MARSHALL,   J. J. NELLIGAN
DR. J. HALL PLEASANTS, LAWRASON RIGGS
MISS JULIA ROGERS, AUGUSTINE J. RYAN
DR. WILLIAM S. THAYER, MRS. MILES WHITE JR.
S. DAVIES WARFIELD, HENRY H. WIEGAND
CHARLES S. YORK,   DR. HUGH H. YOUNG

Baltimore Museum of Art

19

WORLD WAR I AND
EVERGREEN, 1917–1919

Now we must back up a bit. With the outbreak of hostilities in Europe in 1914, America raised its guard. In 1916, at age forty-two, Dr. Bordley was appointed chairman of the ophthalmological section of the Council of National Defense. The United States became involved in the First World War on April 6, 1917, when it finally declared war on Germany. Dr. Bordley joined the Medical Corps, was given the rank of major, and was assigned to be the ophthalmologist for the surgeon general's office in Washington. He became a lieutenant colonel on May 21, 1918. He was placed in charge of developing a national rehabilitation program for blinded soldiers.

The gas attacks occurring on the battlefields of Europe were blinding soldiers. When chlorine gas contacts water, it forms hydrochloric acid. This acid was especially effective in destroying the moist sclera of the eye and the lining of the lungs. Mustard gas was a blistering agent with similar blinding effects. Dr. Bordley wrote,

> There are many types of handicaps which result in economic and social troubles, but I think I can aptly term the blind as the Ishmaelites of this century. They have been driven out of community life, out of industry, prevented from owning their own homes and maintaining them, and for decades they have cried out for a chance and the answer has always been "Charity" … It is simply one of our horrible social mistakes.[16]

Building on experience in Britain, France, and Italy, a program for the rehabilitation of the blind was begun. Not only did they have to overcome the despair of the blinded soldier, but they had to teach the public that a blind person could be a valuable, self-sufficient citizen. A training school for the blind was quickly established in Baltimore. Mrs. T. Harrison Garrett donated a large portion of her estate, Evergreen, for this purpose. It was on the northeast corner of Charles Street and Cold Spring Lane, extending all the way to York Road. Loyola College occupies much of this area today.

A series of temporary wooden barracks-like buildings providing living space and classrooms was quickly constructed. The men's psychological problems related to being blind were dealt with first—they were taught how to function in society as blind people, and all were required to master a basic reading of braille. They learned an occupation appropriate to their own abilities and it had to be one in which they could find employment in their home community. A man could be trained in a diverse number of skills. Industries were approached to work out assembly-line jobs for a blind man. Assembly-line mock-ups were created in the classrooms. One could train for the blind shopwork or receive instruction in commercial or agricultural areas. Chicken farming adapted well as an occupation for the blind. Clerical skills such as typing were taught. Men could learn physical therapy techniques and got work in veterans hospitals.

The Federal Board for Vocational Education was charged with seeing that suitable jobs were found for graduates of the program. The Red Cross Institute for the Blind was created to supply the necessary social and economic supervision after discharge. It engaged the man's family and helped him return to community life. The Evergreen project was a real success—Helen Keller and a variety of national and foreign dignitaries visited it. It helped to turn around the image of a blind person in the community.

In the fall of 1918, Germany was on the verge of collapse, and it signed an armistice on November 11. By April 4, 1919, Lt. Col. Bordley was discharged from the army. He was able to step down from an established program at Evergreen, but the school continued until 1922, when the buildings were removed, and the land was returned to Mrs. Garrett.

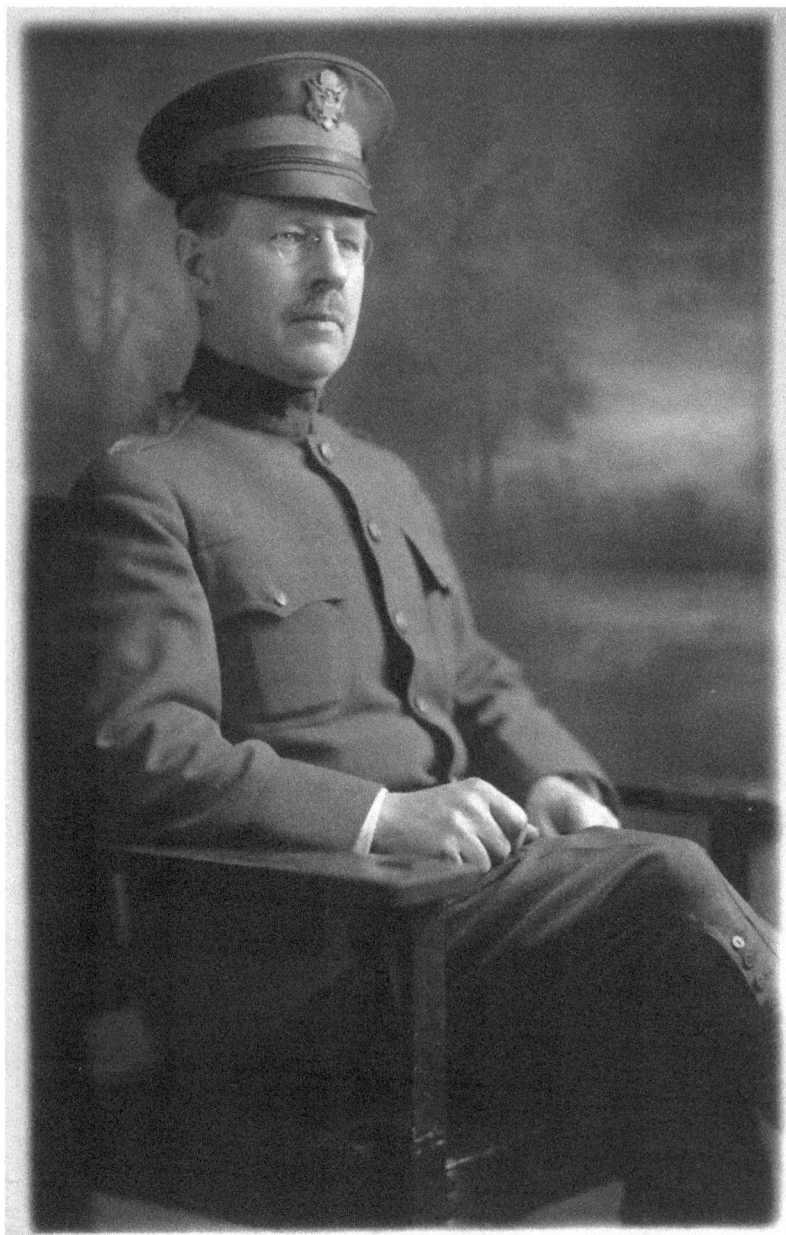

Lt. Col. James Bordley, Jr., 1918

MISSED OPPORTUNITY?

John Bordley, Jim's second son and head of otolaryngology at Hopkins, related to us that following the war, Hopkins asked his father to join the faculty and start a separate clinic devoted to the care of the eye. By now the field of ophthalmology was ready to split away from ear, nose, and throat. Jim declined the offer because he wanted to return to his private practice. However, he recommended his Evergreen assistant, Dr. Wilmer, as a good person for the job. Dr. Wilmer was offered the position and took it. Today one of the Hopkins Hospital crown jewels is the world-famous Wilmer Clinic. Did Jim make a mistake? Certainly he did from the point of view of posterity, but the pay would have been lower than he was earning in private practice. Hopkins requires its professors to work full time and have no outside practice lest they be distracted from their work at the hospital—but their salaries are rarely equivalent to what can be made in private practice. And he went on to many other things: by 1920, he was head of the ophthalmology section of the AMA.

BALTIMORE, 1920–1940

As noted, the Bordleys started their married life in a house at 10 East Mount Royal Avenue. On May 4, 1919, a month after he was discharged from the army, they bought the house at 810 Cathedral Street. It was a three-story town house with a basement and attic rooms on the west side of the street at the northern end of a row of houses. It had a stable and carriage house in the back and an open lot on the north side. Most important, it was within a block and a half of Mount Vernon Square, the most fashionable area of residences in Baltimore in the early twentieth century—they had moved to the "right" neighborhood in town.

It is difficult to know what municipal services were available at the house by 1919. One might suspect that in the most affluent residential area of the city, the arrival of municipal services would not be lagging, but it was on one of the highest areas of town, making water delivery more difficult. By 1904 Baltimore had a municipal water system, but the pressure proved inadequate for the fire department to fight the great fire, even down at the harbor area. The city had been covered with a spiderweb of overhead electric wires before the fire. Improvements to the city during the rebuilding included underground conduits for the wires and a high-pressure water system. In about 1912, a municipal sewer system was about half-completed. By 1919 it was probably serving the Mount Vernon area. A wonderful history of Baltimore from 1912 points out: "With the completion of the (sewer) system now in course of construction, Baltimore will be the best served and drained city in the world, raising her from the bottom to the top of the list of cities in this respect."[17] So we will guess that the house had electric, water, and sewer services with indoor plumbing. By then it would have had a central heating system. We know they had a record player because we still have their 1918–19 RCA Victor Red Label recordings by Caruso. The old 78 rpm vinyl records are cut on only one side; public radio broadcasts began in the mid-1920s—what a dramatic change this represents from just twenty years earlier!

Telephone service is harder to pin down. The first telephone patents were granted in 1876, but these were for very simple systems. By the turn of the century there were some limited exchanges; the use of telephones gradually expanded and developed over the next twenty or more years.

In 1911 Baltimore had three-hundred and fifty miles of cobblestone road. There were still fifty-eight miles of unpaved roads in the city, and it was just starting to replace or cover the cobblestones with asphalt or macadam. By 1919, when the Bordleys bought their new house, the automobile was replacing the horse for personal urban transportation. Ford's Model T did better on city streets than on the dirt roads in the country. The Automobile Club of Maryland was in existence by 1910. On September 4 of that year, the *Sun* reported on a Baltimore-to-Frederick rally. It outlines the thrills of the trip and challenges of the roads. Later in the same article, it notes, "Dr. James Bordley, Jr., of this city, returned from a 1,000-mile trip in his Cadillac car to Atlantic City, N.J., points up the Jersey Coast, New York, Philadelphia, Pa., to Baltimore. The party enjoyed the trip very much, the roads being fine except some sections in Maryland. The party was away about two weeks." The photograph of the Bordleys that we have here showing them in Atlantic City may have come from that trip. Unfortunately, it is undated.

The new house was commodious, and there was plenty of space for the children. But by 1919, son Jim was eighteen and about to head for Yale in the fall. John was sixteen and a bit of a challenge—he had been to Marsden, a local private boy's school, and away to St. James. He needed a "postgraduate" year at Gilman before he was ready to follow Jim to Yale. Ellen was nine. She became a teenager in the roaring twenties. She added popular recordings to the family's collection, especially the foxtrot. By age fifteen or sixteen she would be going to Westover, a private girl's "finishing school" in Connecticut. Most girls did not go to college in the 1920s—this was something that would bother her later in life. Her brothers were to have distinguished medical careers, but the women of the day were trained to be wives, mothers, and to do volunteer work.

So here are good examples of how much and how fast the world was changing: Minnie told stories about her education in the little brick schoolhouse on Spaniards Neck, almost three miles from Readbourne. In good weather and sometimes in bad—she walked the distance. No finishing school for her. In those days, girls did not usually finish what would be considered high school. The Baltimore Bordleys were in the vanguard of the movement off the farms and small towns and into the cities. Women were no longer burdened with a seemingly endless string of childbearing. Minnie's parents, Richard and Elizabeth Hollyday, had produced ten children. Food preservation was improving. Commercial canning had been developed, so it was not necessary to stock the home pantry with the summer garden produce. Women had much more free time, but society was not yet ready to utilize it.

During the 1920s and 1930s, Dr. Bordley's practice was booming. He moved to a spacious office occupying the rear of the second floor of the Professional Building at 330 North Charles Street.

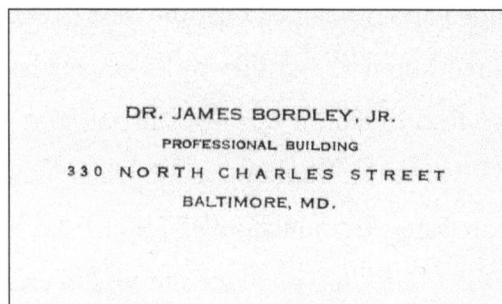

DR. JAMES BORDLEY, JR.
PROFESSIONAL BUILDING
330 NORTH CHARLES STREET
BALTIMORE, MD.

In those days, Charles Street was the finest street in Baltimore. It starts at the harbor and runs north uphill to the Washington Monument on Mount Vernon Square. The office was across the street from Lycett's Stationery store, the Women's Exchange, and Payne and Merrill's haberdashery, where tailors would make a man his suits. Hopper McGraw's was nearby—this was the grocer with everything, including a life-size wooden cigar store Indian out front and a popular lunch counter. Kirk Silver was just a block up the street.

The work of silver maker Samuel Kirk was to Baltimore what Revere silver was to Boston. The Bordleys had Kirk make a set of large silver goblets—these were designed to copy a colonial goblet with clear and simple lines they liked. These goblets could grace a dinner table to hold water. But their premier use was for mint juleps on a hot summer day when moisture frosted on the outside of them, making a wonderful presentation to their guests.

After the war, Dr. Bordley joined the visiting staff of Union Memorial Hospital. It was a not-for-profit, acute care teaching hospital that had opened a new facility uptown at Calvert and 33rd Streets in 1923. This became his main hospital. But he was also on the staffs of the Women's Hospital of Maryland, Saint Agnes, the Maryland General, and the South Baltimore General Hospital. He continued to receive requests for care from distinguished citizens nationwide. The old files still have correspondence from Eleanor Roosevelt when Franklin was governor of New York. She wanted to stop for a consultation as she passed through Baltimore on the train to Hot Springs—it may have been for a hearing problem.

He also enjoyed teaching. He preferred preceptorial to the more didactic type of teaching for his students. Among those who were trained by him in this manner was Dr. Lawrence Post, whose notable career in ophthalmology had its beginnings in Dr. Bordley's office.[18]

COLLECTING FURNITURE

The Bordleys had a deep interest in the Colonial Revival movement.
Jim and Minnie gradually gathered one of Maryland's premier collections of colonial period decorative
arts. In the introduction to his Baltimore Museum of Art special exhibit of eighteenth-century furniture
in 1968, curator William Elder described the first decades of the twentieth century as years of frantic
collecting—the Bordleys were in the vanguard of that group. Much of their furniture was eventually
photographed to be included in Miller's book, *American Antique Furniture*, which is still in print today.
They also had glass, silver, china, portraits, and so forth.

They used local dealers but bought directly from owners when they could. Israel Sack in New
York, one of the country's foremost dealers, knew them. There is a story that one day while driving on
an Eastern Shore back road, they spied a handsome eighteenth-century table on the porch of a Black
family. It supported a washtub where the laundry was being hand scrubbed. In the nineteenth century
when furniture styles changed, it had been common practice for the old pieces to be passed down. Jim
stopped and knocked at the door. After some discussion the owners were delighted to be receiving a new
Sears and Roebuck washing machine in exchange for the old table.

THE MARYLAND
HISTORICAL SOCIETY

Dr. Bordley was a very enthusiastic member of the Maryland Historical Society. He and Minnie were financial donors as well as donors of papers, books, and furniture. They gave the furnishings of the entire colonial kitchen that occupied one of the society's basement rooms in the 1950s. He was for many years a member of the Gallery Committee. In 1944, at age seventy, he was one of a series of speakers for their centennial-year celebration. He gave a very successful lecture on Baltimore furniture makers from 1785 to 1815. His letter to Jim and John, March 11, 1944, discusses it. The lecture is still in the Historical Society's files.

THE HAMMOND-HARWOOD HOUSE

The Colonial Revival movement was in full swing in the mid-1920s. This was when John D. Rockefeller was acquiring the land around Williamsburg for his renovations there. Francis du Pont was collecting the decorative arts that would become the Winterthur Museum. The historic interest led to the creation of Henry Ford's Greenfield Village in Detroit and to Sturbridge Village in Massachusetts. Marylanders were realizing the historic value of Annapolis. Annapolis was unique in that much of the original town and its harbor were intact and in use. The capitol building from prerevolutionary times still functions today as the state capitol—it was where George Washington had resigned his commission in the army.

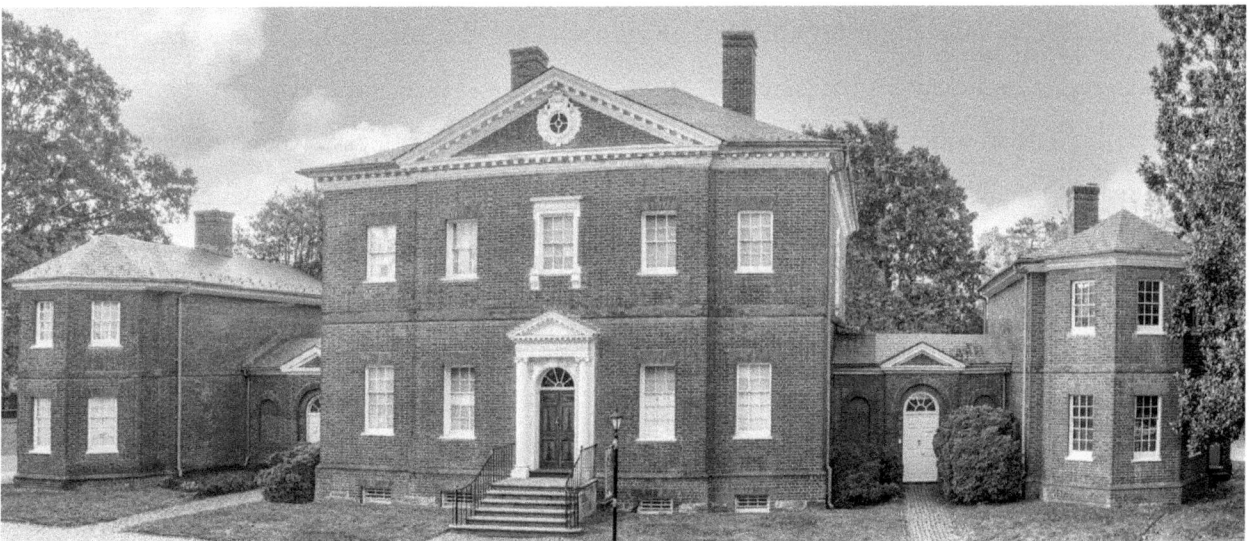

Hammond-Harwood House

The trustees of St. John's College in Annapolis, known as the Board of Visitors, developed the idea that the college should buy the historic houses in town, because these old mansions were at risk of developers who wanted the land they stood on. In 1924, Hester Ann Harwood had died. She was a spinster and owner of the Hammond-Harwood House. This house is one of at least six magnificent Annapolis Georgian mansions dating from prerevolutionary times.[xiv] Because she had no will and no direct heir, the house and furnishings were sold with proceeds going to nieces and nephews. The contents were auctioned in 1925. They attracted a good bit of attention for their historic value. On September 21, 1926, the house was to go on the auction block.

On June 12, 1926, Dr. Bordley was appointed to St. John's College Board of Visitors. He was fifty-two and by now had a reputation for his interest in colonial period decorative arts. He was placed on the building and grounds committee and made chairman of a new special colonial development committee. Other members of his committee were Messrs. Labrot, Hammond, Walton, Woodward, and Buck.

In 1955, Walter Buck wrote Dr. Bordley asking him to recall of the "real story of the purchase of the Hammond-Harwood House." In an article in *Antiques Magazine*, Mrs. Miles White had taken a good bit more credit than Mr. Buck felt she deserved. Jim wrote back to his old friend that shortly prior to the sale, he and Minnie were eating lunch in the Wayside Inn in Massachusetts. The inn was owned by Henry Ford and was a gathering place for people interested in American history. Jim wrote:

> A man came in whom I recognized as Mr. Ford's agent who had visited Annapolis and gone through the Hammond-Harwood House at a time when I was there. This man took a table next to ours and was joined by the lady who ran the lunchroom. She asked what progress he had made in the purchase of the Hammond-Harwood house. The man told her that he had orders from Mr. Ford to purchase it. Mrs. Bordley and I made a hurried exit, and I went to a telegraph office and wired you (Walter Buck) of the conversation.

The thought was that Mr. Ford intended to move the house to Detroit, to his Greenfield Village, where it would have been a real prize. Mr. Buck promptly reported this to college president Enoch Gar-

---

xiv   Others include the Bordley-Randall, Brice, Carroll, Chase-Lloyd, Paca, Peggy Stewart, and Ridout houses.

ey. Dr. Garey immediately took the train to Detroit, got in contact with Mr. Ford's people, and explained the importance of the house to Annapolis. Remarkably, he dissuaded Ford from bidding on it. [xv]

The executive and finance committees of the college met on July 13 and approved a plan for the college to try to obtain the house. With the most serious bidder out of the way, the college got it for $47,000; a mortgage was obtained through the Union Trust Company.

The October 1926 board minutes record that Dr. Garey said, "Without Dr. Bordley's enterprise, Maryland might have lost the house." Dr. Bordley was then asked for a report from his colonial development committee. He extolled the quality of the house and reviewed plans to make it a museum of colonial decorative arts. It was to include some of his collection. He appointed a large subcommittee headed by Mrs. Miles White Jr. to furnish it. He recognized that properly furnishing the house could be a greater expense than purchasing it. Bordley succeeded in appointing a distinguished national group, including Luke Vincent Lockwood, a noted author on colonial furniture, and Richard T. Haynes Halsey of the American Wing of the Metropolitan Museum in New York. They also got Francis P. Garvan on board; he was a lawyer from New York whose wife had inherited a fortune. The Garvans had a large colonial furniture collection and had been buyers at the previous year's Hammond-Harwood furnishings auction. Dr. Bordley wanted a nationwide group to "advertise St. John's among the class of people most desired."[19] He also wanted to make it a shrine for the author of the national anthem, Francis Scott Key, who was an alumnus of the college, but the shrine idea never came to fruition.

In 1927 things were going well. Dr. Bordley opened the year by hosting a dinner for the Board of Visitors in the mostly unfurnished house. An architect skilled in colonial restoration had returned the house to its original condition. There had been no central heat, but Dr. Bordley reported that a modern heating system had been installed; it turned out that Dr. Bordley was the donor.

The chief judge of Maryland's appeals court offered historic judicial documents for a special exhibit—they had an exhibit of colonial clothing. The Maryland Historical Society sent a supportive letter. Favorable articles had been written in the Baltimore and Washington papers. The *Washington Post* said

---

xv   Walter Buck's letter is in the Hammond-Harwood House files. One wonders why Mr. Buck asked such a question so many years later, particularly as he was a principal in this event. It turns out that the ladies of the garden clubs were in the process of eulogizing Mrs. Miles White with a brass plaque for the HHH. Mr. Buck was preparing a letter to remind them of Bordley's accomplishments. In *The Magazine Antiques* in April 1953, Mrs. White had taken credit for overhearing the Wayside Inn conversation. And later in a 1986 article in the *Capitol* (Annapolis newspaper), HHH curator Barbara Brand repeated the story that Mrs. White saved the house in 1926. Mr. Buck may have been wondering if his memory was correct. The St. John's Board of Visitors minutes confirm Dr. Bordley's version.

St. John's would be unique among American colleges in possessing a colonial museum available to its faculty for teaching purposes. There were complementary articles in the *New York Times*.

Under Dr. Bordley's committee, St. John's continued to add to its collection of historic Annapolis houses. The Brice House, another of the five-part colonial Georgian mansion, was purchased for $50,000.[xvi]

In the spring of 1928, the college minutes recorded that "Mr. and Mrs. Francis P. Garvan had sent down furniture that practically filled the (Hammond-Harwood) House, valued at $120,000. Dr. Garey said that he had gone to see Mr. Garvan's representatives in New York, who told him that Mr. Garvan was also planning to send down as much silverware and china as the house ought to have, and possibly some rugs, which he has in his own home." In addition, he had told Dr. Bordley that if they run across any pieces of furniture that ought to be in the house that the Garvans did not have, to buy them and send the bills to him. Dr. Garey also informed the Board that Mrs. Garvan had recently returned to the Hammond-Harwood House the Charles Willson Peale portrait of William Buckland, architect of the house. She had purchased it in the 1925 furnishings auction.

On May 15, 1928, a great celebration was held in Annapolis under the lead of St. John's with Dr. Bordley as chairman. It was "Colonial Days in Annapolis," commemorating the Annapolis Convention of 1786, which had been a forerunner of the Constitutional Convention in Philadelphia. For a day the city was given over to a colonial theme, with citizens dressed in historic costumes. Colonial music was played and historic foods were served—there were many celebratory events and notable visitors. President and Mrs. Calvin Coolidge attended a costumed reenactment of Washington's resignation of his military command but declined to don colonial dress.[20] In the evening, a banquet was served in the state house. The day served to heighten the interest in the city's history and the role St. John's was playing in preserving the historic buildings.

Later in the spring of 1928, the Walpole Society visited Annapolis on a tour of southern Maryland. St. John's minutes record that President Garey had offered a position to one of its members, Mr. R.

---

xvi   Subsequently, the portraits of Thomas Jennings and his wife by John Hesselius came on the market. Jennings's daughter Juliana had married James Brice in 1745 and was the first mistress of the house. Dr. Bordley bought those portraits and gave them to St. John's College to hang in the Brice House ballroom. Later, when St. John's sold the house, the portraits were moved to Carroll Barrister House (the admissions office), where they are today.

T. H. Halsey.[xvii] Halsey was a member of Dr. Bordley's decorating committee and had been cofounder and first director of the American Wing of the Metropolitan Museum. Disliking the administrative work, he was giving up his position at the Metropolitan Museum in New York. He was thinking about going to the College of William and Mary to help with a restoration project at Williamsburg. However, since visiting Annapolis, and at the request of Dr. Garey, he decided to help with the project at St. John's. The Board approved of this. Mr. Halsey was given an honorary doctorate of letters and made professor of fine arts, as promised by Dr. Garey. He joined the faculty at a one-dollar-a-year salary and was given charge of the Hammond-Harwood House. He planned to make it the first college teaching American colonial decorative arts. The Bordley-Randall House was up for sale.[xviii] St. John's bought it for $45,000 and made it available to Mr. Halsey as his living quarters.

By 1929 the college owned the Hammond-Harwood, Brice, Bordley-Randall, Peggy Stewart, Pinkney, and Humphreys Houses. Halsey's curriculum was a success—it attracted students to the college and was gaining it national attention. We have devoted so much space to this subject because saving the Hammond-Harwood House was one of the accomplishments of which Dr. Bordley was most proud. Privately, he was dismayed at losing personal control of it to Halsey, but this was never expressed in the minutes of the board. It came out in the letter to Walter Buck in 1955. Mrs. White's decorating committee had no further role and resigned when Halsey took over. Dr. Bordley remained active on the Board for several more years. In 1932 he headed a planning committee that looked at the whole structure of the college.

The stock market crash in October of 1929 marked the beginning of the end of St. John's colonial revival efforts. The college had an excess of mortgages to be paid on the houses. The Hammond-Harwood expenses exceeded its income, and it became a burden. Then, in the spring of 1932, the whole thing fell apart over a silly power struggle. A new college president, Dr. Douglas Gordon, sent a note to Mr. Halsey that he planned to host a lunch in the Hammond-Harwood House for his fellow Harvard alumni prior to the Harvard-Navy crew race and the St. John's–Haverford lacrosse game. Halsey refused, saying he had been given sole authority over the house and was responsible for Garvan's furnishings. He

---

xvii   This was a society dedicated to the appreciation and study of American decorative art, architecture, and history. Luke Vincent Lockwood was one of the founders. He was a member of Dr. Bordley's furnishing committee. See http://findingaid.winterthur.org/html/HTML_Finding_Aids/COL0386.htm for a good summary of the organization.

xviii   The Bordley-Randall House was built in 1760 by Thomas Bordley (1710–1764), son of Stephen, who came to Annapolis with his brother in 1697.

felt that such a boisterous group posed far too great a threat to the historic contents. A vitriolic meeting of the Board of Visitors executive committee ensued; the board had to support its president. Halsey, who was serving as Garvan's representative, resigned. Garvan took his furnishings and paintings back and they went to the Mabel Brady Garvan collection at Yale.

In 1934, the Board fired President Gordon. Although a brilliant man, he seems not to have been skilled in dealing with people—but it was too late to save the furnishings and Halsey's program.[21]

The house was little used for the next several years. On December 2, 1935, the board decided it must sell the Brice and Hammond-Harwood Houses. Due to the Depression, it could not carry the mortgages. The chairman of the executive committee, Charles A. Cummins, wrote to Henry Ford stating that the college had to sell the Hammond-Harwood House to reduce its indebtedness. Hoping Ford was still interested, he wrote there would be a strong reaction from the community should the building be removed, but he felt compelled to make the best possible arrangement for the college. It was offered to Ford for $175,000, three and a half times what the college paid for it! On December 10, Mr. Ford's secretary replied that Mr. Ford was not interested. Finally, in 1941, the Federated Garden Clubs of Maryland bought it. So the house was "saved" a second time to become the museum that it is today.

From 1928 to 1932, the Hammond-Harwood House under St. John's College had been a beacon of American culture. Under Professor Halsey it was the nation's leading institution teaching the history of our colonial decorative arts. And it had Garvan's wonderful collection to use as teaching material. Then between the financial strain of the Depression and a foolish, egotistical college president, it all collapsed.

Finally, there is an interesting comment in a letter that Jim sent his cousin Mary Brown in 1955.[22] He was recalling the colonial revival effort for Annapolis and said, "The idea was to reestablish the old colonial lives and make a Williamsburg out of Annapolis. We had options on $870,000 worth of property when the Depression struck, and our sponsor went into his shell." Considering that St. John's was buying the finest old buildings in Annapolis for no more than $50,000, this was a huge sum. There has been a longstanding rumor that Henry Ford not only had declined to bid on the Hammond-Harwood House in 1926 but later had become interested in helping restore Colonial Annapolis—the story was that he saw it as an opportunity to best the Rockefellers at their Williamsburg reconstruction. Annapolis certainly had great potential. Glenn Campbell, historian for the Historic Annapolis Foundation, thinks the Ford rumors are unfounded. Our review of the St. John's board minutes revealed that there was indeed a plan and sponsor to restore Colonial Annapolis, but it was Francis Garvan, not Ford.

HOMEWOOD AND WHITEHALL

Dr. Bordley's interest in the rehabilitation of old colonial houses led to two other notable Maryland homes. In 1929, a committee of the board of trustees of Johns Hopkins University formed an advisory committee for the restoration of Homewood, the home of Charles Carroll on the Hopkins University campus. Four men were on the committee: Dr. Bordley, our old friend Professor R. T. H. Halsey from St. John's, and two others.[23] Mr. and Mrs. Francis P. Garvan are credited with funding the work and refurnishing the building as a gift to the university. The work was completed in May 1932, just before the management crisis at the Hammond-Harwood House erupted. Furnishings that Garvan donated to this project are still there.

The other building was Whitehall, which had been built outside of Annapolis on Whitehall Creek. It was the summer residence of Horatio Sharpe, the last British governor before the revolution. In the spring of 1929, Francis Garvan had bought it, probably with the idea it should be saved as part of the restoration of Annapolis. The Depression intervened, and Garvan offered it to the federal government as a retreat for the White House. That was turned down, and it stood vacant until purchased by Charles Scarlett in 1946.[24] I can recall going with my grandfather to visit Whitehall and Mr. Scarlett, a family friend, shortly after he bought it. What a treasure for a nine-year-old! I had the run of the magnificent empty house and the grounds while the grown-ups talked restoration. A second floor had been added, and the discussion was whether to return Whitehall to its original state. It was restored.

CHARLCOTE PLACE

Dr. Bordley continued his lifelong interest in the Maryland Historical Society. The *Baltimore Sun* reported on December 13, 1927, "Dr. James Bordley, Jr., an authority on antiques, spoke last night at the Maryland Historical Society on the houses acquired by St. John's College…Dr. Bordley illustrated his lecture with lantern slides and gave a brief history of each of the houses."

He was a regular user of the Maryland Club, where he played squash. He continued to play golf at the Elkridge Club. In 1933, Governor Ritchie—who knew him through the Board of Visitors at St. John's—enlisted his help in repealing the 18th Amendment (Prohibition). We have no doubt of his enthusiastic support for its repeal.[25]

By the mid-1920s it was clear that a shift in residential demographics was occurring in Baltimore. Electrification of the city was progressing. The automobile had replaced the horse as a means of transportation. Electric streetcar lines were being extended out of the city, allowing mass transportation to suburban areas. Guilford and Roland Park were the desirable places to live. These neighborhoods had been laid out according to the principles of the Olmstead Brothers in 1913. They were much further north than Mount Vernon Square, but they were well served by good new roads and the trolley. They offered well-designed homes on large grassy lots in parklike settings. It was a dramatic change from the tightly packed downtown housing. With enough money invested in the soaring stock market to cover the cost of building, the Bordleys bought the lot at 4 Charlcote Place in Guilford. They hired the architectural firm of Mottu and White to build a large and beautiful Georgian brick home modeled after the best of historic Annapolis. The front door is like the Hammond-Harwood house. There is a large entrance hall stretching to the back wall and opens to the second floor. The stairs come down on the right side from a balcony in the back that crosses in front of a large Palladian window, which floods the hall with light like the Chase-Lloyd House. The house would set off their collection of furniture and other colonial period paintings and decorative arts;[26] it was designed with good flow between rooms to facilitate entertaining.

In 1903, when finances had forced Richard Hollyday to sell Readbourne, the family had saved as much as they could.[27] The eagle cornices in the dining room came along with all the plantation record books.[28] In the attic they found things like the brick molds from the 1740s when the house had been built. So as building proceeded at Charlcote Place, they used the decorative brick molds from Readbourne to make the distinctive brick band at the base of the building. Flooring was saved from an old downtown theater that was being demolished and was used in the front hall. The house had high ceilings and an elegant front hall and staircase. The study was to the left and parlor to the right. There was a spacious dining room beyond the parlor. The basement contained a safe, a wine cellar, and a squash court, as well as the furnace and storage areas. Minnie refused to have a swimming pool. The large house needed a staff, including a maid and a cook—they even had a butler. Domestic help was available and relatively inexpensive in those flush days of the roaring twenties.

The actual construction began in 1929—then the stock market crashed and the money for the house melted away. It was a severe financial blow, but they were able to complete the home and moved in by 1931.

Despite Jim's protestations about not liking to travel, Minnie had talked him into a second trip to Europe sometime in the late 1920s, probably after plans for the new house were underway. We know this because of another family tale. As they toured, Minnie collected ivy clippings from an English cathedral, probably Salisbury. She kept them alive in hotel room water glasses as they traveled. She sewed them into the lining of her overcoat on the steamship home to get them through customs. They survived and grew to cover the walls of the house.

The Bordleys liked to entertain. On one occasion, with a black-tie dinner underway, the guests began to hear a series of loud reports coming from the basement. Investigation revealed that Jim was making beer—this was during Prohibition—and the corks were blowing out of the beer bottles.

Angus MacLean noted that "for many years one of the most delightful occasions of the holiday season was the annual eggnog party given by Dr. and Mrs. Bordley on New Year's Day." And here I indulge in another personal aside: At about age fourteen, while visiting my grandmother during the Christmas season, I was offered a cup of the eggnog, to my mother's horror. It was the most velvety smooth ambrosia that I had ever experienced. After a second helping, the room seemed to be in motion, but I had been unaware of any taste of alcohol as I drank it. It was a formidable old Eastern Shore recipe

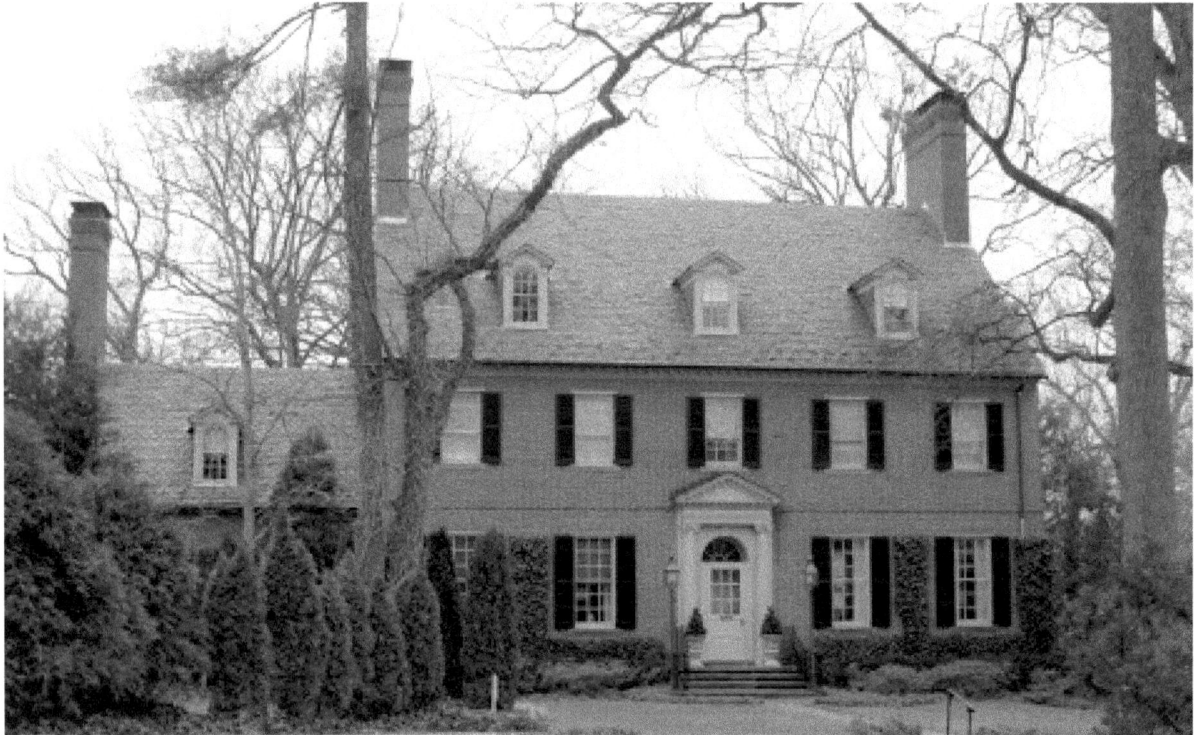

4 Charlcote Place, Baltimore

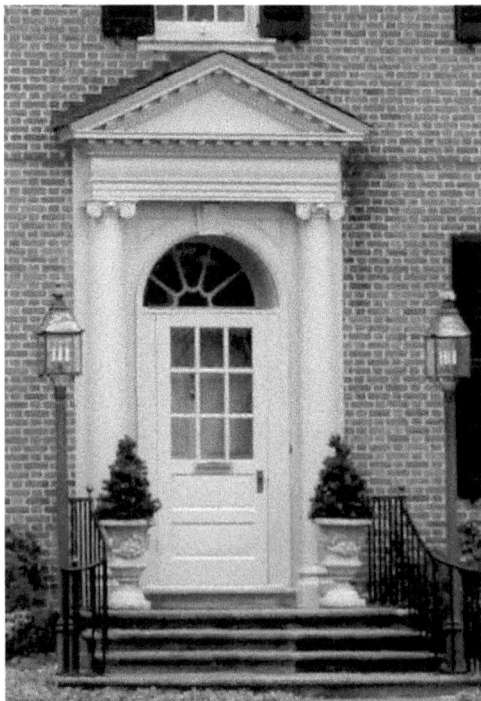

Charlcote Place Door

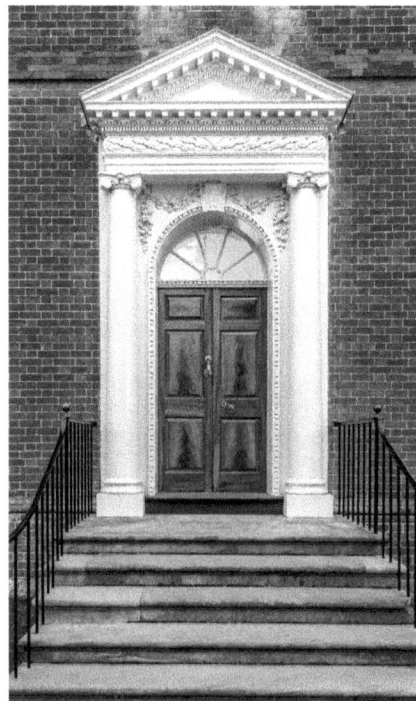

Hammond-Harwood Door

from Readbourne. It required starting early in the fall, a large silver tray for the beating of dozens of eggs (with a silver fork, of course), an outrageous amount of cream, and quantities of alcohol, sugar, and spices. Finally, one needed a cool space and a large earthenware pot in which to age it for about three months.

The holiday season was also time for Albany cookies (sometimes called Albany cakes). They were a tradition in the Bordley house that all the grandchildren associate with the Christmas season. The recipe is in the appendix. The cookie was popular in many Eastern Shore homes and goes way back in time. It can also be found in the cookbook *Maryland's Way*, a classic of recipes from old Maryland homes. We suspect that these small delights were a special holiday treat in early colonial homes, when sugar and spices were hard to come by.

Although the Bordleys usually had a cook, Minnie was quite a good cook herself and often taught the hired cook just how she wanted food prepared. She told granddaughter Brucie that she sometimes used muskrat in place of terrapin for the stew if terrapin was scarce. She said no one ever knew the difference and always exclaimed how delicious the terrapin was. During the war in the 1940s, with meat hard to obtain, the family often ate internal organs. Minnie always had either creamed sweetbreads or kidney stew to go with waffles on Sunday morning, even well after the war. We viewed this as a great treat and still do.

A favorite early memory is being allowed to help Linwood, the butler, who was in a black bow tie and white jacket, prepare the mint juleps for friends who were visiting. I was given a rolling pin and a canvas sack full of ice cubes, which were made at home in the new electric refrigerator.[xix] My job was to place the bag on a brick surface and beat it until the ice was powder. Linwood packed the powdered ice into the silver goblets preloaded with mint and sugar, then filled them up with a very generous amount of fine Maryland rye whiskey. Within a few moments on a sultry afternoon, a thick frost formed on the sides of the goblets—it was a great presentation when Linwood arrived with a tray full of the icy silver goblets and a sprig of green mint sticking out.

When Jim and John finished at Yale, they returned to Baltimore to go to medical school at Hopkins. The brick row house behind the hospital at 1936 McElderry Street was bought for their living quarters.[29] They stayed at Hopkins for their residencies. Jim specialized in internal medicine and joined the Hopkins staff full time; John went into otolaryngology. He joined his father's practice but retained a part-time position at Hopkins for teaching and research.

[xix]   This was a prewar General Electric model with large, coiled condenser on top.

All three children were married in the mid-1930s. Jim married Julia (Dudy) Ross of Philadelphia. John wed Ellen Fisher in Baltimore, and Ellen in 1936 married Charles Webb at Charlcote Place. By 1942 there were six grandchildren. John had the first children, Brucie and Anne. I was next, and then my sister Carroll arrived. Shortly after this, Pat was born to Jim and Dudy. In 1942 Dudy was pregnant with JB IV (really the sixth) when Jim and John left for the war.

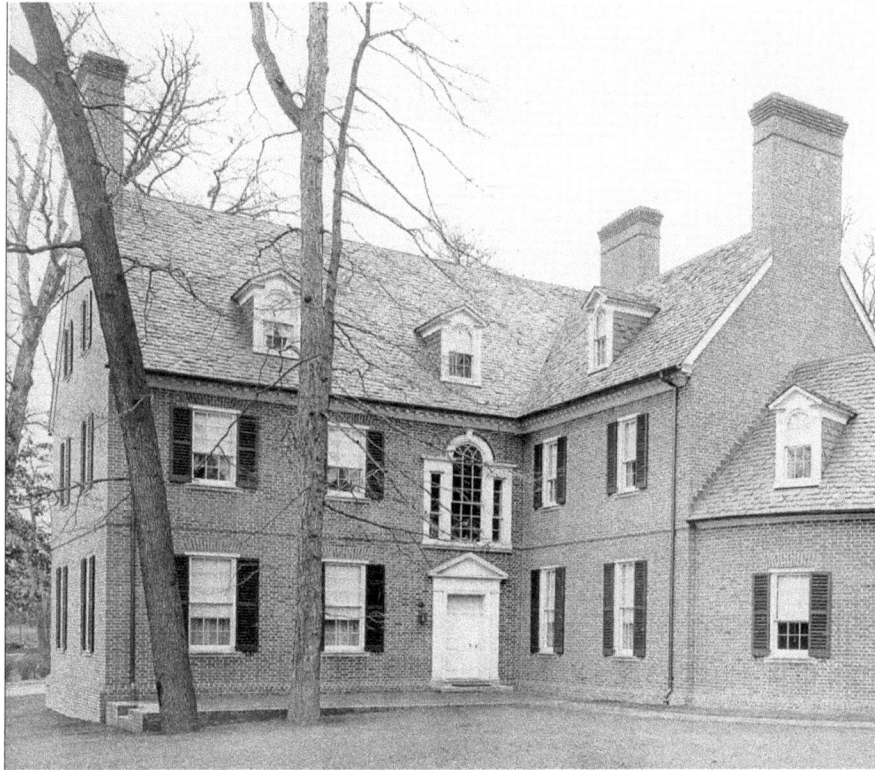

Rear view with tree-shaded brick patio in summer

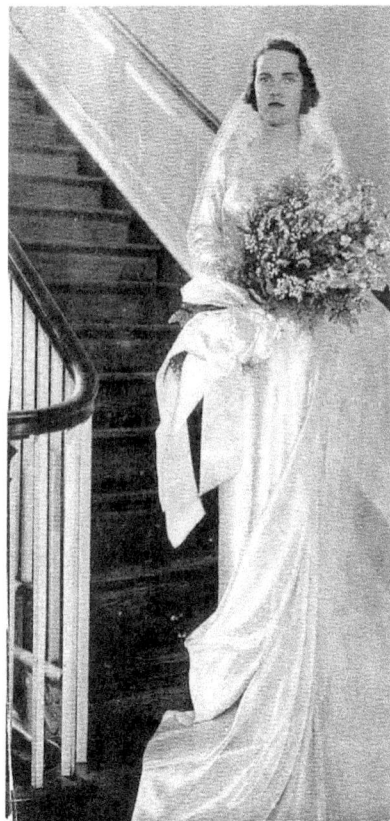

Ellen at Charlcote Pl., 1936

THE WAR LETTERS, 1942–1945

When Germany invaded Poland in 1939, war broke out across Europe. Although there was a strong antiwar lobby in this country, the government started preparing. In 1940, at the request of the US surgeon general, the Johns Hopkins Hospital organized the 18th General Hospital. Originally organized as a thousand-bed unit, it was split by the army into two smaller five-hundred-bed units, designated as the 18th and 118th General Hospitals. In those days, each major city hospital provided most of the manpower for a military general hospital from its own personnel. The younger doctors, nurses, staff, and administration all went as a unit. The older staff would stay behind, continuing to man the stateside facilities. The University of Maryland Hospital had similar units.

When the Japanese bombed our fleet in Pearl Harbor on December 7, 1941, Jim and John had been assigned to the 118th General Hospital. Jim was a lieutenant colonel and second-in-command. John was a major in charge of the ENT staff. The 118th initially went to Herne Bay, New South Wales, Australia—this is on the eastern coast near Sydney. They built a five-hundred-bed hospital that eventually grew to three thousand beds in conjunction with Australian units. By 1943, Jim had become the commanding officer and was later promoted to full colonel. When MacArthur began moving up and into the Philippines, the 118th followed to Leyte with a brief training and organization stop in New Guinea.

In 1941 their father was sixty-seven years old; he was thinking of retirement. John had joined his practice and would have been taking over, but with the start of the war, all the younger physicians in town were off with their units. Shortly after Jim and John shipped out, their father started sending them letters that he typed himself on the office typewriter. One letter was sent to both, addressed to General Hospital #118, APO 1142, San Francisco. All he knew was that they had headed west. It was much later

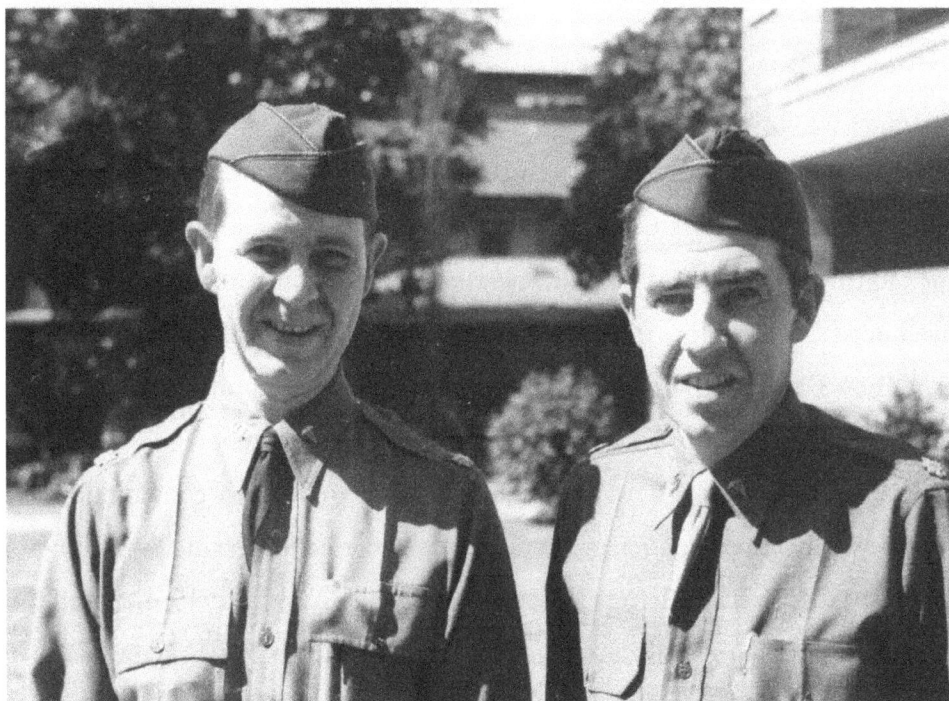

Lt. Col. James Bordley III and Maj. John E. Bordley in Sydney, 1942

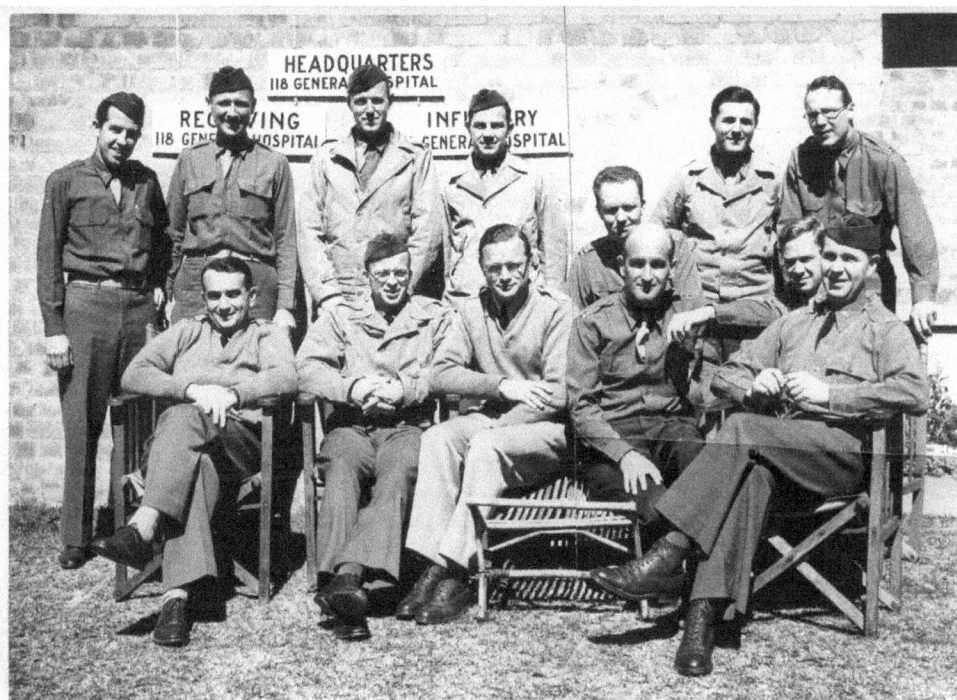

Probably Australia, 1942 or 1943
Back left: John Bordley, J. H. Long, Eaton, W. Jones, Johnston, H. Fox, Billings
Front left: A. McGehee Harvey, unknown, Walter Winkenerder,
J. Whitridge, W. S. Stiffler, Jim Bordley

that he finally learned they were in Australia. The letters are numbered, and dated and a carbon copy was saved.

Those carbons became the stimulus for this biography. After John Bordley died, his daughter Anne (Mrs. Peter Moss) found an old cardboard grocery carton packed with papers and files under John's bed. She recognized they were from our grandfather, but she could neither bring herself to wade through them nor to throw the box out. Finally, she asked me if I would like to take the box. I did, which seemed to relieve her of an obligation. It went on the top shelf of my closet and stayed there, unexplored, until years later. When I retired, there was time to investigate its contents. Out came a cornucopia of history with the prize being the letters, sixty years after they were written.

Dr. Bordley was not much of a typist; the letters are rough in their construction. He would type a few lines or a paragraph between patients. There are many corrections, which stand out on the carbon copy. Yet he managed to get out 214 letters between June 1942 and July 1945. They tell the story of the family, of how the war was progressing, and its effects on Baltimore life. They are full of national news and his political opinions. He expressed very patriotic views, but he was not in favor of Roosevelt's handling of the unions. He thought that the whole country was making sacrifices and was furious, especially at John L. Lewis and his mineworkers' union. He viewed the unions as holding the country up for personal gains with ever-higher wage demands. He thought this was outrageous and the recurring strikes that slowed the war effort were unpatriotic. He was thrilled when Truman finally became president and refused to be blackmailed by a union strike. Truman nationalized the striking workers, risking his own political future.

At the start of the war, gasoline rationing restricted citizens to two gallons a week. Minnie had learned to drive and had a new 1941 Plymouth sedan, which had to be put up on blocks. Jim had to ride crowded streetcars to get downtown. He wrote in horror that "the wildest lot of dames" was driving streetcars. Women were taking over men's jobs—it was the start of the era of Rosie the Riveter. Gas restrictions eased a bit after a while, but one was not allowed to drive a car to the Elkridge Club just to play golf. Arranging to make a house call just beyond Elkridge could circumvent this; he could then stop there on the way home. So he was up to a little cheating, but he rails against the hoarders and black marketers. When he made it to the golf course, there were no caddies and not much of a crew to maintain the course. At home, domestic help had become unreliable to almost unavailable. He and Minnie had to work hard to maintain a very large house.

Hospitals were having problems. The staffs were so limited it was difficult to admit patients. Anesthesiologists were few so it was a struggle to find surgical time. But there were some bright spots in medicine—when sulfa drugs appeared early in the war, he wrote to John about what wonders they could do for nasal infections. Then, towards the end of the war, penicillin became available, and he writes about using it to cure a serious postoperative eye infection.

He describes how Baltimore filled up with war industry workers. Glenn L. Martin Inc. was mass-producing airplanes. At its peak the Baltimore shipyards were turning out a new liberty ship (transport ship) every four days. War-production jobs paid well and pulled in people from all walks of life. He wrote, "There are hillbillies all over town." Not only did domestic help vanish, but farmers were leaving farms either to join the army or to go into a high-paying war industry. This created problems with food production. Jim had two farms—one, which he had probably inherited, was on the Eastern Shore and one in Howard County; lack of farm labor led him to sell both.

Despite the war, the Bordleys managed to continue going to Rye Beach, New Hampshire, for the summer months. The cities tended to close in the summer where possible. Although summertime infectious diseases that had plagued inner cities in the nineteenth century like yellow fever and malaria were gone, polio was a serious problem, especially in crowded places. Operating rooms had no air conditioning. Sweat dripping from the brow of a masked, gowned, and overheated surgeon posed a real risk to a surgical patient. Elective surgeries were postponed to the fall.

The trip to Rye Beach was a tour de force by Minnie. The house was closed. Sheets covered the furniture. Window shades were pulled down. Steamer trunks were packed. These trunks stood about four feet tall and hinged open vertically in the middle—one side had hangers for suits and dresses; the other side had drawers for everything else. The trunks and golf clubs were taken to the Railway Express office at Penn Station several days prior to departure so they would be at the hotel on arrival. During the war it was difficult to get enough gasoline ration coupons for the drive to New Hampshire. The train trip was a long journey done in one day. In New York City you had to go from Penn Station across town to Grand Central Station.ˣˣ There you got on the New York, New Haven, and Hartford line to travel up the coast to Rye Beach. It must have seemed a remarkable trip compared to what travel was like when Jim was born.

---

xx   The B&O railroad also went to New York. One could board an overnight Pullman sleeping car parked at the Mount Royal Station in Baltimore up to about eleven p.m. It was coupled to a train coming north from Washington. Lacking a tunnel into New York, the B&O deposited passengers on the New Jersey side of the Hudson River and ferried them across. The passengers would be on the ferry by about seven-thirty a.m. Taking the ferry across the Hudson River with early morning sunlight on the skyscrapers was a slower but more spectacular entry into the city than the Pennsylvania Railroad tunnel.

The Farragut Hotel was a long rambling wooden building next to the golf course. A couple of blocks from the beach, it was an oasis of cool away from the Baltimore heat. Many old friends turned up there every summer. Letters to the 118th General Hospital are missing for the weeks at Rye Beach—he had no typewriter there. The letters must have been in handwriting without copies. Practical portable typewriters had been designed but were not generally available as war production took precedence.

In 1944 he gave one of the lectures for the Maryland Historical Society's centennial celebration, as was noted earlier. On March 11 he wrote, "I told the history of Maryland from 1785 to 1920 as background and then gave a brief history of the cabinet makers involved and showed some sixty slides of the motifs used by them as points of identification and then illustrated and analyzed two pieces which have been wrongly classified as English, illustrating the differences." He reports the auditorium was packed. After the talk, two journals wanted to publish the lecture, but the Baltimore Museum of Art, which had helped make his glass slides, offered to do the talk as a monograph and they also wanted the slides for their library—he preferred this, and what remains of the slides are still there. But the museum librarian can find no record of a monograph. He was clearly delighted with the result of the lecture, but it had been a lot of work in preparation. It was a relief to have it behind him.

On May 2, 1944, he wrote, "I have been invited to a dinner tonight at the Belvedere (Hotel) and have been tipped off. I will be asked to become President of the Baltimore Museum…of course I will not accept it because I have too many responsibilities now which can not be shelved. I want them to elect a younger man, one with enough pep to build a future…All I want now is to finish what I started."

One of the most delightful sections in the letters occurs in June of 1945 after Germany's surrender. Col. Bordley wrote his father that the governor general of New South Wales, Australia, Lord Wakehurst, would be visiting the States that month. One of his stops would be to visit the Hopkins Hospital to express Australia's appreciation for the medical help that had been sent to them. Jim, now the commanding officer, asked his father to go all out for Lord Wakehurst as they had been treated very well while the 118th was in Australia. His father writes back that because of the rationing (Japan had not yet surrendered) and limited food supplies, it would be nearly impossible to put on a proper celebration. Later he warms up a bit and wrote,

> Hopkins is entertaining the Lord and Lady and their fellow travelers. If they can spare the time, I am going to give them a dinner at the [Elkridge] Club, having as our other guests the returned members of 118 and their wives…To do this I will have to petition the Board of Governors as they have passed a rule stopping all dinners except family affairs…There is no variety of food or drinks and we will have to take what is served on the

day of the dinner. We could not possibly entertain them at home because we have only a second-rate cook, can secure no additional help and have not the necessary food coupons.

On June 22 he wrote,

Well the Gov. General and his Lady plus the daughter and Peter arrived yesterday. Ma and I had them for luncheon with eighteen others at the Kennels.[xxi] If I do say so myself, it was a bang-up affair. It was on the porch. In the background were placed a British and US flag. Place cards were on a little basket at each seat. With the place cards were miniature American flags on staffs except at the Governor General's place where the flag was that of Australia and at the Lady's place where it was the British flag. The table decorations were beautiful, in fact the most beautiful I ever saw. The predominant flower was the pink water lily. In the center the flowers were in an oblong dish about two feet long and at the end of the table in round dishes where they were mixed with white and yellow field flowers. Instead of cocktails we served mint juleps made of fine old Maryland rye. They were served on the lawn with chairs placed in a circle around a table filled with pretzels and potato chips. This function took about half an hour…the first course was melon, then imperial crab served in the shell, like devilled crabs. With it were served broiled tomatoes which greatly pleased the Gov. and Lady.[xxii] Then a salad of Avocado pears followed by an ice…The Governors of the Club turned everything over to us…The Lord Wakefield party went to the Hopkins on an inspection trip at three o'clock; they were given a large reception after which the Governor showed in the Hurd Amphitheatre two long rolls [presumably film] of New South Wales and New Guinea.

The remarkable event at Elkridge, like many other things they did, was surely managed by Minnie, although she does not get much in the way of credits.

---

xxi   The official name of the club is "The Elkridge Kennels," presumably going back to foxhunting days. The clubhouse is a large old wooden building with a spacious covered porch wrapping around its front. It is a wonderful setting for a luncheon on a nice June day. The tree-shaded clubhouse is surrounded by the golf course.

xxii   Broiled tomatoes with a sprinkle of brown sugar on top are a signature dish at the club, still popular today.

SALE OF 4 CHARLCOTE PLACE

The home in Guilford was a pride and joy. However, by the middle of the war years, Linwood and most of the help were gone. Real estate taxes were rising, and the big house and yard were becoming too much for the two seventy-year-old Bordleys to manage. As early as June of 1943, he wrote that he was thinking of moving. "The strain on Minnie was too much."

This was true especially as he was still maintaining a busy medical practice at that age. On May 8, 1944, he said, "For the first time for a long while I have only a hand full of patients and what a relief as I had two operations this morning and it takes a lot out of me...I am losing my desire to work and if you were home, I would quit...I am ashamed to stop while so many men are making so many more tragic sacrifices."

Then in the last paragraph of the April 14, 1944, letter, he casually mentions: "I sold our home last night. Charles Garland, now with Alexander Brown, came over to the house at nine o'clock and stayed until eleven, and left with a contract."[xxiii] Mr. Garland was a squash player, and the court in the basement sealed the deal. "I got five thousand dollars more than the real estate men said I would get. In fact, it was the best price for a house in Guilford in twelve years. While it was nothing like the cost, or, value, it was satisfactory."

They had until October 1 to move. He thought they would move to a nice apartment building and was caught by surprise to discover there was virtually no available housing in Baltimore because of the influx of war workers. On May 8, "We still have no place to live but if we can get priority to put in an oil heater, we will go to the house on Guilford Avenue...This will only be until we can get an apartment

---

xxiii   Mr. Garland was the president of Alex Brown, one of the leading investment houses of Baltimore.

in one of the nicer apartment buildings."[xxiv] So they ended up moving to 2630 Guilford Avenue. It was a row house in a declining area of town and Minnie hated it—the sudden and dramatic loss of the status and beauty of the old neighborhood was not for her. They fixed up the new place well. She developed a nice rose garden in the back. But he had to shovel coal into the furnace until the oil burner arrived after the war—it meant disposing of a good bit of their collection of furnishings. The best they kept. What the children had room for, they could take. But at that time, all the children's families had limited-sized living quarters. A good bit was sold. Despite the real estate comedown, the tone of his letters seems much happier after they settled in.

He developed a woodworking shop in the basement without much prior experience and he really enjoyed it. He learned to do simple repair work on old pieces and made some small things himself. He had a collection of Civil War bone saws that he occasionally used on pieces of wood.

Dr. Bordley typed what turned out to be his final war letter on July 5, 1945. Then he and Minnie were off for Rye Beach. The war would be over before they returned. He continued to express fatigue about his workload but was proud that in his seventies he was still playing golf.

---

xxiv   His younger brother had financial problems and Jim bought the house on Guilford Ave. as a residence for him and his family. With a good war job at Bendix, Worthington had been able to buy a home in Rogers Forge and the Guilford Ave. house was available.

...AFTER THE WAR

After the two atomic bombs fell on Japan in early August 1945, the Japanese announced their surrender. Shooting stopped on August 15. By September 3 John was on a transport ship in charge of seven hundred patients being returned to the States. The goal was to return the staff that had been there the longest, leaving the wind up to the newer men—but Jim stayed in Leyte. Hospitals in Luzon were evacuating their wounded to the 118th. Those hospitals needed to open space to accommodate freed American prisoners of war.[30] Jim stayed until the 118th closed in December and he got home shortly before Christmas.

John rejoined his father's practice and held a part-time role at Hopkins Hospital. In 1952, when Dr. Crowe retired, he became the head of ENT at Hopkins and stopped his private practice.

Jim had reason to hope that he would be the next head of medicine at Hopkins. On June 2, 1945, his father's letter reported that Hopkins had requested Jim's return,[xxv] but he was the commanding officer of the 118th—the request was denied. Just before Jim got back in December 1945, Hopkins announced that one of Jim's subordinates, Dr. A. McGehee Harvey, who had returned early due to hepatitis, was appointed to succeed retiring Dr. Longcope as professor of medicine.

Jim returned to Hopkins and helped set up the private outpatient service. But with Dr. Harvey in the chief of medicine role, Jim had no possibility of advancement. He got an offer to go to Tulane as their medical school dean, but his wife rebelled at the idea of New Orleans heat. In 1948 he accepted an offer to become the director of the Mary Imogene Bassett Hospital in Cooperstown. It was in a beautiful setting in upstate New York. The Bassett was a teaching hospital affiliated with Columbia University and its medical school.[xxvi]

---

xxv   The War Department was then allowing medical schools to request the return of needed faculty members. Dr. Longcope was the professor of medicine.

xxvi   See Appendix for family comments on Jim's move to Cooperstown.

RETIREMENT

There is an interesting letter in the Hopkins Medical Archives. Jim (JB III) wrote, "Early in 1947, my father, who had virtually retired from practice, came to see me one evening, and told me that one of his old and cherished patients, and a friend, had sought his advice about a memorial to her late husband, Thomas C. Jenkins." A consultation was held with Dr. Harvey. It was established that Hopkins needed a biophysics institute. Mrs. Jenkins donated five million dollars for its establishment, with encouragement from Dr. Bordley.

In retirement Jim started writing. He wrote letters to the editor that were published in the *Baltimore Sun* and the *Evening Sun* newspapers about a variety of his political opinions. But his major effort was directed to writing a history: *The Hollyday and Related Families of the Eastern Shore of Maryland*. Minnie still had all the record books from Readbourne and Jim was able to write the history of multiple related Eastern Shore families.[31]

In the late 1940s, the Bordleys bought one of the first television sets. It was a freestanding piece of furniture, a cabinet about three and a half feet tall, with the lower half taken up by a single speaker. Centered in the upper half was a ten-inch screen that showed black-and-white images. It was a technology marvel that had all the family crowding around regularly to see what was being broadcast.

After the war was over, an apartment that Minnie wanted finally became available. They moved to a building close to the Hopkins University campus near University Parkway and Charles Street.

The senior Bordleys stopped going to Rye Beach after Jim moved to Cooperstown. The summers were spent with Jim and the grandchildren in upstate New York. They worked out an arrangement with the Tunnicliff Inn in the center of Cooperstown. It was three or four blocks from Jim's house at 13 Main Street. They got two adjacent first floor rooms—the front room was converted to a living room and the inn dining room provided meals. They spent many pleasant summers in Cooperstown.

After he retired, Dr. Bordley developed laryngeal cancer. Both he and Minnie were heavy smokers. It was such a part of society to smoke in those days that it was almost unavoidable. Today it seems incredible that a physician in an ENT specialty would have done this, but they did not know that tobacco was a cancer-causing agent. He had a partial laryngectomy that left him talking only in a frustrating hoarse whisper, but it cured the problem.

In the summer of 1955, while in Cooperstown, Jim wrote a series of letters to his close cousin Purnell Brown. Earlier that spring, Jim and Minnie had moved to a smaller apartment.[xxvii] Purnell and his wife, Mary, had come up from Centreville to assist with the move. Then shortly after the Bordleys went to Cooperstown, the Browns returned to Baltimore. Mary had a gallbladder attack and needed surgery. Purnell stayed in the apartment while Mary was at Union Memorial Hospital—it was a six-week recovery in those days. Jim wrote a series of letters to them from Cooperstown. The packet of letters was recently found in an old Brown farmhouse in Centreville; one was on the obituary of Mrs. Miles White, who was discussed earlier with the saving of the Hammond-Harwood House. It is what led us to the research of the history of the sale of that house to St. John's College.[xxviii]

The Hollyday family history was just finished at the end of 1955 when Dr. Bordley began to have heart trouble. He passed away after a couple of weeks. His friend Jim Foster, director of the Maryland Historical Society, arranged to have the index done and published the book. Dr. Bordley had also been writing another history, *Bordleys of the Eastern Shore*—this is a typed draft with multiple corrections and additions in his handwriting. It is over eighty pages long and not quite finished. Unfortunately, his parents were not yet included.

In the eighty-two years that Jim lived, the world went through an enormous transformation. He started in the horse-and-buggy era and lived long enough to postulate that in the not-too-distant future, we would have a man on the moon.

Medicine went from a primitive art to a modern, scientifically based profession. He had the luck and ability to ride the wave of this era to a rich and full life—and Minnie must have had quite a trip being married to such a dynamo.

When he died, she asked me if I would be one of the pallbearers. The coffin was surprisingly heavy. It was a raw, gray winter day; the grass was wet. We carried it down the hill from the hearse to the

---

xxvii   The new dwelling was in the Greenway, Apt. 417, St. Paul and 34th Sts.

xxviii   Bordley-Brown letters

open grave at Green Mount Cemetery. So comes the end of our story. The author learned a great deal about a very interesting grandfather and a remarkable period in American history.

APPENDIX

Memories from the Grandchildren
Legal Tender

Researching the Bordley history has led to some interesting but extraneous facts. For example, Jim's father was president of the Centreville National Bank during what is known as the national currency period (1800s to the Depression). The federal government printed notes and sent them to local banks for distribution. They had to be signed by the local bank president and cashier to be legal tender. The bank note shown below is from a series known as "brown backs," as the back was printed with brown ink. It was signed by James Bordley Sr. in red ink in the bottom right. In this black-and-white image, all that can be seen is the "Ja…" of James, but I am told the original is more readable. The clerk's name, J. F. Rolph, is easily seen. It is the only such note known to exist and is in a private collection. It is still legal tender and can be used, but it is worth far more as a collector's item. And think what it would have bought in the 1890s when it was new, compared to how little it buys today—it was a very large bill then.

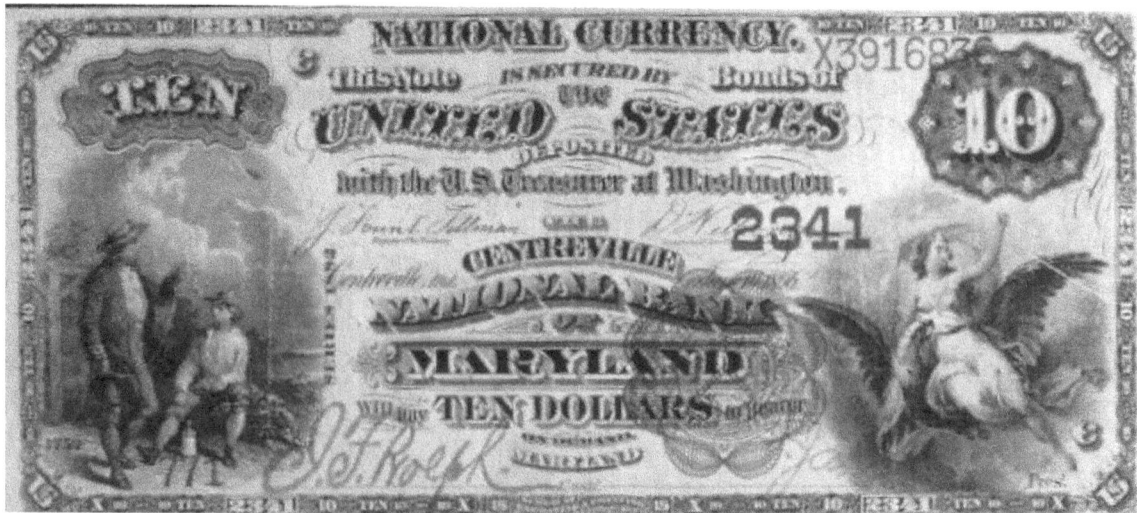

ALBANY COOKIE RECIPE

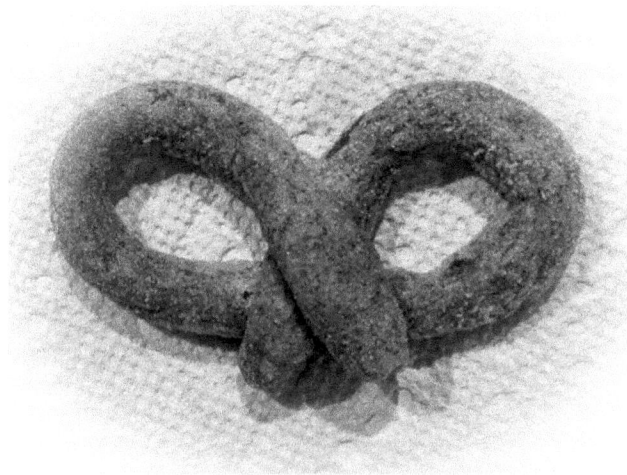

This is the Otwell-Readbourne recipe, adapted to a contemporary kitchen. It is the recipe that Minnie's sisters, Elizabeth ("Bessie") and Clara Hollyday, used. They learned the recipe from their Goldsborough grandmother. Every Christmas they produced these easy-to-make, delightful cookies for the family. There is a similar version of the recipe in the *Maryland's Way* cookbook published by the Hammond-Harwood House.

From Patricia Bordley Wiltse: This recipe came from Otwell, the home of my great-great-great-grandmother (Clara Goldsborough) on the Eastern Shore of Maryland:

- 6 cups flour (sifted)
- 1 lb. dark brown sugar
- ½ lb. butter or margarine (not soft margarine)
- 1 egg
- 1 teaspoon baking soda
- 1 scant cup evaporated milk (about 1/8 inch from top) or 1 cup cream

- 2 oz. cinnamon (10 tablespoons)
- Pinch of salt
- Granulated sugar to roll cookies in

Mix flour, cinnamon, and salt in a bowl. Dissolve soda in evaporated milk in measuring cup. Cream the softened butter, add brown sugar, and beat well. Add egg and beat well again. Alternately add flour and milk, mixing until all ingredients are incorporated. A pinch of salt may help. Put dough in bowl, press down smoothly, and press saran wrap on top of dough. Cover bowl tightly with foil and refrigerate overnight. Dough will keep for several weeks in fridge.

When ready to bake, divide dough into about eight or ten pieces. Take out one piece at a time, pinch off a small piece, and roll on a sugar-coated board with hands till about the shape and size of a lead pencil, coating the surface with the sugar. Twist into a bow or pretzel shape, and place on ungreased cookie sheets. Bake at 375 degrees for twelve to fifteen minutes. Let cool, then tap on underside of cookie sheet to loosen them.

MINT JULEP RECIPE

To paraphrase *Maryland's Way*, **a mint julep must not be entrusted to a** novice, a statistician, or a Yankee. It is a heritage of the old South, a ceremony and an emblem of hospitality. The book goes on for two pages in a similar vein. The mixture is the same as used on the Bordley terrace. A silver goblet is the container. In a canvas bag, pound twice as much ice as you think you need with a rolling pin or wooden mallet until it is a powdery snow. Keep it cold; do not let it get soft. Put one round teaspoon of granulated sugar into the goblet and barely cover it with cold water. Stir and add one or two mint leaves. Sparingly bruise the leaves with a spoon and fill the goblet about a quarter full of fine Maryland rye whiskey—Kentuckians mistakenly use bourbon. Fill the goblet with the powdered ice, sprinkling in a small amount of additional sugar if desired. Now comes the magic. Gently stir the contents, and the moisture forming on the outside of the goblet on a hot day becomes a magnificent, frosted coating that seems heaven sent. Add a sprig of mint to dress it and serve at once.

Brucie Gibbs: We, too, had mint juleps on Blythewood Road [her Fisher grandparents' home].
They looked so beautiful in the frosted silver goblets with mint. Joseph, the butler, came back after a while and brought a bottle of Maryland rye on a silver tray for seconds. However, seconds were only offered to my grandfather!

Don Bordley: Is anybody besides me amazed at what folks were able to drink and still stand up in those days? And a full workday the next day, no less!

Pat Wiltse: Yes, Don, that occurred to me too. Speaking as one who falls asleep after the second glass of wine, I have obviously not inherited Poppy's head for booze!

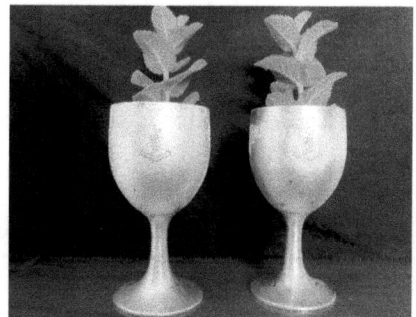

THE WEDDING OF JIM (JB III) AND DUDY

They were married in the Wilderness Chapel at Saranac Lake in upstate New York. It had been built by one of Dudy's Chandler ancestors.

Pat: There are some interesting stories about that wedding. The most famous, of course, is that Dad broke his foot playing tennis the morning of the wedding, and Mom had to drive all the way to Wyoming for their honeymoon (and that was well before the interstate highways were built!). Note the pained expressions on his face in some of the wedding pictures.

Mrs. DuPont, Aunt Mina's mother, was in charge of arranging the flowers in the church, and in the process, she tipped over one of the candlesticks and broke the candle. There were no spares and she was very upset. Someone who was helping her said, don't worry, we'll fix it with DuPont cement. Mrs. DuPont said, "What is that?" Everyone thought it was hilarious that she had no clue about one of the products that had added so handsomely to her family coffers. They did the repair and I think they were lucky they didn't have a huge fire in the church. That stuff was really flammable, which apparently didn't occur to the ladies.

Mom and Dad spent their wedding night at the Lake Placid Club. Early the next morning, their phone rang, and it was Uncle John. He said that he and Aunt Ellen were in the lobby and were coming up to say goodbye before they left for Wyoming. So they scrambled around to make things presentable (Dad couldn't scramble too fast with the broken foot), and then Uncle John called back to say they weren't there at all, but back in Saranac, ha ha!

There was an incident between Poppy and Uncle Don (Ross) on the croquet field. When Poppy thought no one was looking, he kicked his ball into a more advantageous position. Uncle Don caught him at it and said, "Jim, you can't do that!" Poppy said innocently, "Do what?" Uncle Don was quite outraged. Vintage Poppy! Nobody could be mad at him for long, though.

Jimmy adds: By the way—Poppy even cheated at solitaire—he taught Pat and I how to "slip a card" out of the pack if you really needed it. Always practical.

THE MOVE TO COOPERSTOWN

Jimmy (JB IV): I knew about the Hopkins chief of medicine stuff from Uncle John. We had discussed it after Dad's death. Uncle John was still upset about it after all those years. I guess I wish for Dad's sake that he had gotten the job, as it sounds like he deserved it, but I never heard him complain about it. He and Dr. Harvey wrote *Differential Diagnosis* together, then the *Two Centuries of American Medicine*. They were always good friends, and Dad even made Mack an executor of his will. The Harveys spent their summers in Cooperstown, and that's when they did most of their writing. Medical politics being what they are, I'm not sure that Dad didn't think he had the better deal.

The other offer he had at the time he decided on Cooperstown was to be the dean at Tulane in New Orleans. Dad told me that he was ready to take that job when Mr. Clark (an extremely wealthy man who was president of the hospital board) came down to Baltimore personally and persuaded him to consider Cooperstown—how different our lives would have been. In any case, I don't think we would have stayed in Baltimore.

From a selfish point of view, Cooperstown has worked out well for me, and I have enjoyed having a career at the hospital that Dad helped to put on the map as a model rural teaching hospital.

Pat: [adding to her brother's comments] I remember hearing about the Tulane offer from another side: Mom's. She said that Dad had been offered the dean's position at Tulane and that she had absolutely put her foot down and told Dad she couldn't live there. Baltimore was hot enough in the summer, but New Orleans was a hot, humid steam bath most of the year, and she had always hated heat and humidity. And, of course, there was very little air-conditioning at that time. I, for one, am glad, as well, that we ended up in Cooperstown. It was surprising to hear, though, that Mom had stood up to Dad so force-fully about a job choice. So maybe Stephen Clark's offer was a bit more appealing to him after that.

TERRAPIN STEW AND THE DINING ROOM CHAIRS

Pat: We had terrapin stew for Thanksgiving one year as a first course at the house on Guilford Avenue. I think I was about seven or so, so we must have been visiting from Cooperstown. Ma said the children should all try it because it was a traditional Maryland dish. My bowl of stew had a whole terrapin foot right in the middle—it was so grisly looking that I refused to even try it. I also vividly remember that occasion because I had on a short skirt and was sitting on a dining room chair covered with horsehair. It scratched and prickled the backs of my legs.

Anne Moss [from Lankford Creek, Queen Anne's County]: I remember the hard-boiled turtle eggs and various small bones floating around in the stew but never had to deal with identifiable body parts. Every now and then I catch a terrapin in one of the crab traps here, but it is easy to overcome any thoughts of turning it into stew. Ma had redone all those seat covers herself in petit point. We still have them.

Pat [to Anne]: I am surprised that Charlie and Jimmy don't remember those itchy horsehair-covered seats, because little boys always wore short pants for dressed-up occasions at that time. When I was older, and visiting your family on Woodlawn Road, I remember being awestruck that Ma could have had the perseverance to do all those chair seats in petit point...Thank goodness that situation was rectified before yet another generation was tortured by them.

Brucie: Ma told me years ago that she sometimes served muskrat in place of terrapin when terrapin was scarce. She said no one ever knew the difference and always exclaimed how delicious the terrapin was. She never told them otherwise! I found this hard to believe but she promised it was true.

I loved the creamed sweetbreads. That was a very special dish that was lavished on family members on Sunday mornings with waffles!

Do you remember having angel pie—yummy—with lots of meringue and whipped cream; orange charlotte (charlotte russe with orange); Spanish cream; and wine jelly? Even as children we had wine jelly that was made with gelatin, lemons, sugar, boiling water, and one quart of sherry and a little rum or brandy. We were told that all the alcohol evaporated in the cooking. We should make it sometime and see how we are afterward. Of course, all desserts were covered with lots of whipped cream.

JIM'S GRANDDAUGHTERS

Pat: Now, about Poppy and the girl babies: Mother said that when she had me (and was in the hospital for two weeks), Poppy never came to see her. Ma, of course, was there, along with everyone else, but no Poppy. She thought she must have done something to displease him, so she finally mentioned it to Aunt Ellen, who said that she had had the same experience when Brucie and Anne were born and not to worry, he'd come around. By contrast, Mom (Dudy) said that when Jimmy was born eighteen months later, sure enough, he was Johnny on the spot at her bedside! It's very hard to explain, since I remember him as always being very loving to all of us, girls and boys alike. I think it must have been a throwback to earlier days when male children were much preferred. Apparently, as soon as he got to know his granddaughters a bit, he melted!

Brucie: You may think that Poppy didn't visit baby girls. Maybe he didn't, but there is a picture of Poppy and me at Charlcote Place having beer together on the terrace in the back—I am dancing around in diapers! I don't know whether the picture was taken before or after I had my beer. [Editor's note: Poppy had a theory that a small amount of beer was therapeutic for children; many of us got it on occasion.]

RYE BEACH

Brucie: I remember we used to drive up. We were up about four a.m....that is when we heard the milkman rattle the bottles on the back porch. The most exciting event for me was when we went along New York Harbor where all the transatlantic ships docked. I remember seeing the *Normandy* both before and after she burned and lay on her side at the dock. I think that was the beginning of my interest in foreign travel. And we used to stop at Howard Johnson's for lunch, which was grilled cheese sandwiches and green peppermint ice cream with hot fudge sauce. HoJo's had paper mats that we could draw on—that must have been a "first" for restaurants. We'd arrive in Rye Beach probably at midnight because Anne and I were always sound asleep. We loved Rye Beach and couldn't wait to get there. [Editor's note: the *Normandy* fire was 1942. How did they get enough gas ration cards to drive all the way to New Hampshire?]

MA'S ADVICE

Charlie: One of the better pieces of advice I ever received came from my Bordley grandmother. In 1957 I discovered that one could attend a British university for a tuition cost of five pounds per year. The strong dollar in those days made it seem even cheaper. Britain was at the peak of its postwar socialist swing, and even this Yank could get into a university there almost for free. It was an opportunity not to be missed. I got approval from my dean at Trinity College. My father agreed when he learned it would cost no more than the $2,000 he would be paying for my junior year tuition, room, and board. The University of Edinburgh agreed to take me, and I was off. Passage was far cheaper in those days by ship than air. I secured the least expensive third-class bunk Cunard Lines had to offer. None of my friends could be convinced to join me on this adventure, so it was a lonely feeling when the *Queen Mary* gave three long blasts on her horn and backed out of her pier into the Hudson River. But the loneliness did not last long—there were many other young men along, and most of them were on their way to a Rhodes scholarship. What a great group of traveling companions.

Before leaving, a goodbye kiss for my grandmother had been in order. She casually asked me if I was taking a tuxedo. I could not imagine why that would be useful. It was the start of the backpacking era, but it was also the last gasp of the Victorian era. Girls did not travel unescorted in those days. She pointed out that all the girls on board would be in first class with their grandmothers heading off for the European "Grand Tour." We would be at sea for almost a week. After dark, she advised, put on the tux and go out on deck, up the stairs, and over the waist-high railing to second and then first class—there would be no deck stewards after dark to stop me. Find the ballroom and behave like a gentleman.

The ballroom was a product of the gilded age. It was a magnificent space with a twelve-piece orchestra playing Broadway tunes. There were some old men dancing with wives or granddaughters but few young men. The women were splendidly dressed in evening gowns. I picked out a bored but good-looking girl sitting alone with her grandmother. As Ma instructed, I went directly to the grandmother and introduced myself. I asked permission to request a dance from the lovely girl sitting next to her. Before the smiling old lady could reply, the girl was up like a shot, and I was started on a fabulous transatlantic social swirl. Every morning there came invitations from Mrs. Somebody to attend a luncheon in honor of Miss Somebody, a tea for someone else, and cocktails for a third. Those invitations were free passes by the Cunard guards straight into first class without climbing gates at night. I may not have had a Rhodes scholarship, but I had something even better for that ocean crossing: very savvy advice from a wonderful grandmother.

DESCENDANTS OF JAMES BORDLEY, JR. AND MARGARETTA CARROLL HOLLYDAY

Numerals refer to the generation below JB Jr. and MCH

1   **James Bordley, Jr.** b. Feb. 20, 1874, Centreville, MD; m. Centreville, MD, Nov. 28, 1899; d. Jan. 20, 1956, Baltimore, MD

. . . + **Margaretta Carroll Hollyday** b. Aug. 12, 1875, Readbourne, Queen Anne's County, MD; d. Oct. 7, 1966, Baltimore, MD

. . . . .2 **James Bordley III** b. Dec. 7, 1900, Readbourne, Queen Anne's County, MD; m. July 4, 1936, Saranac Inn, NY; d. Jan. 6, 1979, Cooperstown, NY

. . . . + **Julia Peabody Ross** b. May 3, 1905, Philadelphia, PA; d. Jan. 23, 1999, Cooperstown, NY

. . . . 3 **Patricia Bordley** b. May 25, 1941, Baltimore, MD; m. Aug 5, 1961, Cooperstown, NY

. . . . + **Roderic Duncan Wiltse** b. Dec. 10, 1934, Catskill, NY; d. 2017, St. Louis, MO

. . . . .4 **Diana Louise Wiltse** b. Aug. 15, 1962, Cooperstown, NY; m. Sept. 1, 1984, Coldwater, MI

. . . . + **Eric Michael Yope** b. Mar. 26, 1962, Ft. Wayne, IN

. . . . .5 **Madeline Julia Yope** b. Aug. 11, 1990, Grand Rapids, MI; m. July 4, 2014, Grand Rapids, MI

. . . .+**James Michael Gomez** b. Mar. 6, 1990, Flint, MI

. . . . .6 **Winston Michel Gomez** b. May 25, 2019, Nashville, Tenn.

. . . . .6 **Nora Cathleen Gomez** b. Oct. 5, 2022, Nashville, Tenn.

. . . . .6 **Evelyn Diana Gomez** b. Oct. 5, 2022, Nashville, Tenn.

. . . . .5 **Samantha Margaret Yope** b. Apr. 10, 1993, Grand Rapids, MI; m. Oct. 9, 2021, Grand Rapids, MI

. . . . + **Zacchary Terrence Boyd** b. Dec. 9 1992, Grand Rapids, MI

. . . . .4 **Andrew Duncan Wiltse** b. Dec. 3, 1963, Cooperstown, NY; m. July 4, 1987, Coldwater, MI

. . . . + **Tamara Lee Holt** b. Jan. 8, 1965, Coldwater, MI

. . . . .5 **Alexander Wiltse** b. Feb. 28, 1988, St. Louis, MO

. . . . .5 **Nicholas James Wiltse** b. Aug. 10, 1990, Grand Rapids, MI

. . . . .5 **Lindsey Michelle Wiltse** b. Feb. 17, 1993, St. Louis, MO; m. Oct. 10, 2014, Grand Rapids, MI

. . . .+ **Jeffrey Scott Rea** b. Apr. 24, 1993, St. Louis, MO

. . . . .6 **Harper Lee Rea** b. Oct. 22, 2016, San Diego, CA

. . . . .4 **Jonathan Ross Wiltse** b. Nov. 6, 1968, Grand Rapids, MI; m. Oct. 9, 1999, St. Louis, MO

. . . . + **Stephanie Ann Alcamo** b. Oct. 4, 1972, St. Louis, MO

. . . . .5 **Helena Jane Wiltse** b. May 4, 2002, St. Louis, MO

. . . . .5 **Gabriel David Wiltse** b. Aug. 1, 2005, St. Louis, MO

. . . . .5 **Noah James Wiltse** b. Jan. 30, 2007, St. Louis, MO

. . . . 3 **James Bordley IV** b. 1942, Baltimore, MD; m. June 30, 1973, Passaic, NJ

. . . . + **Carol Isabelle Fondiler** b. Aug. 26, 1947, Passaic, NJ

. . . . .4 **Jessica Lynn Bordley** b. June 22, 1975, Cooperstown, NY

. . . . .4 **Seth Bordley** b. Dec. 15, 1976, Cooperstown, NY

. . . . .4 **James (Jamie) Bordley V** b. Apr. 11, 1978, Cooperstown, NY; m. Dec. 31, 2011, Seattle, WA

. . . . + **Marnie Hanel** b. Mar. 3, 1981, St. Louis, MO

. . . . .5 **James Bordley VI** b. Sept. 23, 2014, Portland, OR

. . . . .5 **Calvin Douglas Bordley** b. Dec. 8, 2016, Portland, OR

. . . . .5 **Alistair Dash Bordley** b. Sept. 23, 2018, Portland, OR
*2nd wife of James Bordley IV:

. . . . + **Dianne Marie Redmond** b. Oct. July 12, 1955, Utica, NY; m. Oct. 25, 1986

. . . . . . 3 **Donald Ross Bordley** b. Aug. 1, 1947, Baltimore, MD; m. June 14, 1969, Bernardsville, NJ

. . . . + **Gladys Williamson (Billie) Pell** b. June 15, 1949, Rye, NY

. . . . 4 **Erin Chandler Bordley** b. Dec. 1, 1978, Rochester, NY; m. Aug. 3, 2013, Genesco, NY

. . . . +**Mark Cassidy** b. July 11, 1958, Upper Danbury, PA
*2nd Wife of Donald Ross Bordley

. . . . + **Priscilla Sarah Martin** July 28, 1955, Burlington, VT; m. Oct. 17, 1987, Pittsford, NY

. . . . .4 **Christopher Ross Bordley** b. Nov. 11, 1990; m. Aug. 25, 2018, Rochester, NY

. . . . + **Jacqueline Consul**

. . . . .4 **Kathleen Hollyday Bordley** b. Dec. 28, 1994, Rochester, NY

.....2 **John Earle Bordley** b. Nov. 8, 1902, Baltimore, MD; m. June 3, 1930; d. July 12, 1993, Baltimore, MD

.... + **Ellen Bruce Fisher** b. Apr. 4, 1908, Baltimore, MD; d. July 20, 2004, Baltimore, MD

.... 3 **Ellen Bruce (Brucie) Bordley** b. May 30, 1933, Baltimore, MD; m. June 22, 1957, Baltimore, MD

.... + **W H Holden Gibbs** b. June 11, 1932, Philadelphia, PA; d. Nov. 7, 1997, Sparks, MD

..........4 **Ellen Bruce (Ell-Be) Gibbs** b. Dec. 5, 1958, Columbia, SC; m. Oct. 20, 1983, Baltimore, MD

.... + **Arthur Leon Lewis II** b. Oct. 8, 1953, Boston, MA

.............5 **Eliza Bordley Lewis** b. May 1, 1991, Boston, MA

.............5 **Arthur Leon Lewis III** b. Nov. 21, 1992, Boston, MA

.............5 **John Holden Hartley Lewis** b. Feb. 16, 1995, Boston, MA

..........4 **Anne Holden Gibbs** b. May 28, 1963; m. April 21, 1990, Baltimore, MD

.... + **James Dixon Bartlett** b. Mar. 25, 1962, Baltimore, MD

.... 3 **Anne Bordley** b. May 18, 1937, Baltimore, MD; m. Oct. 22, 1960, Baltimore, MD

.... + **Roland Charles Sherrer, Jr.** b. Garden City, NY

..........4 **Alexandra Baylor Sherrer** b. Apr. 25, 1962, New York, NY; m. Dec. 10, 1990, Richmond, VA

.... + **Craig Wilson Diffee** b. Mar. 25, 1962, Richmond, VA; d. Feb. 21, 2022, Richmond, VA

.............5 **Graham Wilson Diffee** b. May 29, 1993, Richmond, VA

.............5 **Chandler Baylor Diffee** b. Apr. 16, 1996, Richmond, VA

    * 2nd Husband of Anne Bordley

.... + **Peter Bayard Moss**; b. Nov. 8, 1932, New York, NY; m. Nov. 22, 1967 Baltimore, MD; d. Oct. 15, 2021, Charleston, SC

.....2 **Ellen Fassett Bordley** b. Dec. 31,1909, Baltimore, MD; m. Apr. 28,1936, Baltimore, MD; d. Feb. 13, 1971, Baltimore, MD

.... + **Charles Albert Webb** b. Nov. 25, 1898, Pikesville, MD; d. July 19, 1974, Oxford, MD

.... 3 **Charles Albert Webb Jr.** b. Dec. 31, 1937, Baltimore, MD; m. June 16, 1961, Quogue, NY

.... + **Ann Carroll Heroy** b. Sept. 9, 1939, New York, NY; d. Sept 15, 2018, Oxford, MD

..........4 **Charles Albert Webb III** b. Apr. 2, 1965, Charlottesville, VA; m. Nov. 16, 2003, Williamsburg, VA

.... + **Carol Melissa Ezzell** b. June 16, 1963, Newport News, VA

.............5 **Andrew James Webb** b. May 15, 2005, Austin TX

.............5 **Amelia Christine (Alex) Webb** b. May 15, 2005, Austin, TX

. . . . 4 **William Heroy Webb** b. June 26, 1968, Baltimore, MD; m. Oct. 30, 2009 Oxford, MD

. . . . + **Katherine Elizabeth Myers** b. Dec. 12, 1973, Washington, DC

. . . . .4 **James Hollyday Webb** b. Jun 10, 1974, Easton, MD; d. Oxford, MD, July 20, 1991

*Partner of Charles A. Webb, Jr.

. . . . + **Patricia Christine Wilson Fei** b. July 11, 1947, Milwaukee, WI; Engaged. Dec. 25, 2019, Charleston, SC

. . . . 3 **Margaretta Carroll Webb** b. Feb. 14, 1940, Baltimore, MD; m. Aug. 18,1962, Baltimore, MD; d. Sept. 20, 2005, Cambridge, MA

. . . . + **Thomas Noel Bisson** b. Mar. 30, 1931, New York, NY

. . . . .4 **Noel Bisson** b. June 23, 1967, Bala Cynwyd, PA; m. May 6, 1995, Cambridge, MA

. . . . + **Allen Ralph Cooper** b. Nov. 24, 1966, London, England

. . . . .5 **Josephine Cooper** b. Aug. 5, 1998, Boston, MA

. . . . .5 **Caroline Cooper** b. Mar. 1, 2001, Boston, MA

*2nd husband of Noel Bisson

. . . .+ **Clate Dylan Sanders** b. Jan. 29, 1965, Honolulu, HI; m. Oct. 1, 2022, Lexington, MA

. . . . .4 **Susan Tilghman Bisson** b. Feb. 20, 1970, Berkeley, CA; m. Oct. 12, 2002, Cambridge, MA

. . . . + **John Sterling Lambert** b. Nov. 22, 1968, London, England

. . . . .5 **William Tilghman Lambert** b. Sept. 29, 2005, Cambridge, MA

. . . . .5 **Helen Hollyday Lambert** b. Sept. 3, 2008, Leonardtown, MD

JAMES BORDLEY, JR.'S PUBLICATIONS

Medical Papers

1907

Bordley, James, Jr. "Trachoma in the American Negro Race." *Johns Hopkins Hosp. Bull.* 18 (1907): 37–39.

Bordley, James, Jr. "Treatment of Trachoma." *Opth. Record* 16 (1907): 324–326.

1908

Cushing, Harvey, and Bordley, James Jr. "Subtemporal Decompression in a Case of Chronic Nephritis with Uremia; with Especial Consideration of the Neuroretinal Lesion." *Am J Med Sciences* 136 (1908): 484–504.

1911

Bordley, James, Jr. "The Early Recognition of Choked Disc." *Ophthalmoscope* (1911): 282.

1915

Bordley, James, Jr. "Malignant Uveitis Treated with Thyroid Extract." *Trans Am Ophthalmol Soc* 14 (1915): 232–249.

1916

Bordley, James, Jr. "Two Patients with Unusual Corneal Opacities." *Trans Am Opthalmol Soc* 14 (1916): 526.2–529.

1917

Bordley, James, Jr. "Opthalmic Surgery." *Surg Gynec & Obst* 25 (1917): 727.

1918

Bordley, James, Jr. "Plans of the US Government for the Soldiers Blinded in Battle." (1918): 167.

Bordley, James, Jr.. "The Blind as Industrial Workers." *The Annals of the American Academy of Political and Social Science* 80 (1918): 104–110.

1920

Bordley, James, Jr. "Optic Nerve Disturbances in Diseases of the Posterior Nasal Sinuses." *JAMA* 75 (Sept. 1920): 809–814.

1921

Bordley, James, Jr. "Optic Nerve in Relation to the Posterior Nasal Sinuses." *Virginia Medical Monthly* 67 (1921): 144–147.

Bordley, James, Jr. "Ocular Manifestations of Diseases of the Para-Nasal Sinuses." *Arch. Ophthalmology* 1 (1921): 137–146.

1924

Bordley, James, Jr. "Progressive Middle-Ear Deafness." *Transactions College of Physicians* 45 (1923) 427–452.

1926

Bordley, James, Jr. "Report of a Patient with Incomplete Opthalmoplegia." *Trans Am Ophthalmol Soc* 24 (1926): 115–121.

1931

Bordley, James, Jr. "Reeducation of the War Blinded." (1931): 482.

Historical Papers

1928

Bordley, James, Jr. *Historic Houses for St. John's.* Twenty-four-page monograph, copies at HHH and Maryland Historical Society. It is undated and unsigned, but from the content, reference to Garvan, a similar fundraising monograph by Bordley, and his handwritten signature on the front of one copy, it is surely by Dr. Bordley in 1928.

Bordley, James, Jr. *Colonial Annapolis.* 1928. Monograph at Maryland Hist. Soc.

1930

Bordley, James, Jr., "Early American Glassmakers." Lecture manuscript in Maryland Historical Society files.

1944

Bordley, James, Jr. "Baltimore Furniture Makers 1785–1815." Lecture for the centennial celebration of the Maryland Historical Society, manuscript at Maryland Hist. Soc. Lantern slides in the Baltimore Museum of Art library.

1956

Bordley, James, Jr., *Bordleys of the Eastern Shore.* Typed and unfinished manuscript at Md. Hist. Soc.

1962

> Bordley, James, Jr. *The Hollyday and Related Families of the Eastern Shore of Maryland*. Maryland Historical Society: Baltimore, MD, 1962.

Letters to the Baltimore Sun

Dr. Bordley had twenty-two letters to the editor of the *Baltimore Sun* published between 1932 and 1945. These are found by online search of their files. Below is a selection of the topics he addressed. After retiring, he also wrote letters to the *Evening Sun*, but there is no available digital file for it.

1932, April 6: Reverse side of the veteran's bonus march on Washington.

1932, June 22: Some thoughts on radicalism and Gov. Ritchie.

1934, April 7: Where democracy has the advantage over dictatorship.

1940, July 27: Reasons for wanting to aide England.

1941, July 10: Comments on the recently ended strike in the "captive coal mines."

1942, March 10: Suggesting an unofficial draft to get men for the OCD.

1942, August 14: An appeal for a start on the job of world house cleaning here at home.

1943, July 8: Looking towards the peacemaking period, he urges the election of statesmen not ordinary politicians.

ENDNOTES

1   Nathanial Philbrick, *The Last Stand* (Penguin Group, 2010).

2   Shakespeare, *Julius Caesar.*

3   Frederick Emory, *Queen Anne's County, Maryland* (Queenstown, MD: The Queen Anne Press, 1981): ch. XXI.

4   *Star Democrat*, October 22, 2010.

5   "A Law the Doctors Want Enacted," *Baltimore Sun*, January 3, 1890, 4.

6   See Appendix, "Legal Tender."

7   Angus MacLean, "James Bordley, Jr." *Trans. Am. Opth. Soc.* 54 (1959): 5–7.

8   MacLean

9   MCH born 12 Aug. 1875, died 7 Oct. 1966.

10   James Bordley, Jr., *The Hollyday Family* (Baltimore: Maryland Historical Society), 71.

11   Thomas Hollyday, "Readbourne Manor Revisited," *MD Historical Magazine* 85, no. 1 (1995).

12   *Baltimore Sun*, August 26, 1903, 6.

13   E. F. Cordell, *Medical Annals of Maryland 1799–1899*, 327–8.

14   *Baltimore Sun*, January 26, 1906, 9. In 1905, Church Home Infirmary opened a wing with an electric elevator.

15   Bordley-Brown letters, Queen Anne's County Historical Society, 1955. Newspaper articles in the *Sun* document he was away about ten weeks, not four months.

16   James Bordley, Jr, "The Blind as Industrial Workers," *The Annals of the American Academy of Political and Social Science* 80 (1918): 104–110.

17 C. C. Clayton, ed., *Baltimore, Its History and Its People, Volume I* (1912), 360. (Online this is available through Google Books, but is best found by doing a google search for "Baltimore, history of its sewer system" and opening the link "Baltimore: its History and its People")

18 MacLean

19 Board of Visitors minutes, St. John's College, Oct. 1926.

20 Glenn E. Campbell, "Preservation Pioneers: St John's and the CRCA," 1.

21 Charles A. Webb, Jr., "Annapolis Colonial Restoration: The Secret Project," *Maryland Historical Magazine* 115 (2020), 33–61.

22 Bordley-Brown letters, Queen Anne's County Historical Society, July 15, 1955.

23 The *Sun*, May 9, 1932, 3.

24 Charles Scarlett Jr., "Governor Horatio Sharpe's Whitehall," *Maryland Historical Magazine* 46, no. 1 (1951), 8.

25 James Bordley papers, the Maryland Hist. Soc.

26 Edgar G. Miller Jr., *American Antique Furniture*, Lord Baltimore Press, 1937. Photographs of many pieces of the Bordley's furniture are included in this classic text.

27 J. Bordley, Jr., *The Hollyday Family of Maryland*, 213.

28 Hollyday records at the Md. Hist. Soc.

29 *Baltimore Sun*, April 4, 1930.

30 John Bordley, "Under the Dome," Johns Hopkins Hospital, Nov. 1945.

31 The Hollyday records, the Maryland Historical Society.

PART TWO

THE LETTERS OF JAMES BORDLEY, JR. M.D.1942-1945

Written to his sons stationed in Australia during WW-II
Lt. Col. James Bordley III, M.C.
Major John E. Bordley, M.C.
C.O. of the 118th General Hospital

This large collection of letters by JB Jr. were in a cardboard box which also contained copies of talks and papers he gave and the remaining material not given to the Maryland Historical Society for his book "The Hollyday Family". There are several handwritten notes from Eleanor Roosevelt trying to arrange an appointment to see him probably about hearing loss. The box was under John Bordley's bed at the time of John's death, having been saved there after his father died.

The loose style, frequent spelling errors, and smudged corrections confirm they were personally typed. The remarkable thing is that he did carbon copies which were dated, numbered, collated and preserved. In the Oct. 26, 1942 letter he says he types between patients in the office. There are long gaps in the summers when he was at Rye Beach N.H. He says he wrote from there. It must have been by hand, without the ability to do a carbon.

They paint a picture of how the war affected the nation, an affluent family's life, and the medical and civilian affairs in the city. The letters also contain a good bit of chit-chat about the weather, his family, the social news, and his political opinions. Reading these letters reveals Jim to be an energetic, popular and successful man. But there are some quite prejudiced remarks also. It is strongly tempting to delete those letters lest the reader throw this book down and write our subject off as a hopeless bigot. He has unflattering comments about African Americans, Jews, and women. In fact, it represents a common behavior in his day. It adds another dimension to the scene of life in Baltimore in the 1940s and, if we consider it unacceptable today, is another example of how the world is changing.

On June 4, 1942 the 118th left its training area in Florida and deployed to the Pacific. No one knew where they were headed as Dr. Bordley sends the first letter. While the letters are mostly addressed to son Jim, they are intended for John as well since both were together. Any letters the boys wrote back were not saved.

Organization: *There are 4 "volumes." Each ends when they depart for Rye Beach in the summer, and a new one begins when they return in the fall.*

Numbering of Letters: *the first 3 letters have no number. The fourth letter, June 27, is then called number VI. The next one on July 1 is called No. 7 and Arabic numerals are used there after.*

Vol. # I

Notes on Letters to Jim and John 1942-1945

001- Family pictures: the ugly old woman was probably the Charles Wilson Peale portrait elderly Elizabeth Bordley, that we called "Aunt Ugly". It went to Carroll Webb Bisson.

002&003- In discussing his work, it sounds as though he came out of semi-retirement to keep the office going for John's return.

004 Apparently he has been thinking about selling the house (#4 Charlcotte Pl.). It had been built in 1929. While very proud of it, it was far too big and an upkeep headache.

005 The Garrett estate was where the Evergreen unit for Rehab of the Blind (run by JB jr) had been in WW I. The estate with the coin collection went to Hopkins University.

008- July 7,1942 Cam is Dr. Campbell Goodwin, pediatrician who with his pediatrician wife, Mary, ultimately followed Jim (III) to Cooperstown.
-The problem in Ellen Webb's house was bed bugs. (in my bed!)
-Oil on the beach may refer to the subs sinking coastal ships.

The first Sept letter is Vol. II, No. 1 and starts with "Back at the old stand…"
Several letters describe typing between patients. We presume that any August letters were handwritten without copies.

June 4, 1942.

Dear Sons,

        Well another blackout last night. We are gradually approaching a knowledge
of the fact that we are at war. This is further impressed by a rationing of gasoline.
It is quite a remarkable feeling to drive down Charles St. for instance and see no cars
coming or going, to be able to cross a down town street without holding your breath. I
asked my filling station man how he was getting along, he said "I am just taking it and
liking it, I have been sut from 22,000 gallons to 8,000 and if I gave all who hold
X cards (unlimited) what they ask for I would clean up in one day". Among the people we
know, except Charlie Cromwell, the A card is generally held. It gives you three gallons
a week. People are doubling up and really displaying a fine sense of responsibility.
        Anne and Brucy have had birthdays, Anne had a slight cold so no party. Brucy
was fine and had a party. They both look very well and are very happy. I had a long talk
with Brucy a day or so ago. The questions she asked were eye openers for me. She apparently has a real idea of the war, its causes and effects. She wanted to compare it
with the last war and even with the Civil war. She was most anxious to know who in her
family had served, what they did and how they acquitted themselves.
        Pat, too, is fine and full of pep. She and I have struck up a real acquaintance
and are on very warm terms. She now knows our family pictures -- the ugly old woman, the
pretty young girl, the little girl, etc. She also has a penchant for the little boy on
the drawing room mantle. She always wants to kiss it but will have nothing to do with
the boy's companion. She loves the radio and when it is playing where she can reach it
she shoves everybody away and proceeds to dance. She is very cute. She tried to dance
on her all fours yesterday and after some marvelous gyrations she lost her balance and
took it on the tummy. Since then she has refused to try. She sits up at the table and
eats toast and bacon and now and then takes a chew out of her dolls. If her toast is
not ready when she gets to the table, she raises the devil.
        Everybody here isterribly excited by the giant British raids on German cities.
Some people believe the German people can't take it and the war will soon end. I hope so
but don't believe a slave driver like Hitler & Co. has forgotten how to use the lash.
There can be no doubt, however, that the blows will seriously wreck thisprovocation.
        For Johnny I am still making some money. A number of patients and a few
operations. The daily visits go to the general account for Ellen, the operating fees
are invested in War Bonds for Brucy and Anne. Not a fortune but a help.
        Dr. and Mrs. Black arrived from Hot Springs this morning. They will be with
us for a few days before going to Atlantic City for the A.M.A. I would go with them
but I am so busy I feel I must stay home. Not another appointment open for five days.

        Will write again in a few days,

                                Your

Lt.Col. James Bordley,III., M.C.
General Hospital #118,
A.P.O. 1142,
c/o Postmaster, San Francisco, California

Dudy and her daughters are temporarily staying at 4 Charlcote Place with the senior Bordleys.

"For Johnny ..." John had started work in his father's practice prior to the war, planning to take over.

June 12, 1942

Dear John and Jim,

You should see what the lack of gasoline is doing to transportation. You can even park your car at the Belvedere corner, in fact can park it most any place. There is supposed to be a car shortage of some 54%. Reminds me of twenty-five years ago. Paul McNutt took a crack at the doctors before the A.M.A. Say they are not volunteering for service. I wrote him they never did and never will and if he wants them he has got to call them by name. Four hundred and ninety more are requested of Baltimore and if they don't come up they are to be drafted. Well, that is good technique to get out the boys who are staying out to get the practices of those who have already gone. I am all in favor of it.

All the golf courses in the United States held a Red Cross tournament at a dollar a head. I was lucky enough to win at Elkridge with an 82 plus a handicap of 16. My handicap is now reduced. There is not much golf being played except Saturday and Sunday when the crowd is some 50% short of the normal. The difficulty of getting ground keepers, caddies and balls does not make for enthusiasm, then with almost no gasoline and no tires it is becoming an increasing difficulty. I am sorry because I believe that some form of relaxation and fun is essential to an alert mind and out at Elkridge there are many, many loaded down with Government jobs and worries. They should be encouraged to get away from business now and then.

You have possibly heard of the death of Dr. Finney. He was an excellent man and a great loss to the worth while causes of Baltimore. His was a full life so there is no real cause for mourning.

Charlie Larned passed out a day or so ago and to my surprise was seventy-five years old. I always looked upon him as a contemporary but he was old enough to be my father.

You should see some of the nurses helpers that are flowing into the hospitals. I don't know who gives the mentality tests or what the standard, I only know the quality accepted. I guess it is no longer picker and chooser.

Crow operated on Anne on Tuesday. I saw her yesterday and except for a little stuttering I would say she is in fine shape. I did encourage Ellen to keep her in the Hospital an extra day in spite of her good form.

About the other children there is nothing to report. Pat is standing alone has got the idea of the radio sufficiently to try and turn it off and on. She is also eating a bit of real food and looks like a million dollars.

Charlie and Carroll invented a new game, so Guinea Williams told me: eating small stones and then sticking a finger down the throat to induce vomiting. It worked all right with Charlie but Carroll could not vomit so she still has a liberal amount of stones in her gizzard.

Another letter in a day or so.

With love from,

Your

June 18, 1942.

Dear Jim and John,

      Well we had a practice for the noise makers in the down town district
yesterday.   With one of the devices on the top of the B. & O. Building the people
inside failed to hear it.   The one on the top of the Gas and Electric Building sounded
like a fellow talking through a megaphone.   With the windows open we could hear it.
One of the radio announcers said the other night: "How many people are aware that a
Messerschmidt 109 flew over New York City at noon today and dropped leaflets. Well,
it is the truth, but, it was flown by an American pilot and was captured in England".
The first part of the statement was excitin and if he had stopped there we would now
be installing adequate sirens.

      The soldiery put on a full scale show at the bowl on three or four
nights.   It was a wonderful show, exhibiting all the different engines of destruction
so far invented. The proceeds go to the Army relief and totalled about $75,000.
To me the most exciting part for the air plane. They were in various formations
and were so low they just missed the trees in our yard.   Such speed you can hardly
imagine. There were no accidents but a great deal of excitement.

      Dooty has had a slight cold which I think was excellent for her because
she went to bed for several days and got a good rest.   Now she is fine.   Pat has
been very well and is developing by leaps and bounds especially in her demands on me.
She has the idea that I am just a flunkey and maybe I am but, if so I thoroughly
enjoy the job.

      It was very interesting to hear the stories about where you are, were
going and then had gone.   You were in Alaska, South America, India, South Africa,
Ireland and Australia.   Everybody had"first-hand information" from either a General
or a mother-in-law.   Sometimes when you traced out the sourse at least six people were
involved and not one with a scintilla of real information.   The same stories are
going around about General 18 and with no better sources.   It really is wonderful to
listen to the stories that goaround.

      I am too busy, in fact, back working like I did formerly.   Operations
are flowing in and practice keeps me flowing out.   I must say I have enjoyed it more
than I expected.   It means I will stay on the job during the summer.   Maybe next
Fall I will run away for a couple of weeks if the tax assessor will leave me enough
money.   So far the weather has been so nice that I have felt fine.   Every night a
couple of blankets feel good.

      Well another letter in a day or so. We got your cables -- two -- and
were delighted to hear.

                  Yours,

84

July 7, 1942.

Dear John and Jim,

Well with Rommell stopped we feel a bit more comfortable here. He certainly went through Libya like a hot shot. This will put a crimp in Germany provided it lasts but Rommell is a sly bird. You know he is the uncle of the old Base-ball pitcher, famous too in his time and an all out American.

Well Dudy and Pat have gone to the mountains and it certainly leaves the old home a lonely place. Pat and I are very close friends when I have my glasses on but if I take them off she will not come near me and screams if I make a move toward her. She is the most hungry animal I ever saw. Eats her full meals and then comes to the table for bacon and toast, waffles and any other thing she can beg. Passes her little silver plate and says "ta ta" when she has been supplied.

Dudy is getting along fine and looks very well. She had a going away party, Cam and his wife and Harrison and his, plenty of good mint juleps and a nice dinner.

Little Charlie has come in to spend a few days while they have their house fumigated to get rid of some visitors brought by their old cook. Ellen has a real problem on her hands as the whole house was infected before she knew it.

Ellen Fisher and her children are still down at Atlantic City. The papers published some pictures of the Jersey Coast, showing what the incoming oil was doing at the beach. I hope none at Atlantic City but I don't know.

The rubber collection gained real impetus and now amounts to hundreds of thousands of tons. The authorities are still crying for more which is anproper attitude. Charlie told me this morning he was too little to fight the Japs but he gave the soldiers all of his rubber balls so they could bomb the Japs. I really think he expects them to use the balls in cannon. When I told him I had given his old rubber doll he was so surprised that I had to explain that they were going to make a tire out of it for an air plane so they could bomb the Japs with his balls.

The Jap beetles are back but nothing like as bad on our place as last year. Ma had all the ground soaked with arsenic and none so far have appeared coming out of the grass.

Beale had a three day furlough and was home. Now he is gone but we do not know where. Worthington has about completed his officer training and will be East again in a few days. Where he is going we do not know.

John Brown was in yesterday to get a test. He has managed to hold on to his A 1. rating and is crazy to get into the Army. Came to have me test his hearing and find out if I thought there would be a chance for him to get into some non combat unit if he was turned down by the fighting forces. I did not encourage him amd saw his keen disappointment. He is a fine chap.

Mr. Daniel Willard died today at 81. He had an "embolus". Just where I don't know. He will be a distinct national loss.

The doctor business is getting serious and many doctors are getting a bit uneasy at the rate they are being absorbed in the military forces without adequate community provision. It will I hope get straightened out before it too greatly bothers hospitals and medical schools.. It is most important not to curtail their functions.

We received and enjoyed John's letter very much.
Well, another in a few days. Ma and I are well.

Your,

July 10,1942.

Dear Jim and John,

Well such a July. The temperature in my bed room this morning was 64. For nearly a week the temperature has not been over 81 or 2 and down in the sixties every night and morning. I can recall but one such July and that was over forty years ago when on the 4th of July it was cold enough to have fires in the fence corners for the men cutting wheat.

This is wonderful weather for those working long hours in war factories and what production they are getting out. It is, in practically every line, far ahead of schedule the spirit of effort of the community is rising every day. We were a bit slow in getting away from our luxurious life and coming to a realization of the necessities for total war but now that we are arriving I feel progress will be more rapid and its results on the war more positive.

Of course we still have politics to contend with and will have until after the fall election but there are developing strong forces to make out war effort non political and in the end the idea will prevail. Personally, I have had more fear of the effects of politics than of the power of the enemy, but now that the people are becoming aroused I believe the military will soon be military and not political Of course there are a lot of people who cannot see the danger to their own casual ways of life but such people can never be made to see that they fit in the national picture whether they wish it or not. Most of such people are parasitic in their whole contact and war is just no exception. Maybe we grew up in an atmosphere of serious contemplation and are poor judges of those less serious. I distinctly know that I have a real lack of tolerance for the stupid and the frivolous and an equally strong preference for those who have a realistic viewpoint.

Both of you have given me infinite satisfaction because you have shown a serious regard for your responsibilities. While your going away troubled my spirit, deep down in my heart there was a feeling of comfort and joy. Your choice was your own and came I am sure from a desire to perpetuate what you appreciate in our own way of life. Applause is a fickle child but duty well done is a source of perpetual satisfaction. You know it and so do I.

Dudy writes that Pat fully enjoyed her journey to the Adirondacks and is taking the change with good grace. She is developing so fast that I am sure when she comes back she will take charge of the house.

Mother and I continue well.
With love from
Your

July 17, 1942.

Dear John and Jim,

We were delighted to receive letters yesterday from you both -- several. It makes us much happier to know that you are comfortably located and while we realize that yours is not a joy ride it helps along to know that pleasure is not an absentee in your lives. I really found the break in the routine of my life during the last war quite agreeable. Dr. Black said the thing he missed most in not going into the Army Medical Corps was the complete change from office to field medicine. In one you are supplied with much, in the other you have to use your ingenuity, in one you are a slave to convention, in the other you are in a sense free as a bird.

We had an all night black out with a "complete black" out during the night, with warning sirens and all clears. The main blackout was for houses, the special for everything. They have installed a siren near our house and oh boy! You can hear it down the cellar with the victrola on, in fact it could raise the roof. It makes is feel a lot easier to know we will be able, if the need ever arises, to hear a warning. They have installed a big one on the Maryland Casualty building and with the windows open it was very clear but with the windows closed we would never hear it. One of the joys of the blackout was the housing of the thousand or more dogs in our neighborhood which contributed much to a peaceful, comfortable sleep.

The weather here today is like Rye in September. So far only two hot days. What of the weather where you are? This I know isyour winter but I imagine with flowers in bloom it is not very cold.

The Johns Hopkins is out after two millions of dollars. You might think from the letter they wrote me I wouldgive it to them. But as the Government would only credit me with a small fraction on my income tax I will not yield to temptation. Yes, I said $2,000,000. Indeed, I do not know where they will get it, b cause everybody I know is scraping bottom to keep their homes going. Dr. Dunning told me that out of an income of three hundred thousand dollars, when he finishes settling with Uncle Sam he will have eighteen thousand left and then his home taxes come along and take twelve, so he will have an insufficnet sum to meet his living obligations. Well, when you consider he has three sons, none of whom are serving in the armed forces, I feel sort of glad.

Cousin Frank showed up for dinner last night in a brand new suit -- a bargain sale affair but rather good looking. Your mother gave him a good dressing down because he had not donated the rubber mat in his automobile to the scrap drive. She really went to town so strong I was a bit embarrassed but chuckled inside. He reaps all the benefits but contributes little to the American way of life. Kicks about his taxes but draws an old age pension from the Government larger than his taxes. Ma reminded him we help to pay him off every time he gets a check.

Ma really is doing things and make no mistake she calls the rumor mongers down and never bats an eye. She is thinking of you boys in every move she makes. Some woman at the head of one of the Red Cross working chapters said her son was in the Hopkins Unit but he was too well trained to serve so he resigned to take a job "commensurate with his training". Ma wanted to know what kind of a job and insisted on being told and this before the whole assembly of some fifty women. The woman hemmed and hawed but could not remember. Then she was told that the Hopkins Unit was about the A one Unit and filled with only highly trained men and probably her son was unable to keep up with the pace. I am now commissioned to find out about the young man so a second chapter can be written and I am surely going to do it.

Another in a few days.

Love from Mother and

Your

July 20,1942.

Dear John and Jim,

Well good old summertime is here with a vengeance. Temperature yesterday 99° with humidity varying from 85° - 100°. Makes me feel like going to Rye and maybe I will if I can find transportation to and from which is getting to be a serious question.

Worthington came home by plane from Kansas. He is a junior lieutenant without assignment and is off on a ten day leave. He does not know what he will get but still clings to the cavalry. Beale's outfit holds top honors in the artillery. He is at present in North Carolina.

The tire rationing board struck a hard blow yesterday: no more tires for beer ans soft drink trucks. I don't know what the political boys will have to say but I can imagine.

Everybody istalking second front in Europe, that is, everybody except those in authority and from them comes no encouragement. It is an odd situation but I can see no remedy if more ships cannot be found. It will take a lot of transportation to move and supply a sufficient Army to lick the Germans and it would be foolish to undertake an invasion doomed to failure. With Germany so much occupied in Africa and Russia it seems a pity not to make an attempt buy my faith is in the wisdom of General Marshall.

We had an "alarm" yesterday morning while at breakfast. The reaction was funny. Apparently no one knew what it was all about and no one knew what to do. They have been holding blackouts and at odd times trying out the siren system so nobody was prepared for a genuine alarm. It seems that a plane passed over the Eastern Shore from east to west without announcing its intention as is required -- and no civilian planes are now allowed in the air along the Coast -- a spotter saw it and failed to make out the markings so he sent the alarm direct to Baltimore instead of through the "filter system". The alarm was sounded and thirty-six thousand officials and helpers were called automomatically to duty. If it had been real officials would not have been caught flat-footed which shows some progress in organization and training.

Ellen came over for some bonds I have been collecting for the children. She looks very well as do the children.

Sis' house was struck by lightning on Saturday. Fortunately, it is covered with lightning rods and a stone roof, so there was no damage. She and her children are all very well.

More later. Love from Mother and

P.S.--I see Miss Everist is contributing another "Sun" paper.

July 22, 1942.

Dear Jim and John,

Well I am persuaded to take a rest.   Yesterday, with a temperature of 97, was a
bad day for me and while it is delightful today, I am frazzled out.   Guess I am getting old
and just don't know it (and just don't like it).

Mother and I will go Aug. 1st to Rye Beach.   Maybe we will see a different kind
of undersea craft from the usual one.   If so I hope it goes down to stay.

There is much gossip about making five thousand big air ships similar to the one
Glenn Martin made for the Navy.   It may bemore than gossip as a conference is to be held by
the President and some very substantial industrialists areurging the plan.   Martin says
five thousand of them can be turned out in a few months, if six of the ship-yards are utilized
and he is willing to farm out all of his rights.   It will mean ships that can go to Europe
and back the same day on their own fuel from here. Means five hundred thousand men can
be carried every two days to Europe; means the end of submarine menace; means a great army
fully equipped can be landed behind the enemy. It looks good but it is still gossip.

I have seen none of your friends outside the family lately, not even on the tennis
court or the golf course and after today I will probably see them less often as the new
gas rationing goes into operation tomorrow morning.   It starts with four gallons a week
but with no promise of continuing that high. This time you are examined as to the necessity
 for excess gas.   The last time you only had to ask for a higher card, but no more.   A lot
of the people who have not been curtailed in their driving will have just about enough to
get to town once a week.   I have cut off a lot of my own driving by not going out to see
Ellen and the children and by going to the Hospitals on street cars if possible. John's
work has sent me to the Church Home and the Hopkins occasionally but not so often as to
add much to my mileage. Mother goes down to the market twice a week and seldom gets into
her car except then.   I have been taking her down town and she gets home by street car.
We are really trying to help but many are not, I am afraid.

There is a big drive on for various kinds of scrap and if you help and at the same
time buy War Bonds you are given a sticker for your front window.   I think the rubber
collection was much better arranged than the metal.   You are told to take the metal in and
if it is too heavy call on a neighbor.   My neighbors are Dr. Ames and Mrs. Mc hail You can
visualize my difficulties with about t o tons of large metal objects to deliver.   In fact
I can't deliver them. I guess they will get wise to the necessity of calling for the
material as many people deprived of their cars, many households run entirely by women and
old people have no chance of contributing.

My work is not as heavy in the last few days, due largely I think to transportation
difficulties, real and imaginary.   I suppose as time goes on, the out-of-town patients
will largely drop off. I have been surprised to see it continue so heavy.   The hospitals
are busy as bees and with reduced staffs the boys really are working.   When the next medical
contingent is called there will be real trouble. We have never before had a real man power
shortage and it will take some figuring to make ends meet.   The Detroit "Free Press" had a
very interesting article yesterday showing the necessity for medical conservation.   It
was well expressed and a timely warning.   It ended "When aviators are needed it takes a
few months of training, evenline officers can be trained in ninety days but when it comes
to physicians we must remember it takes years and we want only the best."

I was interested to hear over the radio the announcement of the arrival in England
of a large detachment of the U.S. negro aviators.   The Colonel in charge said watch these
men they are among the very best and will be hears from.   I saw some of the negro air
men in action in the movies.   They made a very impressive showing and I hope they will be
as good in real life. They are good prize-fighters, jockeys and athletes and there is no
reason why they should not make excellent aviators as their ancestors have driven everything
from a bull to a steam engine.   They must have inherited something in some centuries of
training.   Well, more later,

Love from Mother

and

July 27, 1942.

Dear Jim and John,

I see on my desk another "Sun" which Miss Everist has provided, so I send it along.

The great source of conversation is gas rationing. More excuses are being found than you can ever imagine. Loprete was in and you would have died laughing hearing his story about what sad stories his friends are using. He, of course, condemns every evasion. The thing is people cannot get through their minds that rationing is for and their duty to uphold the spirit as well as the letter.

A young aviator came to Washington to be decorated -- he was from either Midway or Coral. I did not hear all of his introduction. He was asked if he had anything he would like to say; he said, without hesitation: "Yes! I would like to say that my buddies who are trying to win the war for you people can't understand what important war subjects are made secondary to politics. Why are you hesitating to put a ceiling on wages and farm products. It is rotten to leave any stone unturned to help win the war and my buddies will never understand any other attitude." It certainly created the proper atmosphere as everybody has apparently heard about it and agrees with the sentiments.

Brucy went to Richmond for a wedding on Friday. Ellen says she was as excited as if it were to be her own. Anne and Ellen came over to spend yesterday (Sunday). I never saw Anne look so well and so pretty. Charlie came in and he and Anne were like a pair of lovers. Hugging and kissing every little while. They play together beautifully and seem really devoted, which tickles me because I want my grandchildren to love and respect each other. It makes for a continuation of our happy family. Anne is as strong as an ox. She handles Charlie -- who is right wirey -- as if he weighed about two pounds.

Mother in looking over her photographs found a picture of John. It could just as well been a picture of Anne. I showed it to Charlie and he said without hesitation "it is Anne". Ellen Fisher wanted it, so mother gave it to her. Now mother is looking for one of Jim which looks like Pat. No luck so far but she is persistent.

We are having the house painted as it may be the last chance until the war is over. Paints, brushes and painters are about the scarcest things in the country. The house needs it badly and by the end of the war much of the wood-work would be gone, I am sure.

I have been writing you every day or so since you left. I hope some of my letters have reached you.

Well this is the last until the next time.

Love from Mother and

Vol. #II

Notes on Letters to Jim and John 1942-1945

038- Mary is Dr. Mary Goodwin.
See family tree to identify all the relatives discussed.

045- line 16 "I am in favor of the "Rum1" plan … (whatever that stands for)

048- 118 is the 118th General Hospital in northern Australia where Jim and John were.
Dr. Sam Crowe, head of ENT at Hopkins.
The Merchant Marine lost more men than the Navy in WW II.

050- Uncle Charles is probably Charles Earle Hollyday, Minnie's oldest brother, who would have inherited Readbourne had it not been sold. He had 2 sons, Charles Jr. (1916-1958) and Milton (1922- ?)
Letter head on reverse of #050 p.2

September 10, 1942.

Dear Jim and John,

Back at the old stand with patients galore. Well I will need them when the old tax bills begin to roll in. I can work for the Government right here, the more I make the more it gets to buy bullets with. If I could just marksome of them for the fellows I want to have them I would gladly work twenty-four hours a day.

Have no worry about our keeping warmthis winter. We will get about seventy-five percent. of last year's oil and with our open fires and electric heaters we have no worries. I only feel sorry for those who cannot buy the extras. Our house is insulated and we are putting on storm doorsand extra windows to conserve heat and we will be perfectly comfortable.

Pat is a great little trick. She is developing so fast and is really beautiful, easily the best looking baby I ever saw. She has a bag of tricks that keep you laughing all the time. She knows everybody in the house and all their peculiarities -- and plays on them. We have a grand time every morning running from room to room seeing the sights. She is a great comfort to Ma and me.

The President stretched the Constitution a bit the other day and told Congress if it did not get busy he would take over their function by executive decree. I hope he means it because living costs are going up pretty fast and the value of the dollar is dropping. It will mean a very hard winter for the poor without something is done of a very drastic nature. There has been too much time lost. Government is too far behind both industry and people.

There is a man by the name of Kaiser building ships on the Pacific Coast who is trying to persuade the Government to let him build 2oo ton cargo carrying planes. He is one of those fellows who love to do the impossible and always does it with glowing success. So far he has been blocked and much time has been lost but last night it looked like he would be able to putit over. He wants his planes to have fuel capacity to go anywhere and back without re-fueling. It sounds like a good way to beat the submarine.

We had a caddy strike out at the Club. They wanted two dollars a round and four dollars for doubles. They were turned down but are back on the job while the Board considers a raise of twenty-five cents which I hope they will not get as every boy now gets a guarantee of a dollar and twenty cents for car-fare. The course is splendid but my golf is rotten.

Ellen has taken Anne and Brucie down to the ducking grounds for a week. The firstthunder storm for a couple of weeks pulled off yesterday and boy the mosquitoes down there will give them an active time. Ellen said if they were too bad she was coming home.

Ellen Webb left yesterday with her flock for a week at Rehoboth. Another place famous for the little biting bugs. All the children and all the mothers are fine. Dudy looks like a million dollars and is taking great care of herself.

I really believe there is developing an idea that we are at war. I see a few signs among the people. Not strong but at least suggestive and if we had strong leadership it would develop into enthusiasm, but leadership is lacking. In fact, the people apparently have to stimulate the leadership.

We had a primary election and the State House and City Hall boys pulled off the usual stunts and gave us a bag of pretty poor game. About 20% voted.

This is all until another.

Love from us all,

Your

Lt.Col.James Bordley,III.,M.C.
Major John E. Bordley, M.C.
General Hospital No. 118,
U.S.Army - A.P.C. 927
c/o Postmaster, SanFrancisco, California,U.S.A.

September 14, 1942.

Dear John and Jim,

Since I came home I have been very busy not only in the office but outside. The war has added complexities which require attention and thought. The way of life is rapidly becoming different even in our well organized home. It is more a matter of inconvenience than of serious import. In other words it is hard for an old dog to learn new tricks but it can be done.

I am enclosing Miss Everist's Sunday Sun. It has some pictures of a pair of John's favorites which I am sure will interest him much. They sort of balance leaving the organization about 50% intelligent.

Labor Day was truly a historic occasion here. About two hundred and fifty boats either launched or had their keels laid on that day. Before the New Year comes we will have added many hundred merchant ships and a pretty good score of war vessels to our list. The buildings are faster than the sinkings. When the sinkings are stopped we will have a good total and a wonderful merchant marine after the war and my how badly it will be needed!2

Ellen and the girls have been down at the ducking shore for a week and were due to arrive last night at ten o'clock. Joseph says they are all very well and were then having a good time. I will see them this afternoon.

Pat is fine and says she is looking forward to a play mate very shortly. So far she has expressed no preference and neither have I. Uncle Dick was at the house yesterday and he was carried away with her. She flirted with him all the afternoon. He put up the gate at the steps in the third floor and made a first class job of it. I know it makes me a feel a lot more easy as Pat is a busy young lady and on the go every waking minute.

I see Wink's wife nearly every day I go to the Club. She and Ellen and a few more army wives go out there for tennis and golf. She looks very well. I understand she is spending the winter in the country as apartment are hard to get and very expensive.

Julia Baker has gone to the University of Virginia to complete a law course she started before getting married. She has moved her family to Charlottesville. The girls all think it a good move for her as she is interested in that sort of life.

Donald Nelson, at the head of war production, made a splendid speech last night and among other things said that since Pearl Harbor production has gone up three hundred and fifty percent. Not enough he said but a good warming up preparatory to an all out effort. He was a wise choice for the job.

Well this all until the next time.

Love from Mother and

September 16, 1942.

Dear Jim and John,

Yesterday the President appointed as rubber boss, the President of the Union Pacific. This is a splendid move if his hands are not tied by politics. It should have been done six months ago or longer. He has a hard job but one no more difficult, I imagine, than running a big railroad through endless Government rules, regulations and taxes.

I told you about seeing the movie depicting the Fourth of July celebration in Australia. The movie man cut the film and gave me the portion with your pictures. I had it enlarged and Jim is at salute with his left hand. It is odd looking to an old soldier but the likenesses are excellent. I had enough printed to distribute among the wives of those recognized. They all wanted them.

Mother is distressed that none of her letters have been received as your letters of Aug. 13th told us. She is not a very active correspondent but has written eight so far.

I understand that Perrin Long has been made laison officer between the United States and British Medical Army organizations. I do not see how it is possible because there are so many military problems involved. I heard yesterday he was dressed in his uniform and waiting to be assigned. The job is probably a confusion or maybe just gossip.

The weather here has been as hot as Hell. The weather man says this is "nothing out of the ordinary" It does feel like it however. On the golf course yesterday it was just 99. Not too hot for a seasoned veteran but intense for the novices who wander around in the nineties. Poor fellow I feel sorry for them. Tell Wink he better keep in form as we fellows who play around in the seventies are hard to get away with.   Mayb I will decide on the sixties before he gets home, if so I may let him carry my bag -- if he will wear his uniform.

It is interesting to see how women are taking the jobs of men, even in the St. Paul Garage. They park the cars, run the offices, etc. Down at Glenn Martins there are about five or six thousand. Mentzer is looking for one as a mechanic or a helper. They nearly all wear slacks. I saw one the other day about eight months' pregnant wearing a sailor suit. She made a most unusual looking sailor.

I am sending a picture of the left hand salute.
Well more later.
Love from Ma
and

94

Sept. 21,1942.

Dear Jim and John,

A real scrap drive for metals and rubber comes off tomorrow. Four hundred trucks and two thousand men start a city-wide canvas. Everybody is asked to put the stuff on the side-walk. Yesterday, mother and I spent the entire afternoon looking for stuff and what a mess we found. It is a good thing this collecting of scrap, it opens an avenue for a real house-cleaning. I suppose we easily have two or three tons of iron and steel alone to say nothing of copper, lead and zinc.

Well, I had to stop this and since the above was written the metals drive is over and I am proud of the way the City turned out the stuff. Twelve thousand tons were collected. This is way over the estimate. It was a funny sight to see the stuff over the pavements throughout the City. Every conceivable size, shape and object. Iron, steel, lead, zinc, copper and aluminum. There were five centers and today they are piled high with stuff. We were told that a full set of golf clubs supplied the scrap necessary for a pursuit plane and an old iron stove enough for a tank. Well, if all this stuff is used for planes and tanks the Nazi and the Rats are in for a real bad winter.

We are all excited over the Russians. Their fight at Stalingrad is a truly re-markable bit of fighting. I think it shows up a real weakening of the German war machine. Last year they carried on a successful campaign over a sixteen hundred mile front and this year a questionable success over less than three hundred. If we could have gotten a thousand fighting planes to the Russians all of the military commentators say that the campaign could have been turned into a terrific Nazi defeat, at the best they have done little except expend a huge amount of material and a vast personnel, they have not destroyed the Russian resistence and have gained no oil their two objectives. To destroy a city means little in this war so long as the army is left intact and the fighting spirit of the people remains high. Our greatest job is to induce action by our Government. It is too slow. Today, Congress and the President are claiming priorities ever labor and agriculture. What we should have is am immediate show down as to farm prices and wages. Food is getting too high and wages are, in the essential industries ridiculous. Politics is the principal Nazi fifth column in this country as it as in France. The people are getting tired of their procrestination and are speaking in loud voices.

Pat is a nuisance: she makes me wear my hat even at the dinner table, not only that but I wanted to change to a felt hate because it is cold and she threw it away and made me put on my straw. very time she sees me she paddles off and finds my hat and brings it to me and stands in front of me and chatters until I put it on then goes about her business. Every few minutes she steps around to see whether I have got it on and if I have not she goes around like a Kildee protecting her nest.

Anne and Brucie came with Ellen to have dinner yesterday. Anne spent the day with Joanna and Brucie with us. They are getting ready for school. I confidentially asked Brucie what Anne thought of school and she told me Anne had no particular enthusiasm, was sort of afraid it would interfere with her way of life and then Brucie ventured the suggestion that she kind og agreed with Ann's notion. She has surprised me the last few times I have seen her by sitting quietly in my lap and asking me to tell her stories. She is very affectionate too, now and then hugging and kissing me. This shows the effect of war in the disposition of children.

Worthington's Ann is a nurse now in the U.M.H. working on a fellowship o the U.S. I had never heard of that way of spending taxes but am glad as long as the money had to be spent it was on Ann. The poor girl is worried because the U.M.H. no longer teaches psycology. I should think it would be a strain on her because of her general aptitude for the obstruce. Personally, I thought she would profit as much from a first reader.

Ma is helping at the St. Paul's Parish House in the entertainment of the soldiers, sailors, marines and the merchant marines. It is really a fine thing that lacks only some good beer and a high ball or two to make the youngsters appreciate the glamour girls -- your maiden aunts and their contemporaries. Really it is a fine gesture, the

women are working hard and the boys seem to take to it like ducks to water.   They have a
little scheme of writing a card home, telling parents and wives that the boy called, if he
willgive them a little sto y. they include it.   I imagine this is appreciated by a great
many parents, especially when they see a church address.
      Well, so long and I hope you will enjoy Miss Everist's Sunday Sun.
            Love from Ma, and

September 23, 1942.

Dear John and Jim,

Well the heating is O.K. We are adding one of the slickest things you ever saw to the oil heater. It is called a coal booster. It throws a flame like the oil and takes onehalf of heating operation. It is all automatic and even the ashes are taken care of by paying a dollar a ton extra for the coal. They will have to be removed only once a year as so little is left by the combustion of the coal. We have been promised three quarters of our normal oil stock so we will always have a surplus. Richard Hollyday has installed one and had Bessie and Clara put one in their apartment house.

Things are getting harder to buy. Such for instance as bacon, stockings and certain canned articles, to say nothing of rubber goods and gasoline. Still I don't feel we have been called upon to make any real sacrifices because for all we lack there are suitable substitutes. There are, of course, some "bellyakers". They are mostly those who have volunteered nothing and who much prefer their own luxuries to the safety of their neighbors' children. They give me a pain and often bad enough for me to freely express my opinion. Personally, I feel we could be doing much more if the Government would get a bit more tough, especially with labor and agriculture. These two factors are having entirely too much wet nursing. It is funny, too, because the bitterest criticism I have heard of the Government has come directly from these sources because they are dissatisfied with our war efforts -- they are not progressing fast enough.

I heard over the radio last night that besides the Army quota of planes which is ahead of schedule we are turning out over two thousand Navy planes a month. It was an authorized statement so I suppose it is O.K. to quote it.

We have a good natured moron about six feet tall as a housemaid. Pat expresses the general opinion every time she appears. She throws her head back and shouts with laughter. It is the funniest thing I ever saw as she never misses the opportunity. Whatever started her no one knows but it certainly shows psychological understanding.

Yesterday Pat was sitting at the breakfast table when I asked her: "Pat what are you?" Without hesitation, she replied "Pappas Pat". It took us so by surprise, especially Dudy. Dudy told me this morning she was so pleased with herself that the practiced the expression all day. Her teeth are coming through and without much apparent disturbance. She is always good as gold.

I saw Ellen and Mrs. Wink yesterday at the Club. Ellen had been caddying for Mrs. Wink and thus both got exercise. Many days we have no caddies and we just take three or four clubs and walk around. I rather enjoy it and it saves money. If. Ellen becomes proficient I may offer her regular employment.

We all watch and listen to all reports from Australia and the surrounding Islands and when the Navy or Army has been particularly successful it is a great source for conversation and speculation.

Well more later.

With love from Ma

and

September 28, 1942

Dear Jim and John,

Mary Joe was at the house last night. She has a book in which she is having all of Bruno's friends write him letters for Xmas. Brucie wrotehim one of the cutest. I wrote and urged him to get in an economic argument with the chief rat - Hirohito. I suggested it would be a real contribution if he did not stop short of stepping on his head if he disagreed.   I can imagine Hirohito in Bruno's grasp. The trouble is Bruno might argue himself into a dual conclusion.

Wellpatients flock in.   Anywhere from three to seven new ones a day. A great many from our new war industries -- the only plutocrats left.   Now and then I get pretty tired of the rush but I try to make it like the grinding of the mills of God.

There are long controversies concerning the shortage of Doctors. Most of the trouble and controversy comes from the New Dealers headed by Parran. The attempt to socialize medicine is too clear to be overlooked. Hervey Stone took a crack at them in the Sun this morning.

The President and Congress still do not see eye to eye on the farmers' problems. First round -- the President, second round -- Congress. The third round is going to be the peoples if I am not mistaken.   They are flooding Congress and the President with protests over the factors involved and want the questions settled and all controversy ended.   The damned lobbies are the cause of most of the trouble, they really dictate too many of our policies and wield entirely too much political power.   Congress had to settle in favor of the President or the lobbies and strange as it seems they backed the lobbies. I often wonder whether Congress knows we are at war.   Certainly they give precious few signs except in their alacrity to levy taxes and create new civilian jobs. The public is not far ahead of Congress when it nominates such cattle as Hamilton Fish and a few others of the same stripe.

Pat has learned to walk up the steps and has to be watched all the time to keep her from practicing.   Charlie came in to spend the night while his father and mother went over to a foot-ball game in Washington. Pat thoroughly enjoyed his visit. She does not have the opportunity of playing with kids very often and she likes it.

Most of John's patients are cured since he left.   Some were in pitiful shape but I had little difficulty and getting them back on their feet.   They seem very appreciative of first class medical service.

We are in dount as to whether you are in your permanent hospital or where you are even now if not in yourpermanent location.   I suppose such things are not tellable and if they are not we do not care to know. Rumors have had you flitting all over the Pacific Southwest but we always listen with deaf ears.

More later.

Love from Ma and

September 30, 1942.

Dear John and Jim,

Well Congress is licked on the farm bloc proposition of no ceiling on farm products. The people have spoken by the hundreds of thousands. I suspected they would take a hand. Our estimable Senators voted against the administration control of prices. They are on my black list forever. It was a smart trick which took no account of the housewives or the war and was doomed to failure. The whole bunch belong under the banner (or umbrella) of Chambrlaine -- just placating the farm vote for the coming election.

Cold weather has arrived ahead of schedule and tomorrow we start our fuel rationing in all of the Eastern States just because Congress and the administration did not want to antagonize the railroads and steamship companies by building a pipe-line up from the Texas oil-fields. With eight months' notice of coming shortage they waited until last month to build a line from Texas to Chicago. This will help by January or February but the delay has cost the house owners millions of dollars because they have been obliged to convert from oil to coal. And now the coal miners have declined to adopt a longer week which is essential.

Well these things were to be expected in a democracy where every man is the captain of his own ship and charts his own course. In the end except for expense and inconvenience we will be O.K. but it does seem terribly stupid to have a Government which can never think through today into tomorrow.

Gradually we are getting into the spirit of the war and strange as it seems the principal inspiration has come from Russia and the magnificent defense of the people. Who would have ever expected this country to follow Stalin's lead. Of course sacrifices are inevitable but so far they have not inconvenienced us, it is more the thought of the sacrifice than its actuality which keeps many on edge. If we can keep the sheriff out of our home we will fair well and be comfortable. When I look around at our lovely antiques and the energy and money expended on their collection I wonder why. They seem utterly insignificant except they represent to me the civilization which gave us all for which we are fighting -- land and our way of life. Now even that seems a bit out of keeping in a world at war. Nothing really matters except liberty.

We have always lived in a fool's Paradise. Selfishness, personal and national is the reward of the affluence which has been built up in our hundred and fifty years of existence. If we had shared a little of both our spiritual and material with our neighbors maybe we would have had no world war but we have been taught to think only of ourselves in the present and have been tragically short on our future. We have had too many opportunities and too few Lincolns and Jeffersons. Jefferson gave the politicians one hundred and fifty years to destroy our nation of the people, for the people and by the people. He was a little too short on time.

We are all well and send love.

October 5, 1942.

Dear Jim and John,

If you are tired of my drony old letters say so and I will stop and give you a rest. This October the first will be writ high in our history books. It marks the first great turn in our individual liberty and makes us more definitely a servant of the State. It brings us closer to what we are fighting against than we have ever been before. Today our meat ration is placed at two and one-half pounds a week; gasoline is rationed throughout the nation; the speed limit is set at thirty-five miles an hour with confiscation of the gasoline rationing book if you violate the edict; this morning marks the end of oil deliveries except on Government permits and thenonly 66% of your requirements; the seller is no longer able to sell in a free market, nor, purchaser to dicker with the seller -- Uncle Sam seesthat the store posts a price list based on the long ago, a price list that regular customers can confirm or deny: soon farm products will join their brothers as the Senate had to reverse itself to the tune of 84 to 0 in favor of the president's demands.

Well does that not sound like we are in war? If I am not mistaken both the Pharisee and Saducee will know all about it before the robins come again

You know there is almost no gossip around except new babies expected. Dudy said she made a trip down town and was embarrassed not the least because every other young woman she met was going to have a baby. Well that has always been one of the fruits of war, a sort of natural compensation.

John's patient, Ned Salafie joined the Coast Guard. After study in New Orleans and being transferred to Newport and then to a ship had the misfortune of having his right ear discharge in the presence of the surgeon. He was put in a Hospital and kept there three months being given large doses of Sulfadiazine three times a day for his entire stay. No blood examinations during the treatment but he is still with us and the ear is still discharging. He is broken hearted because they put him out of the Coast Guard. I think he was really lucky to get out of the Hospital.

I had a nice game of golf with rs. Wink yesterday. She has changed her style of driving and has increased her drive by yards. I suppose playing with someone to encourage instead of someone to nag helps too. Ask Wink if this is not correct.

When I first started playing with the girls I felt that I should carry their clubs asw have no caddies most of the time. I have change a bit now and feel they should carry ine. What a war! It certainly knocks hell out of ones point of view.

If we never open a window or door in our house after it is heated I am sure it would make the one heating last for the winter. The windows are corked up. the outside doors are sealed and storm doors on the outside, every window and door stripped and the house insulated. Where the fresh air will come from, it is a hard question to answer. Then we have as much oil as we used last year. By cutting out the oil hot water heater we are given an extra allowance for the boiler. We have a "bucket a day" hot water heater which runs by coal. Besides we have two large portable electric heaters which have hot water radiators, two small bath-room portable electrics and an open fire-place in each room. If you wished more heat you would have to live in a baker's oven. It is a comfort though to know that you are prepared. It will probably be a mild and balmy winter.

I wish the Man Power Board would really get busy and get some help for the farmer. My tenant phoned me this morning he would be unable to put in any wheat because he could not procure any labor for plowing. He said that all around him farmers are quitting and there will be no harvests of wheat or corn next year. The labor has beenpermitted to go to the cities for higher wages. This should not only be stopped but labor should be made to return to the farms. It will, of course, after the election which means after the wheat planting season has passed.

Little Charlie told me yesterday that he had enough chewing gum for eight boys. I asked him why he had bought so much and he said, "Well maybe they will ration chewing gum and I bought enough to last until they can get more sugar to make more." This was his own inspiration because his mother is so strict in carrying out the spirit of

conservation that her husband says she has "gone religious".   But it is a spirit that has
a large following and I am afraid.

Well, the President has appointed Justice Byrnes as the keeper of our economic
existence.   It is he who will have the final say over wages, production and consumption.
A mighty job and a very ordinary man.   As a Senator, he was the great pacifier.   As
economic boss, he will have to strip to the waist and take off his gloves.   I hope he
can do it.

We are all well and send love.

October 12, 1942.

Dear John and Jim,

This is a harvest season for former boot-leggers according to published reports. They manufacture and sell gasoline tickets, sugar, etc.   The thing that gets my goat is they find anxious customers, people who to satisfy their desires for profits and special comforts are willing parties to schemes for upsetting the government's war plans. These ladies and gentlemen are not confined to the Jews, or, the ignorant, among them are many who do know better.

The necessity for individual sacrifice is slow reaching the vitals of the Nation. Most people think in terms of national sacrifice and do not particularly include themselves. They are willing to be rationed, to have cold homes and work longer hours but it never occurs that they should be out looking for ways and means to help the government. They are willing to follow but never seek to lead.

Of course, we are upagainst a new experience for all of the present people and like a baby learning to walk we must find someone else to hold on to, some other to guide. As a nation we will find our way, but, the progress from affluence to rationing will be slow and painful. It means the end of the upper middle class. One by one reastaurenteersm farmersm shop keepers, etc. are closing up -- and I think -- forever. This will end our times of luxury and special benefits, will indeed change our point of view of life and its values. Maybe we have been profligate, selfish and have lived in a Fool's Paradise, but nevertheless out of it has come industrial and social progress never dreamed of before. We have built a great nation and will our changed status maintain it? Only time can write the answer.

Miss Willets is going to Glenn Martins and leaves in a day or two. I have secured a first class hand to take her place -- Mrs. John E. Bordley. She comes today to get her instructions. She will have to be here from nine to one and will come down in the morning with me. She is anxious to help out and also thinks she can use the salary. Of course, I am delighted to have her.

My work grows no less, what will happen to it -- that is the best of it when railroad priorities are put into effect, I don't know but provision will probably be made for sick people to visit doctors. With the restrictions on automobiles it would seem necessary. The other side if the Government, in its socialized medical inclinations, may insist on people consulting doctors in their own districts. This is for the future do I am worrying.

We are all well, Dudy in particular.

Love from all,

Your

October 15, 1942.

Dear Jim and John,

I have had a patient whose nephew was one of the officers on the West Point when you went to Australia. He was very full of the nephew who is a senior Lieutenant.

Pat and Dudy are home again after a few days' visit to Philadelphia. I am glad they are home as the old house was positively a lonely place to live without the patter and chatter of Pat. She now calls me Pop and is so proud of her invention that she keeps in constant practice. She grows more lovely every day. Yesterday she carried me over to Jim's picture and told me who it was. She wanted me to let her kiss the picture. You might have supposed it was her Daddy in the flesh. When I took her up she spied a letter in my pocket and took it out and said, "letter, Letter Daddy". I suppose Dudy has been telling her about the letters she receives. She cries so seldom that we get excited when she blows off.

Brucie and Anne are fine. They go to school every day and while Anne gets no particular kick out of study she thoroughly enjoys the fun. Brucie is so different. Ellen says she is afraid to play with her friends because she does not know how to skip a rope or throw a ball. She is more interested in the intellectual side of life. She is really a smart girl and a very sweet one

Ellen is holding down the testing machine and says she is getting to like it. She got her first check this morning and seems excited to think she has made her first money. I hope she will not tire of the monotonous routine. I would I am sure.

Your mother tumbled down a few steps about two weeks ago and bruised her leg. I took her over to Bennett who said she had torn a small tendon. She is about well now except for a rather persistent sore spot. She was inspecting a new house bought by John Tompkins and his wife over in Homeland. They are to be permanent residents of Baltimore. Mother is giving them a cocktail party Sunday.

Frannie Cromwell was to move to Mississippi on Monday but Charlie has been put at the head of the Mess and ordered to Indiana for special training for a month. Frannie had already rented her home to a Naval officer but they heard of Frannie's dilemma and told her they would wait for a month.

One by one the young men are disappearing, some in the Navy, others in the Army. When the new draft goes into force few will be left. What a world and what a time! That devil Hitler should be quartered, shooting or hanging would be too slight a punishment.

Our old friend, Wendell Wilkie, is home again. I certainly admire his ability, energy and candor. He is still hot for a second front. I confess I do not know the wise selection but I am all in favor of trusting the judgment of our leaders. It does seem awfully slow but I remember enough of my own army experience to believe it takes time to organize large undertakings.

Well more later.

Love from us all,

Your

103

October 20, 1942.

Dear John and Jim,

I was so busy yesterday, in fact all last week that I could not take the time to write. Practice is booming, in fact there seems no bottom. Not much operative work thank God but new patients from everywhere.

Last week was a bad one, about five and a half inches of rain in two days. Everything flooded including Cumberland and Washington. Fredericksburg -- the lower city -- was seventeen feet under water. As most of the wheat that is to be planted was already in I fear the farmers will have to find other crops if the Manpower Board ever supplies the required labor. The Senate is trying to put over a slazy trick. Boys of 18 and 19 are to be drafted and to the bill the Senate has hooked an amendment for prohibition in all territory frequented by these youths. It is a perfectly manifest attempt to foist prohibition again on the country. If they have a roll call vote we are told it will pass. The poor boobs have learned nothing, they fail to see that to destroy liquor they must exercise powers that are far more productive of evil consequences. So is politics and the rotten hounds who chase office. This same crew were the isolationists and most everything vile and wicked that has hit our country. They cannot see their own likeness to Hitler.

We are following the reports from the Pacific South West. Meager as they are they tell us a tale of effort and sacrifice in our behalf. We are proud of those who are so willing to take up arms in our defense and we sincerely wish them Godspeed and extraordinary power.

The Yale-Navy game was really a corker in spite of the muddy field. Yale had six of its best men out from injuries in the Penn game. Experts think Yale has its best squad of years but many of them are still green. In spite of the weather about 30,000 sat out the game.

I have just heard that Miss Willets has not yet gone to work for Glenn Martin It seems she has high blood pressure. Why that should stop her from drawing pictures is hard to visualize but I suppose they have certain regulations that are applied to all from deck hands to artists. I am worried because she needs the money but not sufficiently worried to have her back here. I have a perfectly competent lady in her place -- Mrs. John Bordley.

Ellen has been coming to the office with me but this morning she had to use her car and when I got on the elevator to come up to the office, the elevator boy said, "By yourself this morning, I hope your lady friend isn't sick"? I haven't told Ellen yet.

I am enclosing a letter I wrote the Sun and Miss Everist's small Sunpaper.
More later.

With love from us all,
Your

October 23, 1942.

Dear Jim and John,

What do you think of two thunder storms in a week the last of October. The one last week dragged along for over two hours.

Well the boys over in Washington passed the tax bill they have been fooling with since last May. It is a corker -- nine billions -- to be followed with a supplementary one for six billions. The taxes will take about twenty-seven cents out of every dollar of income. While I am dubious how I am going to pay my sharem I am nevertheless in favor of paying for as much of the war as we can while it is going along. If the Government would only drop out about four billions a year they are spending on "social benefits" the burden could be substantially reduced but the New Dealers are intent on spending for votes and as they control the situation, we will have to continue to pay. The so-called benefits are bad in that they keep a lot of people from working who otherwise would have to contribute their labors.

I thought we were going to have conscription of all labor but the President, I think, has made the mistake of putting his foot down on the proposition. He dislikes to take Mr. X from New York where he is not needed and send him to St. Louis where his efforts will count. Of course, such a step would be drastic but no more drastic than taking a fellow from his job and sending him to Australia to face hards ips and death. I never believed in high wages for labor and low wages for soldiers, both should share the hardships and economies of war.

Anne has had a slight cold and Ellen kept her in bed for a day or so. Otherwise all the children are fine and their mothers the same. Pat grows in every way and is very cute. She is given to taking things that do not belong to her and is ever conscious of her guilt. My glasses out of my pocket for instance. Her conscience treats such pilfering lightly. She goes out every morning to see me off and as a last stand she insists on my kissing her hand out of the car window. The one nuisance is that I have to wear my hat in the house and even at the breakfast table. What the idea is I have no explanation to offer

The old golf course is like a deserted village. One or two people take up their clubs and march around maybe two or three days in the week. Tennis is about as bad. The reason is lack of gasoline and wear and tear on precious tired.

It amuses me much to see those who rushed in to buy tires and have substantial stock piles having todisgorge. You are allowed to have but five and declare them under oath with their serial numbers and submit them to two months inspections. If you violate the rules your gas ration card is taken from you and you are not permitted to drive. The smart guys were not so smart after all. Then they are taking away the ration cards of those who got them under the plea of necessity and then spend their time at race tracks and other resorts. Sixty were called in only yesterday as the result of detection at the races and Ocean City. The names are not given but as Frank Chew, who is on the office force of Home Defense, took a week off for a trip to Ocean City, I am wondering how he fared. It would be a joke on him. I must say thought he has been working hard on a non pay basis and never takes his car out except on Sunday as a means of transportation to some free food shed.

Well the Prohibition amendment has been temporarily shelved and the 18 - 19 year old draft bill will not carry it, but prohibition is not dead. The suckers have learned no lesson but the public has and Senators and Representatives were told where to get off. From here it looks like Russia has done a good job with the Nazi. They are the most astonishing people in the world, their efforts will be the prime cause of Hitler's failure and they have done it alone. It is curious the change their efforts have wrought on the thinking of the other allied nations. Even partners inJ. P. Morgan's banking house are making impressive speeches on the glories of Russia and condemning those who criticize her ideology.

We are turning out three ships a day exclusive of our Navy vessels. Baltimore is third in line turning out one every other day. If you could see the thousands of men working in the ship-yards you could understand it. Our trouble is housing all the tens of thousands who have come here to work. Our population has increased some two hundred and

fifty thousand in one year. Fifty thousand more are expected before January 1st and another
fifty thousand before July 1st. There is no loafing around here, everyone is busy.
Still a few parties but small and infre uent and looked down upon.
Well more later.
Love from all.

October 26, 1942.

Dear John and Jim,

  We had a group of the "War Widows", as they callthemselves, for dinner last night: Ellen Fisher, Pickett and Eleanor O'Donovan. They seemed to enjoy the little change and played cards with Dudy until about eleven. The last time Pickett came to dinner she had a puncture and we could not find a soul to fix her tire until the next day. Last night I think she was superstitious and was much relieved not to find a tire down (so was I.)

  Well Madam Roosevelt has landed in England with the intention of "seeing everything". I bet she does and she may take command of the Expeditionary Forces before her return. Of course this is surmise but based on established precedents. I only hope she does not strain the relations of our two countries.

  War, War, War, nothing but War! Who would believe that a civilization based upon the gentleness and patience of Christ could turn into a roaring hell of destruction. Learn? No, we never learn, each generation must make its own discoveries, must needlessly shed its own blood. The world has gone a long way but it has not yet discovered that what we look upon as separate states are mere component parts of one picture, that different languages do not make different humans with different souls. Not yet have we come to realize that contentment must be universal to be permanent and that our luxuries are often the other fellows necessities. Will we ever learn that real fellowship is essential to end wars? Maybe, but I doubt it. The only hope is that through education the peoples of the world will find out that it is more their governors than their form of government which makes for peace and happiness. Even with our splendid Constitution we are led over rough roads by a bunch of scalawag politicians who care more for office than for country. Will we ever understand the value of our own rights and duties? Today in our Senate there are not more than a dozen men to whom we can look for sound government and our Legislature is a mass of broken hopes.

  As I watch the irresponsibility of our lawmakers it makes me wonder how we have come so far and done so well. I feel sure it is more due to our abundance thanour wisdom, more to our ingenuity than our Constitution. I hope you fellows, who are now suffering the slings and arrows of an outrageous fortune, will come home with the real determination to clear the mass and corruption from our governing body. I hoped that in 1919, but, found only a gang who were intent on capitalizing on their service to rob the National Treasury, more intent on profit than of making secure the things for which their comrades died. Don't let this tragedy happen again if you can avoid it and, you can avoid it if you think first and actafterwards. So much is dependent on the wisdom of you fellows, the whole world is holding its breath to see what you willdo, it is now crying for just an expression of your intentions, knowing full well the weight your decisions will have on the establishment of a real new order of liberty, fraternity and peace.

  I had no intention whenI started this letter of writing a sermon on your duties but when youare home and surrounded by the accumulations of thought and material of a long and happy life it gives you a perspective which you do not gain from Army life in a foreign land. I so want my family to do a good job as citizens of our great country that what I have written is just some of my thoughts which have almost unintentionally leaked out. Still they are the expressions of a very sincere hope.

  The only local news I know is that one of Polly Barker's twins was operated on Saturday -- had an eye removed. MacLean found an intraocular tumor and operated at once. They feel pretty confident and I hope their prognosis is well founded. Few children however, in my experience escaped a secondary, not more than one in twenty. I think it was fortunate Halsey was at home.

  I was called yesterday to settle an argument: Brucie claimed that a sore throat made it necessary for her to miss Sunday School. Ellen was suspicious that it was school and not sore throat but she was wrong. A mild pharyngitis which is epidemic was sufficient justification.

November 2, 1942.

Dear Jim and John,

Well we have spent many anxious moments watching the trend of events in and around Guadalcanal. With the change of top Navy officials we all felt that something must be wrong with the set-up and were relieved when the Secretary of the Navy announced the withdrawal of the Jap fleet. Apparently in spite of our losses we held them off of the objective and made them go home to think it over.

We had a little party last night to have John Tompkins and his wife (they have moved to Baltimore) meet some of the younger set. About twenty-five guests stayed from five to nine-thirty. They all seemed to have a good time. Mostly women whose husbands are in the military services. Very few of our young male friends are left.

Well Congress is all wet again, especially the Senate. The Army has asked for 18 and 19 year olders. The House voted in favor without amendments, the Senate added an amendment to keep them in training for one year before their induction into actual service. The Army is kicking and it is believed the President will veto the bill. What a contrast -- Soviet Russia called its eighteen year olders for military training. They know they a e in a war and are preparing for the future, the Senate knows that thi ty of its members are up for re-election and they hope to salvage the votes of some million mothers.

The election comes off tomorrow. I have no feeling of elation even if the candidates for whom I vote are elected. The whole bunch is a miserable lot of tripe from the overnor down. Not one really educated, understanding man outside of the Judges. One of Democracy's weaknesses! Somehow in spite of the handicap we manage to make good, possibly it takes less brains to run a Government than we would think.

At the present moment the Internal Revenue Bureau has a deputation to examine John's books and accounts. Well there is nothing like an established reputation -- they only send one to look over mine. If they should find you owe a few thousand that skipped your mind, I will suggest they take it out of your Army pay.
(Five minutes later). The Revenuers have gone. Said they thought they were to go over an important account but found it "so small they were able to clean up and go in four and a half minutes' time." Well that is better than a bill for back taxes.

Work goes on getting moe and more as the days pass and more doctors go away. This is not altogether a happy thought when you focus your eyes on the coming tax bills and th ir rates per thousand, and to a five percent. gross tax before other taxes. The New dealers were intent on preventing savings and just as intent on destroying capital. Boy, they are having a field day!

I want to get this in the mail, so good-bye until the next time. All the family are well.

Love from Ma and
                                        Your

P.S.--Inclosed - ?iss Everist's Baltimore Sun.

November 5, 1942.

Dear John and Jim,

Just a little frazzled this morning after a very difficult cataract operation. Funny how age makes such a difference. Once I could tackle the most complex operation and leave with a smile, now I leave very tired. Indeed I sort of dread difficult procedures.

Well the election is over and there are some distinct surprises, the Governor of our State for instance. He was supposed to win by at least 60,000 but to date and, nearly all the returns are in, he has less than 12,000 plurality. For several hours last night he was a poor second and in the end carried the City by only 3,000. All over the country th re has been great dissatisfaction with the slowness of our war preparations. The people want to go all out at once and not have it fed to them in small and broken doses. They feel that there is too much discrimination in favor of office holders who do not produce nor fight. They registered their protest at the polls and I look for a speeding up and an end of being told one s ory today and another tomorrow.

Dewey carried New York by s me 600,000 in spite of administration efforts to defeat him. The people were tired of old office holders and were looking for new blood with a new viewpoint. Then Wendell Wilkie's statements concerning lack of energy, thought and pu pose swung many a thousand votes not only in New York but throughout the land. He is today the greatest leader of the American people, a great unselfish patriot.

This is a day later.

The Democrats have had the scare of thei lives. They control Congress -- the House 216 - 205 with 4 independents and ten seats doub ful. The Republicans gained nine seats in the Senate and have taken away five or six Gocernorships from the Democrats. The whole farm belt has returned to the Republican ranks. These fellows claim the Administration has favored Labor ever Agriculture in the protection of Labor. Talking with some of them however I gain the impression that they are sore about the stupidity of the wars conduct. They are for a quicker break on the essentials for an all out war program and are tired of waiting for the Administration and Congress to decide whether it is a United Nations or a United States War, tired of hearing about rationing in the future when they see the need in the resent, tired of hearing about national conscription after the first of the year when they know it should have been done after the first of the present year. There is no dissatisfaction because we are in the war, the only trouble is our war activity and the hesitant ways of a timid Administration. It will take more than a fireside chat to convince the nation it is all out to win,

So much for politics. We now have forces in Australia, Persia, Egypt, Liberia, England, Ireland, South America and the West Indies. It really looks like our people will know more about the world when the war is over. I hope it will broaden the view point of the voters and bring a realization that we have serious international responsibilities If it does not, what will? While I think it silly to discuss peace before we are ready to fight the war, I nevertheless feel that our Governors and the leaders of the opposition should put their heads together and decide on the principles which will be involved, and we should definitely formulate our own thesis indtead of being led by the nose. We may have no territorial objectives but we certainly have moral and social obligations and we should never cease to defen them.

Pat's vacabulary is now about the size of Webster's dictionary. She knows everybody and everything and more than that she fights for her rights (and sometimes for her wrongs). She grows more and more cute as the days go by.

Brucie and Anne are well. I took Anne and Charlie out to see an old patient of mine on Sunday and she had toys and candy and did they have a good time. The old lady enjoyed them as much as they enjoyed the candy.

Dudy is getting along well, everything I am told is perfectly normal and correct. Well more later.

With love from Ma and

Your

November 9, 1942.

Dear Jim and John,

It seems funny in this land of plenty there should be food shortages. Well, we have them. Mother went to five stores before she could find any bacon, six stores and found no coffee and that is the way all down the line. Even ordinary cuts of meat are not procurable and the Government has stopped the canning of a large variety of foods on account of lack of tin and, some things they will not permit even in glass. I wonder how the isolationists, who talked about our self-sufficiency, feel when they can't get what they want to eat.

It holds good too for clothes. I bought a new suit, I could not have cuffs on the trousers, no silk or satin lining, no extra trousers, no lapel on the vest, only a certain number of buttons and only of a certain style and composition, no patch pockets and no lapels on the pockets. It holds as good in metals: only the tools in stock can be sold except on priority orders to help the war effort. I tried to get a pair of iris scissors only to be told they are out for the duration. No more metal weather-stripping, no more razor blades and, I could write on indefinitely because the restrictions are limitless and more in the offing.

One of our great trouble is man-power both in civil and military production. This largely due to the labor laws which permit only forty hours a week. The election is going to change the status of labor to say nothing of the effects of the introduction of women to any and all jobs. Scared by the results of the election two New Deal preachers -- one in the Senate and the other in the House -- are rushing bills to end the Wagner law and to revoke the forty hour law. They have seen the dissatisfaction of the voters. Personally, I am in favor of decent working hours, pay, vacations and conditions for labor and I hope the politicians in their frenzy will not upset the worthwhile in the Wagner Act. It is too bad for a man to work all hislife and have nothing to show for his labors when his time isup and, it is too bad to make a human machine burn up to insure profits for others and, still worse not to have some time for relaxation and fun. Labor is cursed by crooked leadership and crooked political handling, two evils hard for labor to overcome. I believe in the average working man, hisloyalty and patriotism but I recognize that he must shoulder some of the responsibility of his dilemma.

We are thrilled by the Allied attack on and destruction of Rommel's Army. What a show it must have been to watch -- especially a lot of damn German's scurring like rabbits to get away from a hunter. I hope the hunter keeps the scent until the rabbits ar destroyed. This will mean much for our cause and efforts. I make a prediction: If Rommel's Army is completely destroyed as a war machine Italy will make a serious effort to sue for peace and in one year the Germans will be out of the picture. We are told of a powerful Allied fleet now at Gibralter with a large number of land troop transports. The Germans have confirmed this advice. They are there for a good and sufficient reason and the Italians know it. With control of the Mediterranean how can Italy escape terrible retribution. Everyone of its coastal cities can be blown from the map. The A.E.F. has been demonstrating on two or three of its cities from bases in England, what could they not do from bases in Africa and from the Mediterranean Sea.

Another day. Italy had a bad bombing last night from London; Italian troops left stranded in Egypt by their Nazi pals -- left without food, water, ammunition and transportation; the Italian Governor of Italy's possession in North Africa skipped over to French Morocco; the Allied fleet left Gibralter last night. Keep your ears peeled for re-percussion.

We had a sudden alert yesterday at three o'clock. Everybody ducked and the show was well carried out. This is our first daylight alert. The Court fined a lot of people in the last blackout and this encouraged consideration of the rules. Still few people can be convinced we are in any danger.

Mailing day. Well much h s transpired since the last notation. This nation is thrilled by the landing of a large force in Africa. You can never imagine the

real excitement nor the real hope that he h s brought about. It was like an electric
spark and it sets at rest the doubters of the wisdom of our military authorities. If they
carry it through to a successful climax it will consilidate public opinion as nothing since
Pearl Harbor and even more because we are slowly taking part in the show as civilians and
all that was needed was a show of constructive leadership. If the Administration and
Congress will now settle their differences and go all out so will the public. The doubters
now know we are in war and except for anunpatriotic editorial of old McCormack of the
Chicago Tribune there is not a unity of opinion and hope. This old vagabond seeing the
world he has been some eighty years building up, crumble, denounced Russia and England and
warned the public against trust in the Allied cause. Always a baiter of England and Russia
he hates to see their importance and our alliance. He is so old that he cannot recognize
unavoidable trendsin world affairs. Hispower isnil except among the disgruntled isolationists - Nazi followers.

Well I have to wear my overcoat along wit my hat now. Pat is so afraid I
will satch cold that she drags my overcoat to me ev ry time s e sees me without it. It is
a nuisance that 1 rather enjoy.

Charles Hollyday, Jr. brought his bran new baby to see us yesterday and at
had a fit over it. She saw the baby on Ma's lap and insisted on holding it but as she
wanted to keep her hands on its head all the time it was thought unwise to sit her on Pat's
lap. Charles has been sent to New York by the Glenn Martin Co. to supervise the plans for
a new Navy plane. The Otis Elevator plant is the cite of operations. Charles h s full
supervision, his salary has been greatly increased, he is supplied a home and all expenses
concerned therewith and all traveling expenses. He says he is not capable of filling such
an important ob. I told him that was his father's attitude and the reason he never got
anywhere.

More another time.

With love from Ma and

Your

November 10, 1942.

Dear John and Jim,

We have put in the cutest little hot water heater you ever saw. It takes one small shovel of coal and is an air-tight affair so the generated heat cannot escape and the water gets the entire benefit. It will carry us through the winter with as much and as hot water as ever and at half or less the expense. We too have learned that a 70° temperature in the house is a nuisance. We live in about 66° and thoroughly enjoy it because the work I have had done on the house eliminates any drafts. No one has so far had a cold and I think the temperature has helped.

Roy Gill, whom you may remember, tried to beat priorities and stored a lot of gasoline in his home. It caught fire and blew up. One of our firemen was killed and several injured. He has been indicted for manslaughter and the fireman's widow is suing him for $50,000. I am glad he isin trouble because he wilfully disobeyed, not only the law, but, the spirit of conservation. He is not the only one, some others have been caught and some have so far escaped. The meanest are those who stole the copper and iron accumulated in a very successful drive. I hope they are discovered and either shot or given life terms because they are enemies of our country.

As the news of the African adventure piles up it makes one stand on the side line and shout. It is wonderful and everybody associated with it has done a first class job. The timing was perfect and the deception used left Hitler and Mussoline flat-footed. Hitler announced in a speech that it did not worry him and he, unlike the late Kaiser in the last World War, would not run away. Evidently he had such an idea in mind and thought perhaps someone might read his thoughts. God knows where he could find asylum even if he tried to get away. Certainly no country inEurope would take the responsibility of his protection and if it did no attention would be paid to the effort. His doom is fixed in the stars and his soothsayer has probably told him of the discovey — if he needed telling.

The whole war picture has changed. Heavy fighting may be necessary and, will be, but as sure as day follows night the defeat of the Nazi is assured. America was the additional weight necessary on the scales of justice and it is bearing down hard.

Ellen is getting along very well in the office and seems to like it. It is a great help because I don't know where I could find anyone else half so good as the girls prefer jobs calling for slacks and other odd devices. I must say the women are getting along famously and their accomplishments are worrying the men laborers. They are beginning to ask how soon after the war they will quit. Personally I don't believe they are going to quit without employers drop them and that is not likely if they deliver the goods. Their stay will greatly enlarge an already overcrowded labor market (I mean for peace-time work.) I remember how worried employers were during the last war when the question of employment after came up for discussion. They knew there would have to be curtailment and they were afraid of repercussions. Well there were none, except, an unemployed labor pool of some 15,000,000 within fifteen years. Of course the prophets say that no such thing can happen again because Moth r Hubbard's cupboard will be bare and it ill take the combined efforts of worl labor to catch up in a generation. I wish I believed it, but, I don't, because I cannot see where with taxes and other normal expenditures Mother Hubbard will have opportunity to more than replenish bare necessities for generations to come. I look for no easy time or glorious spending.

I had a young aviator, on his way somewhere, in to see me. I asked him which he considered the best fighting plane in the world: "The Flying Fortress by all odds. We can't find a vulnerable port to get at without sure death". He belongs to a fighting command but says that none of them can take it like a Fortress. I asked him how he felt in combat. He said, "Well after the fine training we get and the fine planes handed us if we can't hold our own it is because either we are dumb or the other fellow is smart and I don't believe a German or a Jap is any smarter than we are and so far I have found it works out that way."

Practice still goes buzzing along. Now and then one of John's poor derelicts comes in for relief. Not so many now. Whether the others are still living or have just given up hope I don't know but suspect both.

I am removing the tonsils in the 11th of one who escaped his watchful eyes. I think he treated him for some sinus condition. The poor fellow is enthusiastic over the certain cure that is now offered him. He asked in a rather wistful way wheth r was a possibility of John's getting back before I had chance to cure him. He is still wearing the broad smile of realization.

I have been much interested in hearing about your lectures and talks even though the titles seem to be secret. Interested also in the Radon Clinic but don't understand where the children come from for treatment. Is John doing any work outside the Army personnel? Over here they have stopped it as it was being greatly abused.

Well more next time.

     Love from Ma and
      Your

November 16, 1942.

Dear Jim and John,

We had a weird day yesterday: a warm rain in tropical fashion, ending with a thunder storm and a high wind and this morning it is clear and cold.

Pat never stops for the rain, so yesterday the nurse started out with her, andjust about a square away the Heavens opened and the wind started so she was brought back and did she raise the devil because she could not stay out in the rain. It took much cajoling to get her mind fixed on another subject. She is crazy about going out under all circumstances but bad weather is her choice.

More changes: All Charles and Fayette St. buses are to be taken off. Wherever a bus parallels a street car line the buses go. These buses will be used on shorter hauls to Martins and the ship-building plants. The move will save 4,800,000 tire miles. This we are told is just the beginning. Another cut in fuel oil with the amount not yet determined. I am surprised at t is because hundreds of thousands of people have converted to coal and hundreds have adopted heating adjuncts to save oil. I hope the Government will realize the effect upon the peoples morale of inadequate warmth inthe homes It will create more unhappiness than too little coffee or sugar and more wide spread in its effects than too little gasoline and tires. We are living up to requests of the Government in conserving fuel but we can cut no further without real distress. We are told that tank cars have proven inadequate to fill the requirements.

Anne has a little cold but is to go to school today I am going to work on this family and clear up these colds. When one gets it th other follows. I am starting on Mamma Ellen's throat. She has a lot of nodules and I am not sure that she is not harboring and passing something along. Neither of the children has been much sick but for two or three years it has been a continuous show and when you come home I want t em to be well. They both look very well in fact I never saw Anne so rosy and healthy.

Things are moving here in much better shape. Building ships in from t ree to seven days. One of the shipyards launched three destroyers in one day last week. I feel the African campaign has really set the machinery hustling.

Of course Congress is acting like a spoiled child in spite of the election but there are signs that it is coming to. It is ridiculous how many asses we send to Washington to make our laws and it is tragic how many of them do not yet know we are at war. It takes weeks to pass a law which should be done in hours. Stillpoliticians throughout the ages have been ponderously stupid.

We are watching with baited breath the Japs formation for an attack in force somewhere. We have every confidence in our leaders down in the Pacific. They have done a good job under many handicaps and we are rooting for them again. The boys over in Africa are doing a first class job and may God be with them in their plans. It really is wonderful that at last e can go on a limited attack aft r all of these months of defense. I know we will succeed, the U.S. has never lost and this will be no exception.

The F.B.I. have located a Black Market in gasoline and tires and fell on the offenders Saturday. It is a widely extended business but unlike prohibition the purchaser is co-guilty with the seller and a few dozen sent to jail and fined a fe thousand dollars will put a crimp into such irregular practices.

John Tweedy is the only one of the younger set out at the Club (except Tom -- down at the Safe Deposit and Trust) who has not gone into the military service. Poor John has had to be restrained and Glenn Martin has given him an important job. I don't know what the trouble was but Jennie told me: John has been made to see the light and has consented to go to Martin's". She seemed to think I knew about John but I knew nothing. I have a sneaking suspicion that he tried to get a military rank but was not encouraged and he could not keep his family on a private's pay and having lost his fortune he had nothing to give them.

I have played golf only once in a week. Between patients in the office and at home and in hospitals I have had little time to spare. I don't feel much like

golf either after a hard day's work but 1 miss the exercise.
Well, no more until next time.   I am enclosing Miss Everist's Sunpaper.
Love from Ma and
Your

P.S.--Dudy is fine and looking forward to a little trip very soon.

November 19, 1942.

Dear John and Jim,

Another week filled with good war news: Guadacanal victory, African campaign going well, Rommel still on the run, Germany withdrawing troops from the Russian front, eighteen and nineteen now available for the draft, war production going much better, scrap drive bringing in ten million tons of scrap, etc., etc. We are looking up!!

The home front too is about to increase production. Dudy hasbeen told that she may expect a change of location at any time and everything going well with her. Maybe another young soldier if you fellows do not win a war to stop wars, or, I might say win a war to change human nature. I cannot imagine a permanent political peace, nor, can I imagine the Haves being willing to share with the Have-nots, that is as long as selfishness remains a human characteristic. A lot of dreamers are dreaming wonderful things but I am still a skeptic when I think of the good old politicians looking for an issue. What could be more potent than a suggestion of robbery on the part of the ins, and how many ins knowing of the issue will be reluctant to divide the holdings of their supporters with China or Germany? Well we will see in due time whether Roosevelt will last longer than did Wilson if he tries to be altruistic.

Work is progressing harder and harder. Yesterday, I got home at seven, the day before at six. Today, I am going there at five or bust. I must say I am rather enjoying it and except that my old bones get tired after about ten hours I would have no complaint. •

I have just hada very interesting case -- John Requardt. The worst strep throat I have seen in many years. With no rooms available in the hospitals he had to be treated at home. I was loathe to give him any sulfa where he could not be watched as his history is poor, but I did use John's sulfa spray every three hours. In twenty-four hours his temperature was normal, the ulcerated mass had healed and the tremendous oedema had markedly lessened. His brother died of the same thing some years ago.

Perrin Long was given the Southern Medical Association medal for scientific work. I don't know where he now is except that he isin the Army. The Sun had a fine editorial commending the award.

Ben Tappan's sons was awarded a cross or medal for dropping a torpedo down the smokestack of a Jap carrier. He operated off the carrier on which Bill Fisher performed. A cable and letter from Bill shows himO.K. which is a great relief particularly to his mother who isin the Hospital having been operated upon sometime ago.

Anne is all right and at school, Brucie is fine and Pat is a veritable chatter-box, as well as a perpetual Jumping Jack. All the girls have taken on eight and so has little Charlie who now weighs almost fifty pounds - a pick upof twelve pounds in about eight months.

How did you like the colored films? We thought they were fine. More later.

Love from Mother and

116

November 23, 1942.

Dear Jim and John,

Mrs. Roosevelt says we parents should not write our soldiersssons of the limitations which are being placed upon our articles of food, etc. She is afraid it will have a depressing effect. Well, young my sons, would hardly feel depressed at discovering your mother, for instance, is now limited to a pound of sugar a week, two pounds of red meat and a half a pound of coffee, and her usual and ordinary diet. Poor mother has succeeded well for many years on less than she now feels she should eat to satisfy Government privilege.

I do not feel that the people in our stratum of society have been asked to make a single serious sacrifice except tires. For many this is serious because their lives have been built around easy transportation and they have strayed far from business and markets and schools. Fuel for some homes can become a very serious item if e have a hard winter which so far has not materialized.

Ma Roosevelt has suddenly developed a sympathy which has not been one of her characteristics except for certain people.

We are thrilled at the war news but there have been no outward manifestations of unreasonable joy. We know the peaks and valleys in war ne a and I see no signs that anyone looks upon our good news as final and fixed. Even the senate wastes days in an idiotic fillibuster over such an item as poll-taxes and lets such an important item as man power wait its pleasure. This is disgraceful and shows the mental quality of our law-makers. Fighting for democracy and limiting a man's right to express his opinion is hard to understand (even if he is only a negro.)

Sam Crowe brought over John's letter with the picture of a part of the Unit. He was evidently much tickled and wanted to share his satisfaction with us which I thought extremely nice. He looks very well.

The children are all well and Ludy is still with us.

With love from Ma and

Miss Everist's Sunpaper is enclosed.

117

Nov. 25, 1952.

Dear Jim,

By the time you get this your son will be
nearly grown but I want you to know some of the
particulars of his advent so here goes.

He was born -- weight 7 pounds -- at 9.20 p.m.
November 24th after a labor of about two hours.   In
fact Dudy was in the Hospital less than an hour and
a half before the show was over.   She is a spunky
girl, filled with intelligent toughness.   In the
afternoon she and Ellen Fisher had lunch down town
and went to a movie.   She had her hair washed and
"set", got home about five-thirty, played with Pat
and was ready for battle about seven.   Mary Goodwin
says, "Dudy makes it look so simple".   Mary was at
the finish and came downstairs in the greatest excitement, threw her arms around me and kissed me and said,
"She did it, you have a fine great big grandson!!!! "
You see what it takes to make an old man popular.

Dudy arranged every detail and has forgotten
nothing.   Wires, telephone calls and letters.   Fixed
everything concerning Pat and her own return home.
She is a systematic woman and a very lovable one.

Johanna told Pat the story when she took
her up.   She was having breakfast with me sometime
after and when Ma came down,without suggestion, she
told Ma "Pat's baby brother".   Just how much she
understood I don't know but she is a wise little miss.
Dudy is in fine shape and had a very pleasant sleep
after the function was over.   Harrison told me he
was very happy over everything including my grandson "Jim".

With congratulations and best wishes,
affectionately,

November 30, 1942.

Dear John and Jim,

Now that no more heirs are expected we can get back to the common place and, well it is, if we are to conserve our sanity. I bet that within two days we had more than fifty telephone calls of congratulation over the birth of Jimmy. (Oh yes! certain similarities to Apollo made his name a matter of fact).

Well, it is nice to have him, nice to have his mother doing so well, but, one at a time is enough if you prize your digestion and sleep. The funny part is that everyone has settled the kid's fate before he is dry back of his ears. "Doctor", they call him. "Keeping up the Bordley tradition"? "What plan has big grandpa for the future"? I tell them I am not even a silent partner in the ownership and the kid really belongs to his father and mother. Everybody only laughs, laughs mind you, just as if I had some sinister intentions on his future. How ridiculous!!!

It is very interesting to watch the tenacity with which people hold to their old ideals and customs, how they have every desire to carry out the wishes of the Government but reluctantly yield their gasoline and sugar. I often wonder whether a new point of view is being born -- nationally; whether the war will keep up long enough to make its effects permanent by choice; how much the old carefreeness will give way to serious thinking; how much Jazz and Jitter bugery will be replaced by a definite philosophy. I am not so optimistic, nor do I care to be, as to believe we will sever our ties with the past, as Justice Holmes said, it is not a matter of choice but a necessity that the continuity be continued.

When you think of the peace table it makes one dizzy. Here we are fighting to end all governments which are not representative and to the table will go kings and queens and potentates of dubious democracy. What can such a heterogenous congress finally decide without bias. How can ideologists of different faiths ever agree upon ideals which will cover all? My optimism cannot carry me beyond the belief that the changes in the world will be no more than the changes in degree of the existing order. I cannot visualize India and China and Russia being happy over any solution which could fit and please England America.

So far as I know this war was started to lick Hitler and Hirohito but specialists and social one trackers wan to add an appendix. They are already forgetting the cause and looking to what may be salvaged out of the mess for their private hobbies. I just hope they will not forget the Devil while they are putting Hell in order.

Have any of my lettes ever been cut by the Censor? It is a big job to keep out things which should not be told. I try to help them by not talking shop

We have had some very cold weather, just a little ice on the pavement this morning. I trust no more this winter if I have to keep up the pace I am going now.

Ogden Nash has a new volume of poems, just out. It is the same funny stuff with only one serious story which seems asmuch out of place as a giant in an orphan asylum. If you would like to have it I will send it to you.

We are all well. John's family sent the day with us yesterday. They are looking fine.

                    With love from Ma, and
                              Your

Miss Everist's Sunday Sun enclosed.

December 4th, 1942.

Dear John and Jim,

The weather has turned bitterly cold and what a howl the oil users are putting up about their quotas. They still expect to have as much and be as warm as last year without taking any precautions to conserve heat. It can't be done, so they are kicking. Maybe they don't think about the soldiers fighting their battles as much as they should.

Well the heir, much apparent, is in his palace having left the Hospital instate with his footman and coachman. He is a dandy boy with as fine a pair of lungs as they make. He has but two ideas in life: food and sleep and both he does to perfection. He has made a nice gain inweight. Dudy looks fine and says she feels that way. Pat held Jim on her lap yesterday and tried to tell me about it this morning but I was too dense to catch on until Ma spotted a couple of words.

I went out to Ellen's yesterday and the first thing Charlie asked me was "How is little Jimmy?" When Carroll came down she asked me to go with her and in a whisper she showed me her doll, thenlifting it up she said, "This is a brand new born little baby like Aunt Dudy's." I asked her where the child was born and she replied, "In the hospital of course." You see what an impression the birth of the King has had upon the family.

Honestly, I don't realize how many people were interested in my getting a namesake. Scores of people have called up, or, come in to congratulate me. You might suppose I had borne the baby myself. They could not be more solicitous over my feelings. When Dudy got ready to leave the hospital it started to blow, as it seldom blows around here and, snow with it. It had all the appearance of a great blizzard getting under way. She was sunk but in a out fifteen minutes the sun was shining, so she left according to schedule. Her apartment with the reduced use of fuel is still so warm that to date she has had but one radiator on. We keep the thermostat set at sixty-four and turn the furnace off as soon as the radiators get hot. With the house corked up the radiators retain their heat for hours. It certainly has opened my eyes as to heat economy. We have been given a 60% allowance of last year's oil but I don't believe we are going to use it and the house is more comfortable than ever before and not a soul has had even a cold.

I saw Dr. Bill Fisher yesterday, he told me that he had a ~~cable~~ *Caledonian* *extra* from Billy from one of the Islands near Australia, the New ~~Nebrides~~ I think. He hopes, but does not know, Billy will get home for Xmas. They are much relieved as they have not had direct word for sometime.

Everything here is war, all conversationis so directed so there is little gossip I can write you. Ellen Fisher is to have dinner tonight at Mrs. Winks and to meet an Australian war correspondent whom Wink asked to look up Mrs. Wink -- I don't know his name as I am careful about inquiring into the personallife of my employees. She is quite excited over the hope she will get some direct information about how you are getting along.

The West -- that is the politicians -- have been raising Hell about rationing gasoline. Why they should expect to be treated other than the Eastern Seaboard in the conservation of tires I don't understand. It is a terribly mixed up affair with three departments rationing gas. How long it is going to take to straighten it out God alone knows. We have settled down to the inconveniences and you never hear a kick among our friends.

The gentleman out in Roland Park who tried to beat the law by storing gasoline in his cellar was found guilty of manslaughter in the death of a fireman. It carries from five to fifteen years and I hope he gets the limit.

Monday → Well the election has at last opened the eyes of some of the blind and changes are really taking place. The old P.W.A. has been scrapped, one man has beenmade Manpower Chief, we at last have a food chief, the tire business has been put under one head and we have a new over all gasoline coordinator; the youth movement has been scrapped and C.C.C. is a thing of the past. It looks like a real new deal for the people.

     I must stop temporarily.

                With love from Ma and

                    Your

Miss Everist's Sunpaper enclosed.

December 11, 1942.

Dear John and Jim,

No more volunteers for the military services without they are under
eighteen or over thirty-seven. All from now on will be drafted and the man-power boss
says he will discriminate between military and civilian services. This is good because to
get an occupation you will be placed by the National Employment Board which I hope will give
some relief to our farmers. They need it if we are to have food. High wages and bright
lights plus military installations have cleaned the farms of labor and even tenant farmers.
Of course this should have been done months ago and it will require some figuring to take
up the slack.

We face rationing of butter, eggs and milk. The first cuts me right
in the stomach so I am beginning to taper off so as to be prepared for the worst. Coffee
seems to be the commodity to call forth the most conversation. One pound every five weeks
is the allowance and it does not give one full cup a day. Yesterday a good old Jewish
friend brought me two containers of Maxwell House. Said a friend gave him a full case
before rationing started and as he does not drink coffee he is giving it to his friends.
You can8t beat the Jews for looking ahead, that is one of the reasons they are so successful
in business.

The African campaign has set this country up. Yesterday, they froze all
mariners, froze the workers in the Detroit plants, froze the lumbermen of the north and
west and started a big drive for quicker ship construction, although only day before
yesterday they launched sixteen ships including six major war vessels and beside the
Presidentsrequest for 8,000,000 tons of shipping by Jan. 1st is already completed and we
are still turning out better than three ships a day.

We get another cut in gasoline in a few days, pleasure drives getting only
two gallons a week. This is to further conserve rubber and increase transportation for
fuel oil. Before long non-essential driving will be stopped. This will not affect the
allowance for doctors or war workers in industrial plants.

I think the administration is doing well in the war effort but I would
like to see a lot more of its non-essential driving stopped. It is just as persistent in
some of its peacetime foibles as Hitler is in his war terrors. We could save a billion
dollars a year and never miss one single item. I want the country to be relatively sound
financially when the storm is over. We will have enough legitimate debts, taxes and poverty
and we will require retrenchment if we are to help in the rehabilitation of the world. One
can eat his cake with enjoyment but the fund is over when the cake is gone.

Well I have held the king in my arms and been looked upon with a sort of
idle curiosity. Pat has a picture (Xmas card) of Mary and the Child. She knows the
child's name is Jesus and she knows her brother's name is Jimmy. She confuses the two
babies at times and frequently calls Jimmy, Jesus. She realizes her mistake and to correct
herself she usually combines the names into the funniest phrase you ever heard. Jimmy still
gains weight (and on the side and in confidence, so does his mother). Both look very
well. Pat is no exception except that she has the best in looks. She grows more lovely
every day.

I have not seen Anne and Brucie for some days as I never get home any
more until dark and their visit is over long before. One of my employees who is more or
less familiar with their movements, tells me they are very well and much taken up in preparation for some sort of Xmas show at school. Anne, I think, is getting impatient to wear
her costume and do her stunts.

I just had a patient of John's with a profuse hemorrhage from his nasopharynx, something I have never seen occur spontaneously. He says John only treated him
for a sore throat. How did he bust a blood vessel so high up. His name is Hall and he
works at the Fidelity.

Sometimes I think it was a pity the South did not join the independence. When I view its Representatives and Senators and hear their diatribes I feel it would be better if we were free and had a realUnited States. If it were not for the two Virginia Senators and one or two of its representatives plus Senator George that whole section would be represented by the only complete group of nimcompoops in this land. They rant against labor and its strikes and dues but they insist upon a poll tax and go on strike and hold up important warbusiness to prevent the passage of legislation that the balance of Congress and the country approve; they pin the flag to the sky and hout themselves hoarse about democracy and then prevent fifty percent of those entitled to vote. Their lying and conceptof the Southern politician makes one wonder how they are permitted to represent the land of the really great Lee, Jackson and Johnson. It is hard to imagine the latter in a garbage can. There is a very general opinion that the next general election will bring a complete political change. I am not so sure that the country will want to change without the war is over. It is I have no doubt about the result because I am not sold on the international intentions of this land and its will to lead the fight for a bettr world at the sacrifice it ill cost. I hope so, but I have my doubts.

Love from Ma,

and

Your

December 14, 1942.

Dear Jim and John,

I don't know who is raising Pat but her morals have got to have a good shaking up. Yesterday she sat down on the floor too hard. She got up, pulled her dress over her head and presented the hurt spot on her rear for me to kiss and, in the presence of guests. I call that almost a moral lapse.

Jimmy isfine. Katherine Bordley says he is undoubtedly a Bordley. Her guide is his nose and high forehead.

Yesterday Charlie and Ellen went over to Washington to see the play off for the professional football championship between the Chicago Bears and the Washington team. With the temperature around twenty it took more nerve than I have. In fact professional football has no attractions for me.

Practice in the past few days has dropped off. Not a house visit nor a patient in the hospital yesterday. Friday and Saturday only fourteen patients per day. This is really a relief because I have been going too hard for an old man. I cansee what the transportation difficulties will eventually do to my practice. The railroads are corking down and want to know the reason why before selling a ticket, shortage of gasoline keeps automobiles and buses from taking up the slack and today we have a street car and bus strike in Baltimore which is an unparallelled outrage.

Congress adjourns in a day or so. A good riddance I think, as it too is filled with filibusters, poor logic and rotten politics. My what a democracy has to stand for from "the representatives of the people" and not infrequently from the people themselves. Still it is better than the product of Hitler and Hirohito so we at least have a sound right to sleep in our own beds and cuss our neighbors out loud.

Ellen and the children are fine.

With love from Ma
and

Miss Everist's Sunpaper enclosed.

December 17, 1942.

Dear John and Jim,

Well the farewell speeches have all been made in Congress and the lion sleepeth until the New Congress convenes in January. This one has done a lot, some bad, much good. It has declared a war, conscripted man power, put women in the arms factories and in the military services, rationed our food and clothes, taxed us to the last drop, insulted our intelligence with picayune politics, driven the country from the Democrat Party, shown great cowardice in its contacts with various blocks of highway robbers. It has done many things good and bad which will have their repercussions though as yet unborn generations but after all it has largely reflected the publics whims and what more could a democratic republic ask of its chosen representatives.

Many men go back home for a spell, some for good. Some will be missed for their works were good, some will just go back to the void from which they came, in which they have always existed. The two outstanding losses are Senator Norris and a negro Congressman from Illinois. While I did not al ays see eye to eye with them I was always convinced of their honesty and progressive spirit and had I lived in their districts I should have voted for them.

We have had much bitter cold and windy weather. What people on short oil rations are doing is not hard to guess. As for our house we have not the slightest complaint, in fact I think with the lower temperature we have all enjoyed better health. I am convinced that drafts are the root of most discomforts and with none a low temperature can be well stood. It islike a person putting on a thin Bird cloth coat. It keeps out the drafts and the weather makes less difference in one's comfort. Up t the arrival of Jimmy, Dudy never had more than one radiator on and now only two out of seven.

From time to time we are made to think about the war. Blackouts and alerts are handed out just in case ---. I think I told you Pat was caught out with Johanna and had to spend a half hour in a grocery store. Johanna never violates a single rule. She really is the most sincere person in her devotion to what she assumes, or, istold, is a duty.

I am not orried about not receiving letters. Just keep on writing your women. They are not only sentimental about it but they gro a bit uneasy if a letter does not arrive in time. They are very good about keeping me posted.

Mother is in her old Christmas struggles and ends every night among her packages I am doing work during that period on my family history which probably will never be finished. The Maryland Historical has asked me to take part in a lecture program they are o king out. If I do I will talk about the origins of furniture decorations. I have n ver seen nore heard of a similar attempt and it will be fun. I have in the course of the years accumulated much material and this may be a ood time to use some of it.

Well all of the wives and children are ell and happy and the latter looking forward to Christmas. May it please God that this pleasure will be extended through their lives. What could be worse than have a dictator shoot Santa Claus. His own life would not be worth a farthing but his loss would be no compensation.

Love from Ma and

Your

December 21, 1942

Dear John and Jim,

We enjoyed your letters of quite recent date received ten days after sending. There is no dispute about the name of the ne baby and no substitute names are being considered. He will be honored by permission to use the passport into the ancient and honorable clan of Bordley. What more could one who came too late for the honor wish for his nephew?

Well we are in the midst of the coldest spell f r Decembr ever experienced by Baltimore. Out my bed room window last night it was zero. The ground is covered with snow. The old home is as warm as toast on fifty percent. of the oil used last year.

We had much excitement last week when the price administration stopped all sales of gasoline to private car owners for twenty-four hours, it included doctors. This morning it was partially lifted by reducing the coupon value from four to three gallons. I am not kicking, have never, and will never. I am for anything essential to win the war if I have to wear my overcoat to bed.

Peggy was down for the week end and seemed to enjoy the new baby or Jimmy as Pat calls him. When she got read to leave yesterday afternoon no taxi com any would answer thetelephone so I got out the old bus and ploughed through six inches of snow to the bus line (without chains), then the bus driver carried her do n town and had to bring her back, she missed her train.

I have got to go out in the country to see the Sullican girl. I told her I would come if I could travel in my automobile. I came to the office by trolley and have to go several places on foot but when I think of the boys on the Solomons I feel I have no cause for kicking. What a hell of a life they must be leading! It just makes everything else look easy.

The gasoline was stopped by a hurry call from North Africa and they wanted to avoid the submaries off the Gulf Coast so they took one which was not even a fair exchange. We can dowithout it and they can't.

I am so rushed I will have to make this short.

The children are all set for Christmas but even they sense a difference in spite of the fact we have made a real effort to keep them from it. I think it is a damned outrage for the Government to charge for the goods received from the military forces. I am going to air my views in the Sun and try and get the editors to feel s i do.

We are all well. With love from Ma and me, and enclosing Miss Everist's Sun,

Your

December 23, 1942.

Dear Jim and John,

With a prospect of you of 100° temperature, we have a prospect of being just a hundred degrees colder. The weather has been atrocious and the roads double that. For two days I have not been able to take my car out because the snow and ice is so heavy in the lane I could not get through without chains and have no one to put them on and it is easier to go on the street car than put them on myself.

The street cars too are a mess. They are jammed from door to door but with a good natured crowd who understands why. When the busses are off Charles St. it will give the street cars a tremendous load. We now have motormen and conductors on many of the cars. I started out home last night on such a car and the power plant blew up and put the line out of business. I had to walk from Charles to Guilford Ave to catch another line. This morning I had to reverse and walk from Guilford Ave to Charles, but not from a lady motorman, that time a man.

Pat gets more and more cute every day and is in the full swing of her sex. Never stops talking a minute. She can say anything and apparently understands the meaning of her words. She does not seem a bit jealous of Jimmy, just takes him in her stride, if he interferes he is put in his place but she likes to touch and kiss him. Sometimes she calls him"Pat's little brother", but most of the time she sticks to Jimmy.

Well in two weeks we get our next ration cards -- fats and greases, including butter. Soon we will get our clothes tickets, as there will, by June, be only one suit and one overcoat for every third man. My how I gloat over the fellows who used to say we were self sufficient. The only "sufficient" apparently is hot air and politics. I hope none of the isolationists find sufficient food nor clothes.

Rickenbacker's episode I suppose you know about. His plane had to land on the ocean and for three weeks he floated about on a rubber raft and then was found and saved in the nick of time. He made a speech over the radio Sunday, a timely speech. He said it was a shock after he landed, to hear conversation monopolized by talk of rationing of such things as gasoline and sugar, especially when he had just come from the Solomons where our defenders were wallowing in mud and grime without a single kick about their hardships and dangers, where lack of production in this country endangered their lives and made their perils more grave. I was glad he took off his gloves, it is what we all need as there is too much self complacency. I often wonder just how deep the feelings of our people are and just how much the realization of the seriousness of our situation. Of course it is hard to visualize so intangible a thing as remote danger, hard to believe that a life of peace and satisfaction can be lost forever by a far away war. When I look at the average person on the street and see the same old paint and powder, hear the same frivolous conversation, know that the night clubs are jammed with merrymakers, it gives me pause. Perhaps in their hearts there is worry and anxiety but it is hard to believe. It is a shocking thought that only such reminders as bombs and casualty lists can stir up a national consciousness of stern realities. Maybe I have spent too much time with Washington, Jefferson and Lincoln. Perhaps their views have prejudiced my mind against what I see and hear in this middle of a changed century. But I gather a certain satisfaction from their companionship because they have convinced me that the foundations of our way of life are very firmly fixed in the hearts and souls of man, that everyone loves liberty.

I am sorry you will not be home for Christmas. It has always been a season of great happiness for mother and me, because it meant the gathering of our little flock. I will especially miss your helping hand in trimming the tree, a pleasure I have gladly shared with the members of my family realizing as I do the sacrifices I make for their happiness. This year I will take up the old and untiring custom invented if not by Satan certainly by one fully acquainted with his schemes to defeat salvation.

This is mother's time of deep happiness because nothing with her compares with the opportunity to serve the whims of her children and her children's children, and,

I might add, her husband's pleasure.

I hope you will have a pleasant time and that the fellows, men and women, in your unit will find some real pleasure. We think and talk of them often and love them for their every service to our cause.

With love from Ma

and

December 28, 1942.

Dear Jim and John,

Another Xmas has come and gone. It was a queer affair. Just not normal and could not be made so. Even the Xmas tree lights were stricken out. That is no outside trees permitted and everyone requested not to use lights on the indoor trees. The request I fear was not very well bserved except by Ma. Ahe would not even put the lights n the tree for fear someone might turn them on.

We received the usual amount of liquor (now th t I never t uch the filthy stuff). I want to thank you, one, for the Time subscription and the other for the story of Paul Revere. Both w. ll bring me much pleasure in the coming year and I will need it to overcome the tax depression.

Yesterday it was announced we are to be put on the point ration plan on some two hundred and fifty commodities. It meets my hearty approval and I think it will bring about a much more e uitable distribution. We have an abundance in this country and hen yo hear that some large community is without such an essential as meat it just makes you stop and ponder. Of course, now that it is known in advance -- and it really had t be -- the old hoarders will probably get to work if the stores permit. But they have learned at least one lesson when they had to return eleven million tires and at a substantial loss. The point ration tickets will be issued only after a full statement, under oath, as to your holdings. This will put the fear of the law, if not the fear of the Lord, into many hearts. I hope so or else I hope they open the prisons to all violators. You can bet on one who will have no trouble even if we go hungry -- Ma.

What do yo suppose thet gal did for me. Way back last June she decided I would not buy a new overcoat this winter so she ordered a Burberry from ngland because she knew I liked them. Well it arrived just b fore Xmas and a perfect fit except the sleeves are a bit long. That was one of my five Xmas presents from her. I am well stocked with things to keep me warm if the oil gives out, which of course it ill not. This started as a mild Fall but the early winter has been pretty cold. We have the heating down to a science. We were cut forty percent. from last year but we are going to make it in comfort. My, how we used to waste oil. This is a good lesson, not only in economy but in conservation. I am sure I have wasted hundreds of dollars and then w thout half the satisfaction we have had in health and comfort this season. I hope the food game works out as favorably.

Well the hand of Fate has barred all golf balls and clubs. What a fortunate thing a good patient gave me a half dozen for a Xmas present. To tell the the truth I have played golf but three times in the past month. I have been too busy to fool with it but I confess my digestion and sleep miss the exercise.

The Russian picture looks pretty good. Just think what we formerly said about Stalin! What a Godsend he has been to our cause, what in fact could we have done if he had jumped across the fence. It makes one pause and think how close the call to our rights, privileges and greatness. Joe Stalin may have been a devil when we did not like him, but, now he is the leader of the gang and, more power to him and his people.

We got the cable on Xmas Day with its good wishes. Everyone was delighted to hear from you. You could not have pleased Ma and me more by any act or deed.

Pat thrives and the boy weighs nine pounds. Both look fine. We spent the afternoon yesterday wit Brucie and Anne. They wanted to show us their tree and presents. Ellen read us John's latest letters and the damned dog was kept out of the house so altogether we had a very nice time.

Well, I must see some patients.

     With love from Ma and

      Your

Miss Everist h s added to her Sunday Sun

December 31st, 1942.

Dear John and Jim,

Well this is a new New Years Eve. What the New Year holds for us all even a crystal gazer could not prophesy. It is not to be an easy time and for many it will be filled with trouble and sorrow but for the world at large it holds great possibilities for a better world. I am not one of those who suffer from delesions of grandure, I see ahead no change in human nature, no less selfishness, no more altruism which springs from a willingness of self sacrifice for the greater good. But I do see a war weary world come to a realization that must, to survive, keep a workable sivilization;to have less pain we must be willing to take a larger dose of preventiveness. Out of this, if not blocked by stupid criminal politics, we may build a great r future. It will be slow tragically painful but our past sufferings have been so many that e may grasp at least temporarily for a straw to keep us afloat to solid ground.

The attitude of our people is a pretty fair index of what the world isup against before the sun will really shine. They are willing to do everything asked of them, willingly, cheerfully. The willingness is not altruistic, it is a self helpful proposition. They all want to know whether their neighbor is hit as hard. If so they are sheerful, but with the slightest insinuation that others are better off, they demand toknow why. They are followers and offer little cons ructive suggestion as to how they can sacrifice more for the common good. All of that must change before we can construct a federation of helpful nations. If we cannot expect helpful sacrifice the world's picture will not be greatly altered.

Pat and Joanna went up to Philadelphia by train yesterday to spend New Years with the Rosses. Pat was as quiet as a grown woman but knew all about it. On the way to the train she told me: "Pop, Pat going on big train to see Grandma". The little rascal is really beginning to talk in sent nces and h r vocabilary is astounding. She knows the name of everybody and thing in the house and has a complete command over all. If she can't win wit a smile she tries out the rough stuff, anyway she usually wins. She is v ry nice to Jimmy and shows no jealousy, she is even willing to share with him, sometimes gently and, sometimes not uite so much so. She gets more lovely every day. Ma and I are thinking of going to court for a legal adoption. It is quite definite that her stay is permanent. What we could do without her I don't know. Jimmy will share her fate I am convinced since he smiled at me for the first time yesterday.

Ellen and the girls have had a little of the cold that is on the rampage here. Today they are all straightened out and feeling fine, and getting ready to eat some of Pop Ficher's wild ducks. Bill Fisher, Jr. isin California, whether he will get home they don't know. When his ship went down sometime ago he lost his clothes and telegraphed home to send him a suit. He h s to have an outfit made before he can travel. One of his buddies has been iven a cross for his works -- a Baltimore boy.

The first German (I wish they would change the name) takes place toni t. The oth r one was not held and see li tle sense in this one but I suppose youth must have its fling and the dowagers must have their exalted positions maintained. The Assembly is called off.

It isfunny to see so many women wearing caps and trousers. They are everywhere and are not half as attractive as in hort skirts.

The isolationists and prohibitionists ha e been assailing the Army for drunkenness and lack of morals gen rally. "War Information" un er Elmer Davis made a uiet extensive survey. The results were published today and show this rmy the most model in our history and the only real trouble im camps is in dry territory where boot-leg whiskey takes the place of the beer in the wet sections. Elmer handled t e critics without any glovew and showed they were trying to make the populace dissatisfied and unhappy. He called

the gang fifth columnists of a very putrid order.   I think this exposure will drive
some of the vermin to cover until they can invent something new.

A Happy New Year! One that will end the war and bring you home to
your little families.

Love from Ma
and
Your

January 4, 1943.

Dear Jim and John,

Just to give you an idea what rationing means over here and its serious need Mother went all over town trying to buy any kind of fowl for New Years' dinner and ending up by giving us cold roast beef (a very great delicacy).   Not a bird of any kind for sale. She can seldom buy over a quarter of a pound of butter and the stores sell as much to a household of two as to a household of ten.   This will all be changed when rationing comes to full fruit in February.   Today, the whole procedure is a public scandal, but people only laugh at their troubles.   They are really wonderful and play it like a game.

I had a man in the office today who told me that he had to turn in a tire as he had a car that carries a tire in a rack on both front mug guards and he wasonly permitted to keep three.   The tires are special and cost him fifty-six dollars a piece The Government sent him two twenty-five cent defense stamps in payment.   He said he was satisfied when he found out that Eutaw St. crowd had to turn in about twenty new tires a piece all wrapped in wax paper which had cost about eighteen dollars each and for them they averaged a dollar and a half.

We have to have our tires inspected every three months and when they reach a certain stage they must be re-capped but if you cannot get a priority you areout of luck because until you serve the verdict you can get no more gasoline.   It works a bit screwy but a dictatorial government is a hard customer to deal with.   Thank God it ends with the war,

Today the value of oil coupons drops from ten to nine gallons This means further conservation or less heat to most people but it will not hurt us because of the precautionswe have taken and the amount of oil coupons we have been able to save.

Don't think the home front is not doing its part, indeed it is and with cheerfulness if not with a full understanding.

We had a very pleasant New Years, taking off Friday, Saturday and Sunday from work.   We closed the office so all could get a rest, as we have been on duty since the fifteenth of September without a break and going hard most every day.   I am rather proud of myself to think that at nearly seventy I can get up at six thirty and take care of my little coal heater, fix the furnace and then go all day, generally until eleven p.m. I feel fine, in fact have enjoyed the exercise.

Pat is coming home today after a New Years vacation in Philadelphia. My, how we missed the little rascal.   Jimmy is too young yet to substitute for her and then he cares not a damn for anything but food and sleep and he does both to perfection as you will know when I tell you he weighs nine and a half pounds.

This must be short as I have to be up town at two and it is now one-thirty.

With best wishes for a happy year and a soon return, and with
love from Ma and

Your

Miss Everist will enclose her Sunday Sun.

132

January 7, 1943.

Dear Jim and John,

Well hell has broken loose. No gasoline for pleasure driving in the Eastern States. That means no more parties and that means hell to a large number. If you drive to a movie, theatre or a hotel for a drink, you lose your ration card and will be subject to arrest and fine (as high as $10,000.). It should have come months ago as nothing has been as badly abused as the unnecessary use of gasoline. Now we have a Black Market in the stuff which is getting to be like old prohibition days. That holds good for sugar and even meat. Mother had engaged a pound of butter and when she went to get it yesterday she was told that high-jackers had held up the shipment and stolen five thousand out of the six thousand pounds on the truck, so she got a uarter of a pound. I am in favor of a firing squad for such gents. It will put the fear of the law in their minds. Just small fines and a few days in jail will do nothing to stop the traffic and after all we are at war and any man who interferes with its progress is a traitor and indufficient food will be a serious deterrent.

The new pipe line for oil from Texas to Indiana is finished but there are no pumps so far to pump the oil. We are hoping for better luck next year or the year after, by that time Washington will realize that we are in a war.

Well I saw 500 more patients last year (1942) than in 1941. I have always expected to be far back at sixty-five and about through at seventy so I am rather pleased with my showing. I know what does and should happen to old doctors and I have never had any illusions about my super staying powers, I have had a wonderful life , a regular flower garden of perpetual bloom with a very occasional weed, so why should I upbraid the fates who have been so kind to me. After all that should bring more pleasure than even a few grateful patients who perhaps see in you what does not exist but have no realization of it. If you have pulled your own load you have done your duty and I have always tried to do that, Perhaps my fault has been trying to pull some of the other fellows because he seemed too slow.

We have a new Congress and I hope it will function better then the last, will assume more of its Constitutional authority than the last. If we are to maintain our democracy we must keep a tripartite government. Dictators in Washington would be no better than the same ilk in Berlin and Congress is our only preventive. We can kick Congress out in two years but a dictator never until he ruins our ways of life and peace of mind.

Well the children are fine. Jimmy asked me the other day how soon he could vote and I told him it depended entirely on how long it would take his Daddy to lick the Japs. He is writing you about it in a day or so.

With love from Ma and

Your

133

January 12, 1943.

Dear Jim and John,

Well I missed my Monday letter for the first time since you left California.   To tell the truth I got a bit tired last week and decided to stay in bed all day Sunday and get a good rest.   It made me a bit late getting here yesterday and with the whole day loaded I never could spare a moment.   I am going to take off a week at the end of this month and get a long rest.   I will have to stay home but how I would enjoy some of your good old summertime.

It has been snowing in this man's town off and on since October and the streets are never free from ice for more than a day at a time.   I am getting to be a perfect dare-devil, driving on pavements th t I have not driven on for years. Just have to because of th tremendous changes in transportation.   To give you an idea: 1938 Sunday Jan. 2nd, 181,000 people hauled by the streets cars and busses of the Street Kar lines; 1943, Jan. 3rd, Sunday, 796,000 hauled with two hundred more street cars and eighty less busses.

Well, we are in the midst of a rapidly changing nation.   They say we cannot conceive the battle front, well it is equal because those on th t line can never conceive the changes on the home front and the one changes about s fast as the others.   Who could have conceived Americans standing in line to buy a uarter of a pound of butter, public schools closed for lac of fuel, Baltimore Street at noon without a single automobile in si ht, parking places around theatres and movie houses without a single car, Pop getting up at six-thirty to stoke a furnace and Ma asleep at his bedside.   Don't tell me that the populace is not fast learning the story of total war.   Still we have homes to live in, food to eat and no police sticking their noses into your business.   In fact most of the troubles are due not to lack of any essentials but ju t transportation.   Ou great railroad system is taxed as never before and in spite of eleven million tons of shipping built in a single year we lack boats to haul the greatest industrial production in the history of our nation.

Well, the kin s are well and the mothers likewise so e have somethingto make us very happy.   I must get back to work.

With love from Ma and
                    Your

Miss Everist will enclose
her Sunday paper.

Dear Jim & John

V-Mail Jan. 15. 1943
Series 11 - m. 34

D This will not go to-day but this week is
so packed that I will have to make a
start.

To-day is cold & last night it was
bitter out with a howling wind. This has
really been a hard winter. May be it feels
a bit colder because you know so many
people who are having a hard time to
keep warm. Some of these people could
spend a few hours in movie houses but
now if you go you must walk or
wait on the corner for a street car until
you are about frozen. Things are really
getting tough, not so much for people
who have been wise providers & have looked
forward a bit but for the rank and file
whose thoughts seldom reach to the present
it has been a bad winter. Still you hear
more wise cracks than complaints.

I am afraid Congress is going to raise
some disagreeable discussion over Lend-Lease.
Some of its members are going to crawl
over Hopkins who heads the business, more
because he lives in the White House than
because there have been moral lapses. It
is a good political talking point when

135

You can not go to a store & buy what you are
in the habit of getting, because taxes must
be raised to supply the necessities of our
Allies. Personally I think our Allies by
holding the fort while we slept have earned
all we can give them at any cost in money
or sacrifice. As for the food we send
them after all it is to keep their men
in good fighting condition which saves much
of our armed forces & without which we
would have to expend many more of our men.
Still politics & politicians have no
hesitation in hitting below the belt. They
know the short memories & selfish
disposition of most men & they play such
cards as they can pull regardless of the
ultimate consequences. The President
to forestall such damage has now proposed
a vast extension of our "social benefits" &
the Administration is making ready to
socialize medicine so as to make it free
to all. This will be its first move. The bill has already
been drafted & only awaits the psychological
moment. I am not surprised & have looked
forward to just such a move for a long
time. I believe the rank & file of the

3) profession is going to throw a fit when they are offered # 3 75⁄100 per head ~~for every~~ per year for every patient they list & then get # 1 87⁄100 per day visit & # 2 12⁄100 for night visit. The ~~Obstetricians~~ will get it in the neck according to the schedule when # 55 is made to cover every expense – hospital, nursing, medicines & doctor. ~~It will~~ and this will cover the entire time & two weeks after birth. It is supposed that the doctor will get about # 21 for his part. May be but knowing hospital ~~practice~~ I doubt it. We are told the schedule may be slightly increased but the schedule will be the limit of a legal charge & nothing can be recovered at law beyond this.

No anaesthetic is covered & no present arrangement I understand will be made in ~~to~~ any operation procedure & the hospital may be called upon to supply the ~~service~~.

This ~~story~~ is too long to write but as soon as a ~~no~~ clear explanation is published I will send it to you. I send you life ~~city~~ & from it I hope you will get the full story before long.

the seem to think has lessened the fatalities. It seems to me from those I have seen we are to look upon them as merely unusually bad colds & some of them not very bad. An initial fever which lasts for a day or so and not often over 101° & then complete complete subsidence of all visible symptoms. Occasional one has had an initial temperature of 104° but mostly in very young subjects. The thing is so darn insidious it make me want to have some competent entomologist see every case with cold & temperature. I feel a bit uneasy taking care of patients with symptoms I have always looked upon as meaning nothing.

Murray Holliday jr has sent in his application for the Hopkins Medical School. He gets his A.B. at the University of North Carolina in December & the first class at the Hopkins starts the same month. Halsey Barker is on the Admission Board & tells me he will look after Murray's admission. Drop him a line if you will.

Love from Ma
& Dad

Dear John and Jim,

        Just a note today. I have been so rushed I am getting weary and war or no war I am going to take a few days off and rest up. This hurts my feelings but I know in the long run it will be the wises thing. Don't get the idea I am ill because I am not, I am just tired of work and responsibility and believe me I have had my full share of both.

        The Administration got a blast over the radio yesterday as a result of the disgraceful coal strike which is spreading. For the life of me I cannot understand such dilatory action when the north east portion of our country is freezing. Labor is losing friends by the hundred of thousands and before long the public is going to blow the lid off and labor will find itself back in the 1890s which will be a crushing defeat for our social progress. This is not the only strike there are many of them and now railroad labor is asking for a tremendous increase with a threat to strike and tie up all transportation. Mr. Roosevelt's chickens are coming home to roost and he finds out how much gratitude some of them have for his selling the country out for their betterment.

        I went out to the Club to salvage some of my equipment. Jimmy told me my car was the first member's car out there in two weeks. A few people had gone out on the trolley but it is not a popular trip.

        The streets f Baltimore look like those of a deserted village. You have to have a pair of binoculars to find a car, and even friendly visits to one's home are a thing of the ast. You are allowed to go to your family in a car only if there is sickness or death. You can go to market in an automobile if you are not on a car line; otherwise, no.

        Well I must run to keep an appointment.

                    Love from Ma and

                        Your

V ° Mail

Dear Jim and John,   I have been off for a week. Got real tired. I didn't have a very good time as I had nervous indigestion which always leaves me pretty flat. It did, however give me a good chance to work on my history. I hope when it is finished it does not show the effects of my indigestion.

Except for the fuel question the country remains in tip top shape. Its lack of fuel, oil and coal, has forced many people out of their homes, into more comfortable public shelters in New England. Unfortunately the winter has been pretty tough. The past week we had the worst ice storm in Maryland's history according to the weather man. It did the Bordleys not the slightest damage but it sealed up every window and door in the house and we had to telephone for a man to come dig us out. They were frozen tight. We still have a lot of snow.

Before this reaches you, you will know that the prospective Ambassador to Australia has asked to have his name withdrawn. He saved the Administration much embarrassment. There was a very definite national protest.

What do you think of our sporting President? No one ever thinks of his physical handicaps and neither does he apparently. It was quite a trick for him to go to and from Africa but I hope he undertakes no more such journeys, they are too risky. Five years ago I would have thought it an excellent idea but not now.

The military has asked for the confiscation of 8,000,000 automobiles and all spare tires. So far this has not been granted and with the fight now on I think probably will not go through. The military says it would enable them to build fifteen thousand extra planes above the present prospect. The man in charge of tire rationing and the transportation chief think it will too much curtail the transportation of war workers and essential civilian business. Complete food rationing goes in March 1st. I am watching for the repercussions. They are bound to come as we still house a great many selfish and thoughtless people. I do not believe there will be much protest from the great majority. We will be allowed a capital of five cans of food per person to start with and them come the food tickets. Butter, meat and ice-cream will become luxuries. Some will certainly be caught and I hope so as it will help the cause to jail a few. Boy how this will hit the hoarders.   Jim grows apace. Still eating his quota and gaining weight. He looks fine and is beginning to laugh out loud. I asked him the other day if he wanted to be a doctor. You never saw such enthusiasm. You would not believe me if I wrote a description of it, it seems so fantastic. Had a letter from Bruno. Said he misses John like everything. Their first real separation for years. Says he is on the Garden Spot of the entire world, but did not further day. Brucie and Anne were not tied up by the sleet storm but how they got to school I have no idea. Most all the schools were closed for two days. I don't know any news. Nobody ever comes to see you, you are not worth the gasoline. Sometimes I just sit down and laught at the complaints of the Dowagers. They thought money bought everything and they strongly resent the fact they were wrong.

                    More later,
                         Love from Ma
                                   and
                                        Your

Major John E. Bordley, M.C.O-403012

General Hospital No. 118

A.P.O. 927, c/o Postmaster

San Francisco, California,

Dr. James Bordley,Jr.

330 N. Charles St.,

Baltimore, Md. U.S.A.

February 11, 1943

Dear John and Jim, I have failed for the first time to get off at least two letters per week. I have really been tied to a post -- work.I wonder how I stand it, but I do and am thriving. Still I am not doing as much as I did when I was at the peak of my practice but of course I am a bit older. Things are on the rampage here. The President has increased the weekly hours of labor to forty-eight and that brings a thirty percent increase in wages as the last eight carry time and a half for over-time. This in the face of a grave probability of inflation. Of course, we have a sho tage of labor and the extra day will mean much for production but why the extra pay is a mystery to me. Not altogether a mystery either when I see how fast the Democratic party is falling behind in the estimation of the public. The war effort is too little and the public wants less politics and more work. Of course those in power are responsible and they will have to shoulder the responsibility. Three pairs of shoes a year. Another sacrifice (?) for me when I never bought more than one pair in three years. If it is necessary to conserve leather why not conserve it and stop little driblets! That is the sort of stuff the public is sore about. We have a thriving black market in meat and the offenders who would be shot in Russia or China or Germany here get a fine of a few of their ill gotten dollars. These birds thrive on the restaurants and hotels and buy up beef cattle so fast and at such a price that the legiti- mate dealers who have a ceiling on their sale prices cannot even compete. It is wide spread and dangerous in its implicati ns but the Government just plays along instead of using a mailed fist. The public has had to curtail its use of gasoline some forty percent in the past two months but the civilian workers in the Government have used as much as ever. Why war workers in factories are chased below the civilian workers in Government is hard to figure out. I can't. I can't drive two miles to the golf course but Government workers can drive to California. It does not make sense. Rickenbacker has been touring the country making the stronge t kind of public protest and he is getting the goats of a lot of officials. He is even mentioned as a Presidential possibility for the Republicans because he has so stirred up the public over the short comings of labor and Government. That gives you an idea of the public mind. The worst offenders against our real efforts are the labor leaders. The workmen are 90% faithful but such Roosters as John L. Lewis whose only perspec- tive is gained by looking down the single barrell of personal power are a real menace to our efforts. He not only causes trouble but keeps the public upset by threats of things to come. The changed complexion of Congress bodes no good to the real cause of labor. Already bills have been introduced which are full of potentialities and I must say with very substantial public support. Labor leaders have the power of dictators and the working men are in the position of serfs. There is no more Democracy in labor organizations than in Hitler's Germany -- even there they let them vote one way. The children are well and thriving and not worrying about shoes. Brucie of course is tremendously interest in the war and keeps abreast of everything. She is real smart about it. The other kids except Charlie are unconscious of everything, stern or bad. Thank God.

Love from Mother

and

Lt. Col. James Bordley, III., M.C.

General Hospital No. 118

A.P.O. 927, c/o Postmaster

San Francisco, California.

Dr. James Bordey, Jr.

330 N. Charles St.,

Baltimore, Md.

February 15, 1943.

Series II., No. 38

Dear Jim and John,

We are in the midst of one of the coldest spells we have had for years. The thermometer playing around zero since Saturday night, sometimes below, sometimes a bit above, a heavy wind but clear sky. We had a heavy snow Friday but that melted about as fast as it fell. The house is nice and comfortable and in spite of a hard winter we have twelve hundre gallons of oil left. We have really worked hard to help save and have been rewarded with success. My red-headed grandson, if you can speak of the little he has as hair, is a bouncing baby. No not talking yet but trying very hard. Between Dudy and his doctor Mary he now weighs over eleven pounds and still going strong. Ma has resigned from her regular job and helps Dudy concoct disagreeable things to do for Jimmy especially when I am in the mood to play with him. They are nuisances so Jimmy says. Pat is a very superior lady, condescends now and then to look Jimmy over, even at times tries to pat him with what amounts to a Joe Louis upper cut. There isone thing certain whenever I start to play with Jimmy she invariably wants me to read "Life paper" to her. I suggested to h r the other day as she knew all there is to be known about the English language it would be wise to start n Russian. I bet she would have it in a couple fo weeks. She is as smart as the Devil. I have not seen Brucie and Anne for about a week as I have been too busy to stop off. Ellen tells me they are in good shape. Charlie and Ellen brought their crew in yesterday for the first time in weeks. Ellen will not violate any rule enunciated by the Government and she thinks coming to see us if using gasoline for pleasure driving. She has no servant and it is some job to look after a house and two strenuous kids. She never makes the slightest protest. Worthington has been given another promotion. He is doing very well and if he comes through the war I don't believe he will ever leave the Army. He likes the life and the associations. Beale is in England we think. At least, we know he was there He made application for the air service and successfully passed his examinations. Just what has happened to him I don't know. Madison has made application for the Navy ir Service. He came to see me and talk it over. The Glenn Martin people want him to stay put but he is getting very restless. Besides his training classes he has charge of model airplanesmaking by the school children in Baltimore. The powers that be have just put on an exhibition of Madison's own models, some sixty-five, th y are supposed to be very perfect models. His calsses have prepared hundreds for the Army and Navy. I could not urge him to continue but I told him I thought he should let those who are on the inside decide for him.

More later,

Love from Ma

and

142

Major John E. Bordley, M.C., O-403012

General Hospital No. 118,

A.P.O. 927, c/o Postmaster

San Francisco, California

Dr. James Bordley, Jr.

330 N. Charles St

Baltimore, Maryland

February 22, 1943

Series II., No. 39

Dear John and Jim,

Well, the blow has fallen and the public went down for a nine count but they are up and fighting. The point ration system was put into operation and one month's allowance gives you forty-eight points just enough to buy two pounds of prunes (that is a fact). I am glad I don't eat prunes because for my forty-eight I can get two cans of peas and one of tomatoes. In other words we are allowed a little less than one-half of what was consumed last year. Any extra cans on hand must be reported and come off your allowance. We have about a hundred cans, I think, while our allowance is thirty-five for seven people (including Jimmy). I tell your mother we are at least certain of our hundred and that is more than most people will be. My boy! what the hoarders will get in the neck and I hope so I hear that some of them have put in cold units and filled their cellars and attics. I hope they catch them and send them up for life. We have less than one third of our yearly average for twenty years and much of that is the supply that Judy brought when she moved in. Mother is not breaking any laws or regulations but she is worried for the first time. Of course, meat is not yet rationed but it comes the first of April I understand. Now there is a boot-leg market with all the evils of prohibition. I don't believe, however, it will long get public support. If it does we who want to play the game straight will soon be out of luck. I am banking on help from the F.B.I. I am in favor of capital punishment for the offenders. I think a few first class executions would go a long, long way.

The people were a bit depressed by Rommel's thrust in Africa but it is beginning to simmer through that it was only a thrust through a thin line. If not "too late", it was too little. This is not meant as criticism, I have confidence in our military authorities and even more confidence in our soldiers. I have never criticised them and never will. Congress has changed a lot since the last election. It has acted wisely in not freezing top executive salaries as it has not frozen labors' wages. I don't see what the President expects to gain by limiting salaries to $25,000. I am in favor of letting any man increase and multiply his fortunes if it is based on a corresponding increase in his usefulness. It was that prospect which developed the greatest asset this country possesses, the right of self advancement. Congress has thrown the Executive order out the window and rightly. I heard over the radio last night a thing which greatly surprised me: an organization has been formed "for drafting the President for another term". The surprise was "drafting". It implies an unwillingness. I don't think Churchill's "democracy" has so contaminated the President's political ideals as to require "drafting". But it sounds good for a starter in the Spring of 1943.

The kids are fine. Brucie just came down to have lunch with Ellen. She has gained several pounds in the past month and looks like a million dollars. Anne did not come but she always looks the husky. Pat and Jimmy are fine. Jimmy pokes his head up when lying down and keeps a perpetual grin. Pat is beginning to take real notice of him in an affectionate way. Don't worry about them, they are all well clothed, housed and fed and will so continue. Love from Ma and

Your

143

Lt. Col. James Bordley, III., M.C.

General Hospital No. 118

A.P.O. 927, c/o Postmaster

San Francisco, California, U.S.A.

Dr. James Bordley,Jr.

330 N. Charles St.,

Baltimore, Md., U.S.A.

February 25, 1943

Dear Jim and John,   Series II., No. 40
        One lady in applying for her ration card acknowledged to 4,501 cans of
stuff stored in her pantry.   She was told that she could et no card before 1964. There is
not a store in Baltimore carrying in stock that much canned goods and she and her family
would require several years in its consumption. What an ass!   Compare her with a good
fellow in the ship-yard here who, since his gas ration was cut three months ago, as a patriotic duty, has walked eight miles each way a day and has never been late.   I had an
interesting young woman in here this morning. She was the first woman in war production at
Glenn Martin's. She is not a husky, just an average girl.   I was surprised that a girl of
her build could work on metal both as a riveter and punch operator.   She is well educated
and a sensitive sort but has missed no time in over a year.   Had never done any manual work
before.   I heard an employment agent of one of the large industrial plants giving advice to
women who want to work. He laid great stress on the damage done to the mens morale by sweat-
ers and too much primping. Said it decreased production. Suggested if women were to be of
real help they must not be too pretty or too much primped.   Boys will be boys you see even
in a war factory. There is great dissatisfaction in Congress over the Administration's
handling of preparations for war.   I hope it will not bring about a deadlock but it has
ominous signs.   Just now "man power" is the all absorbing topic of controversy and it looks
to me as if Paul McNutt were on his way out. Too littl and too late has he undoubtedly been
but he has a hard job and many self interests to please.   Labor wants one thing, agriculture
another.   He has hesitated to throw both out the window which would have met with full public
approval.   He has I am confident reflected the President's desires but the President enjoys
an immunity above that of any other man and his mistakes must be carried by his subordinates.
This is why Congress is mad, it has had to stand some dirty cracks itself as a result of bad
administration advice.   Damn politics. It is a cancerous disease in the body politic and its
practitioners have no sense of decency nor honor.   Hitler says he "has taught the world a
lesson it will never forget; that the country comes first and its leaders should be only leaders." Seeing as he is the king bug in the potato patch, he should know. A curious change has
taken place in this country. It is not the physical alterations but a certain sense of mental
suppression which has brought it about. Gaiety and frivolity are looked at with a wicked eye;
in home life the question is whether it is doing all it should and apologizing for things it
is doubtful about.   If you go off on a perfectly legitimate mission you stand ready to explain
the use of your car; if you go to the movies you wonder who is watching to see.   It is a
curious twist but it is spreading as sure as a prarie fire.   It may be the cause ultimately
of curbing selfishness of our people, through its feeling of shame.   Hard boiled babies are
no longer hardboiled, they come with their hats in hand and are afraid of their own superiority.
I often wonder whether we are developing a new mental complex out of which we will get real and
permanent social benefits. I only know that since Plato human nature and human selfishness have
not changed, perhaps we have a stimulous never before applied. Who knows the answer! I am preparing an article comparing our wartime sacrifices and those of our Revolutionary grandparents.
Ithink it will be timely and illuminating to those who think George Washington and his ragged
band went out and licked the British while the folks at home enjoyed their balls and foxhunts.
I will send you a copy and you send me your criticisms.
        Families still on top.   With love from Mother and
                                                Your

144

Major John E. Bordley, M.C. O-403012

General Hospital No. 118

A. P. O 927, c/o Postmaster

San Francisco, California

Dr. James Bordley, Jr.

330 N. Charles St.,

Baltimore, Md., U.S.A.

March 1, 1943.

Series II., No. 41

Dear John and Jim,

Just a note today. I started at six a.m. and have never caught up and the accumulation is getting greater. I enjoy it up to a certain point. We had a most remarkable storm a night or so ago. The afternoon was positively warm and warmer in the evening, then it started to snow and in about fifteen minutes the thermometer dropped below freezing and in a half an hour after that we had a thunder storm. The weather man said while not unprecedented it had not happened before for many years. The next day the temperature was around 18° and the wind high and biting and the pavements a mass of ice.

It looks to me like a political cyclone is going to strike at the next election. I am no prophet nor can anyone be when a successful battle may completely change the public attitude, but it will take just that to keep the Democratic Party in power. I have felt all along that the voters would not change parties in the middle of the war but there is increasing dissatisfaction at the war and preparation therefor. Then with black markets and absenteeism from work on an increasing scale the public is getting blue in the face. Even the Senate leader for the administration -- Senator Barkley exploded a few days ago and voted with the opposition (he doubtless had heard from home).

Rickenbacker is playing an increasing role in the opposition and is the most candid of all the attackers. He is hardly of the caliber for the Presidency but his name is more and more often spoken. This change is not due to sacrifices called for but because more are not asked.

The families are well and everything runs smoothly. We are watching with increased interest the Jap concentration around Australia but feel confidence in our Commander there. We know he is not going to be taken by surprise. Things are shaping up in Africa after a very discouraging start. Some people can expect only victories and defeats are for them hard to understand. I have every confidence in our Army and Navy.

With love from Ma

and

Major John E. Bordley, M.C., O-403012

General Hospital No. 118

A.P.O. 927, c/o Postmaster

San Francisco, California

Dr. James Bordley, Jr.

330 N. Charles St.,

Baltimore, Md.

March 5, 1943

Series II., No. 42

Dear John and Jim,

It may surprise you to know that the mortality rate for the country is 50%
under normal expectations and that includes battle casualties. The insurance people attrib-
ute the drop to two things - the Sulpha drugs and no epidemics. I saw by the paper a day or
so ago that in the British Isles the civil mortality there had struck an all time low. This
seems very remarkable to me when the disjointed way of living is considered. We have had
too much sickness here but of a minor nature. Two definite epidemics of a mild strep nose
and throat infection with but few serious results, even ear complications. So many people
have had to live in cold houses and work under strain and anxiety that it is surprising we
have had a drop in the death rate. Maybe we are leading more healthful lives and don't
know it. More bitter cold weather and snow and icy pavements and more predicted. So far
I have not had a chain on and have driven over more ice and through more snow than for
twenty years. I am really getting foolhardy.

We are losing our maid. She is so uncooperative in our war problems that
Ma can stand her no longer. Some sort of propaganda is about among the domestics making
them believe that are about to be put back into slavery and that the withholding of their
food cards is one of the means of holding them down. This dame of ours cannot understand why
she cannot on her day off take her ration cards and give a party, nor can she understand why
there should be any curtailing of her desires to live as ever. I am not sure which should
provoke the greater sympathy.

The President is definitely out -- that is his friends are -- for election
to a fourth term. The drums are beginning to sound and the cash and credit boys are starting
to toot their horns. It has come very quickly and I imagine it is due to the fact that Congress is kicking over the traces. A President who is going to run for re-election gets less
opposition from his own party. I can see no other reason for the agitation just now. It
is a long, long way to 1944 and many things can and, I hope will, happen between now and then.
I have analyzed my own feelings in the matter -- strange to say -- judicially, weighing the
evidence for and against, and I have not yet rendered my verdict. Against him I can place
the serious curtailment of our constitutional right -- before the war. Such as the seizure
of private telegrams -- for which he elevated Black to the Supreme Bench -- tapping private
telephones, such extravagance as to require taxation which amounts to seizure of one's
property, an executive order limiting salaries of private corporations, his support of a
group of labor crooks who demand and get the right to run the private business of private
citizens. For him I can see a ruthless casting aside of those who would have kept us out
of the war until it was too late, a closer cooperation between us and South America, the high
record in which he is held by the unfortunates of Europe, and a feeling that Hitler and Hirohito may capitalize on his down-fall. Of course he could obviate all the difficulties by
declining to run but his ambitions will never permit such a personal sacrifice in the face
of the great power he will wield at the Peace table. He just is not built for sacrifice and I
feel there is a growing antagonism to him not as much for what he has done as for the things
he has half done in preparing for all out war. We will in due course see what the people think.

With love from Ma

and

146

March 11, 1943.

Dear Jim and John,

This is the first let down I have had for weeks, only ten patients to see today. It is O.K. with me because yesterday I was busy from six-thirty a.m. until twelve o'clock last night. Things are certainly crazy, at seventy (now in my seventieth year) I shoul be getting up at ten and going to bed at nine, but the picture has the setting of blooming youth. This morning I was no more tired than I would have been at forty and not half so cross. I am not the only crazy acting thing. We have just had a complete reversal in our farm policy and none too soon if we are to get sufficient to eat. Farm labor has now been exempted from the draft and pays no income tax. It is too late, most of it has gone either to the Army or the factories. We are going to have a serious time and that I do not doubt. We have followed too much the pattern of England, not withstanding we have the difficult problem of supplying the food for most of the world while England cannot supply even its own food, and knowing that, utilized its man power for factory and Army. We have gone to work to build up an army of twelve million, increase our factory production five hundred percent. and increase farm production one hundred percent. It just cannot be done. If we had started out with a uniform forty-eight hour week it would have released thousands of men, where the forty hour plan has required hundreds of thousands extra. Then we pay factory labor entirely too much money which enables it to lay off a day or two a week and still make twice as much as before the war. The incentive for work is lacking. Few people work for love or patriotism. I know the problem is complicated by all kinds of difficulties but the ground work for its solution has been built on the quicksands of the New Deal.

A move has been made by business men and bankers for a four hour day for themselves in industry. The volunteered for any kind of industrial work regardless of pay. At first their plea to help was not listened to and whenthey came out in the papers with interviews and advertisements and some attention had to be given and they were affronted with the suggestion they were trying to dodge the draft. It happens when they organized and made their offer they specifically stated their employment was not to interfere with their draft status; then they were told they would have to join a labor union. The whole thing is sickening. The country's effort requires additional help but when offered it is repudiated and the help insulted. It is plain that the whole infernal thing was a political obstruction to our war movement engineered from Washington to prevent business men having an intimate acquaintance with labor. They were fearful of losing a political ghost when voting time comes around.

The whole country is riddled with stinking rotten politics from the great White House to the corner saloon. Of course, the President is not involved, that is, no further than the necessary preparations to run for a fourth term. Alexander Hamilton was right when he said "one day a demagogue will arise who by fooling a sufficient number of people will perpetuate himself permanently in the office of the Chief Magistrate". It behooves us to stay on watch and not have our ideals of government turned over by the personal ambitions of any man.

The President has just sent to Congress hispost war plans "to insure the four freedoms." It covers hundreds of pages and will have none of the free enterprise through which we have so greatly prospered. He makes capital and labor partners and the Government goes in business with them. In other words the Government and labor will control business, will set itsstandard and cop its profits. In the place of ability it will substitute the John L. Lesises and the ward bosses. Medicine is to be completely socialized and under the domination and dictation of politicians "so that when the boys return they will have a better country in which to live". His plans spell the death of ingenuity, self setermination and man's right to make his own place in society. His plans outdo those of England and in my judgment will find the sledding a bit rough both in Congress and the nation at large as soon as their implications are understood. It is his great bid for re-election and will doubtless carry the votes ne'er-do-well, the loafer and those who want a change regardless of its costs, so long as they are guaranteed a living without effort.

You know what the old California Doctor (Dr. Townsend) proposed as old age pensions, well he got a lot of votes. This out Herods Herod and perhaps it will draw so many more votes.

I am fearful of my country's future and I am suspicious of the governors. Maybe I am wrong but I believe implicitly with Thomas Jefferson "the greatest enemy we will ever have to fight is the personal ambition of our own leaders". Why should we change the system which has made us the most prosperous nation on earth -- ever -- which has permitted the widest scope of individual initiative, which has erected the highest standard of happiness and of living ever enjoyed by any people. True there are people among us who would work but who cannot find jobs, people who prefer help to effort, people mentally and physically incapable of sustained self helpfulness. Will Government control of industry and business and the professions change this? Will taking away the profit of the industrious for distribution among the lazy and incapable ever compensate for control by a highly centralized government with its effects up the lives and habits of our people? Never, I am convinced. Hitler started the same way. He played labor against capital and then tricked labor into complete submission and where is his nation and what of the happiness of its people. Many thought we would never go to war, that we had within ourselves the only necessary support to make us survive a world catastrophy. Now we are told that the succeeding steps of our civilization have led us nowhere and that e must junk its lessons and make a fresh start along a path not untried but always a failure. High sounding phrases will never change the fact we are asked to substitute for our peoples government, government by word and pathologically ambitious politicians. The governors who profit from government soon become tyrants and this scheme of the Presidents will create such governors.

Maybe John's "pot bellied devil" is knocking at my door and I don't know it or maybe I am afraid of change. But one thing I am certain of and that is France has paid an awful penalty for turning its government to be divided by a lot of Jackal politicians, that if the Germans, who took their government into partnership, survive with a nation it will be alone through the generosity of its enemies. I still believe and no argument has shaken my mind that a government should be the servant and not the partner of the people.

Well Dudy left this morning for Philadelphia and took away the kids for a month's stay with her father and mother. Ma and I will missthem very much but I believe the change will do them good. Dudy will have a new nurse in a day or so and her visit will relieve her of much responsibility and I feel she really needs the rest. She has worked very hard this winter.

Brucie will please John. She has gained weight and really looks fine. I suggested to Ellen she have them looked at by a physician so she took them over to the Harriet Lane and Dr. Guild. The report came back this morning that it would be wise to have Brucie's nasopharynx Beta Rayed but she was found in first class shape. I knew that from her looks. Of course tough old Anne could not be hurt with being run over by a truck of large size.

Jimmie is coming into his own. A big robust happy kid whose only trouble is lack of food for which he perpetually fights. Dr. Mary comes into see Jimmie and Pat every few days not because they need her but because she has a real feeling of responsibility for their health and happiness and also wants to see Dudy.

I had John's cheerful letter sending me a doubtful sort of congratulations. I can assure him the old gentleman found some surprises even if he failed to bring any.

Well I must get to work.

Love from Ma and

Your

Major John E. Bordley, M.C.   O-403012

General Hospital No. 118

A.P.O. 927, c/o Postmaster

San Francisco, California, U.S.A.

Dr. James Bordley, Jr.

330 N. Charles St.,

Baltimore, Md.,U.S.A.

March 17, 1943

Series II., No.44

Dear John and Jim,

Just to keep you informed as to the progress of the new and better nation to which you in due course will return.

Standard Oil has invented a new cracking process by which they actually convert crude oil into high octane gasoline. This new gas is so powerful that no machine so far invented has been able to carry more than a fraction of its power. It can be transported anywhere and then diluted saving tremendously in transportation. It will enable bombers to more than double their present load, will enable engineers to more than double the present horsepower, will enormously increase the velocity of upward speed and lift of present day planes and opens a new field for the construction of an entirely different type of much faster and more powerful planes and speed boats. The War Department has permitted the announcement and all the gasoline men I have talked to are wildly enthusiastic and predict great things from the manufacture. The Standard has put no strings around it so all the oil companies are building plants. Standard has completed three and is building nine more so as to get in production in a few weeks. One tanker will soon do the work of two and half.

We had a flood at home the other night. The boiler busted, or, to be more exact it cracked. I did not know there was so much water in the Atlantic Ocean, and if you ever saw a crew trying to save a torpedoed ship you have a good picture of the work of my pumping crew -- Ma, big Ann Bordley, Dudy and myself. When we found we were going to sink we made the first sensible move and let the water out of the system by the normal route.

Anthony Eden -- I found a letter from his grandfather, who was out last Colonial Governor, to James Hollyday -- arrived in this country yesterday. It seems from what you hear over the radio and read in the papers that there is not a very clear understanding among the Allies over many essential war and post-war questions and a bit of friction between the U.S. and U.S.S.R. and his visit is to help reach a definite formula. From what you hear it seems a timely move. I am glad he came.

Since I started this we have had more snow and ice but today the atmosphere is like Spring. The day started with a thunder storm. March is living up to a very bad reputation.

John Lewis is promising another coal strike, this time from the soft coal miners. If he pulls it off I hope they will hang him. There is too much loose talk and effort and it is time to stop it and get down to brass tacks.

Dudy phones the family well and Ellen tells me her crew is holding up.

With love from Ma and

Your

149

Lt. Col. James Bordley III., M.C.

General Hospital No. 118

A.P.O. 927, c/o Postmaster

San Francisco, California, U.S.A.

Dr. James Bordley, Jr.

330 N. Charles St.,

Baltimore, Md., U.S.A.

March 19, 1943

Dear Jim and John,   Series II., No.45

Well we have undergone several significant changes. The pleasure driving ban has been lifted and we are to get 1½ gallons of gasoline every week to do as we please with. This is a sensible change as I never saw any sense in letting people buy gas and then keep them from using it. I always thought only those needing cars for business purposes should have been given tickets but if that was not essential then let it be used as best suits the ticket holders. The Senate has done a sensible thing. A Committee of four Senators has been organized to act as sort of a liason body between the Senate and President for both war and the following peace. The President must have the Senate's consent in all treaty arrangements and with this body to inform the Senate on the motives of the President and vice versa it may save the disastrous consequencies of Senate objections to the settlement of the last war. This Committee is equally divided, two Democrats and two Republicans. I am sure this will give our Allies more confidence and dependence upon our motives both now and in the future. This is in striking contrast to what is being done to our new tax law where the President has one idea and his party another and the Republicans with still another and bills introduced into both Senate and House which represent no part of any of the wishes of President and Parties. It is the worst mixed up affair of the war. I am in favor of the Ruml Plan, to forgive the taxes of 1942 and go on a pay as you go. The laboring classes cannot pay both the same year and the day war is over they will be able to pay nothing. Their enormous wages now are a treat to our stability and will give us a spiral of rising prices. It will be better to tax them at the source taking away thirty percent. -- twenty for the treasury and ten as a withholding tax to be returned after the war as a means of bridging over unemployment between war and peace economies. Most of the Republicans are supporting this while the finance committees of Congress are trying to make both taxes stick, 1942-3. Better take the bird in hand, I think, a levy at the source cannot be dodged.

Our greatest trouble now is absenteeism. There are many reasons given for it -- some ten million work hours lost in the past two months -- first, the pay is so large that people want to have the fun of spending; then so many people who never worked for profit are making money that it has lightened family burdens and given impetus to loafing and "good times" then thirdly, there is a large element who are far less concerned about the war than about frolic. I suppose this is to be expected when you analyze our population but it does get those who are mindful of the consequences of war a bit hot under the collar.

We go on meat and butter rations in a few days (including cheese). This is going to hit a belly blow in a land of large meat eaters. Our allowance will be four ounces of butter and 1½ lbs. of meat per week. (Think of Ma with her 8 lbs. of roast beef and 12 lb. ham for a sitting). We are in training at home because we have had two meatless days a week for a long time. If don't care if it helps to feed our Army and Navy and our Russian and British Allies. They need it more than we. Congress thinks this no time to prepare for social benefits -- post-war. No one knows what kind of a world we will have to deal with, so how can we prepare? I am glad of it because we do not concentrate sufficiently on war now and if a lot of wild disputes are started it will drive us further away and split us wide open.

The families stay well. Love from Ma and

Your

150

March 26, 1943

Dear John and Jim,

At last the family has produced a genius, an artist. Charlie has just painted and, with house paint, one of the most perfect faces, with large blue eyes. You would have been astonished beyond belief. It was his sister's face. Her vanity called for decoration and Charlie responded with the only paint at hand. Ellen lackes appreciation, probably induced by her effort to restore her daughter to normal and, the effect of the turpentine on her newly manicured nails. At least she did show sufficient appreciation to amply reward Charlie and probably has forever cast a shadow over his art. Recently, Carroll gave herself a shampoo with a newly made apple-pie at Charlie's suggestion. The poorboy has no other boys to play with and his imagination revolves around his little sister and with a sympathetic response from her.

Well, we are now rationed on all except perishable foods, so many points per each. My fear is the points are too numerous for the supply. There is a real fear of such a thing in the minds of those in power, and yesterday, for about the forty-eleventh time, the President appointed a new crowd to take over the whole of production and distribution. The whole trouble lies in the fact that the Army has been given the green signal to take any and all and knowing nothing about farming and food the Selective Draft drained off all the man-power from the farms. My farmer quit last week. He has had no help for over six months and cannot possibly carry on. While I have a contract with him until January 1944, I could not blame him and certainly not stop his leaving. He will get a war job and make more money with less work but there will be just so much less to eat. He is only one of thousands.

Another big snow last week but today is beautiful spring. I played golf yesterday and the second time in months. I really got no kick out of it. Our foursome was the only one on the links and yesterday a holiday -- Maryland Day. Of course, the gallon and a half a week gasoline ration does not create much of an incentive especially in those who live far away from the Club. How much longer the Club will stay open is doubtful as so many members have resigned, so few ever go there and help both in the Club and on the grounds is impossible to get. The Government wants the Clubs to function for some reason but many of them are using their grounds to grass cattle and others have passed out.

Congress is having a big fight over taxes. There are three bills -- the Administration is trying to make everybody in 1943 pay taxes for 1942-3 in the current year. It will bust thousands and give many others a squeaking sound. There is also a bill to put us immediately on a pay-as-you-go basis and forget 1942. This is a far more practical thing because the great bulk will never pay either 1942 or 1943 without the money is taken at the source. Then if the war ends suddenly and hundreds of thousands are thrown out of work or have to work for much less no taxes can ever be collected from them. The third scheme is a politician's scheme to make everyone happy but in the end make everyone sad. The administration crowd point to the loss of $10,000,000,000 in 1942 taxes. To me this is absurd as it is predicated on the idea that labor will pay its just taxes. Even if they wanted to, they have not saved sufficient money our of their wages of 1942. Their scheme is to assess at the source 30% of the wages now received by all types of salaried and waged people. Already they are assessed at the source 5% for the Victory Tax and 10% for War Bonds. So many of the war workers are living in strange places and under such financial strain that I do not believe a cut of 45% will be possible. Thousands of these workers are not yet aware of why they work and look upon the adventure purely from a financial view point. If they are cut 45% they will stop in droves. The trouble lies again in the fact that these things are in the hands of those inexperienced in the broad ways of the world. They are small people with large responsibilities and are way over their heads.

The families remain well and reasonably happy.

Love from Mother

and

Major John E. Bordley, M.C., 0-403012

General Hospital No. 118

A.P.O. 927 c/o Postmaster

San Francisco, California, U.S.A.

Dr. James Bordley, Jr.,

330 N. Charles St.,

Baltimore, Md., U.S.A.

March 29, 1943

Series II., No. 47

Dear John and Jim,

Anthony Eden was at Annapolis on Friday night and spoke before a joint session of the Legislature. I was not so impressed by him as by Churchill. He has a good delivery but talked like he was watching every sentence fearing something might leake out. He got much applause at appropriate times but added little to our sum of knowledge as to England's war intentions. Personally, I don't see how anyone can figure out the mysteries of the world's future, and if it cannot be figured I see no basis for plans. I am afraid of any flat-footed statement because it will be sure to cause an acrimonius debate which might have serious repercussions on our war efforts. The truth is the isolationist crowd in this country wants to embarrass England and are now demanding she give up her colonial Empire. They want to drive her to a statement of intentions. They are a dirty bunch and I feel have no rock upon which to build a defense. They take defeat not as a good, but, a bad sport. Churchill told the world the other day England wants only to keep its Empire, wants no new territory and intends to give every sub-division the opportunity for independent self-government. It would be a world tragedy, I feel, to break up the Commonwealth of Nations. It is the most powerful force for world stabilization and its dismemberment would leave us to hold the bucket and we just cannot do it if our present effort is a good sample of our abilities.

The good news has just arrived that the British 8th Army has Rommel on the run again. Montgomery is a keen soldier. He reminds me of General Grant, slow, plodding but ever pushing. If he is as successful, the world will be better off for his efforts.

Meat rationing was not taken with very good grace in some parts of the country -- a few riots; around here all was peaceful. Ellen Webb has been unable to get a piece of meat for ten days. My old scout went on the trail on Saturday and came back with a small roast beef which Brucie and I carried her yesterday. It delighted her and Brucie had a wonderful time. I never saw her brighter and more full of pep. Played songs and made up games and I was sorry when the time came to take her home because all the kids were having so much fun. I am going to take her again soon. Anne was at Sunday-school. That hot pepper never misses a chance.

More soon. Love from Ma

and

April 1, 1943.

Dear Jim and John,

Well the war looks better. Whether it is permanent or not remains to be seen. The industrialists notice under its stimulation an increase in effort. It is most needed because while production goes forward it is lagging behind the maximum required.

A Commander in the Navy who was treated in 118 sent Ellen a message about the work of the Unit and said he would ever remember with great pleasure the courtesies shown him by John. I don't know whom it was, neither does Ellen.

I am sure you want to know some facts from home even if unpleasant. Well, Sam Crowe had an extensive abdominal operation on Monday week: Gastric ulcers. A week after the operation he had a very serious set back but today he has pulled out and is going forward satisfactorily. There was no malignancy only a very extensive duodenal ulceration. Bill Reinhoff operated. Sam collapsed on the post Monday and on Tuesday had a hemorrhage with loss of pulse and feeble respiration. They were not sure he had not picked up a clot also. Today he is very disagreeable about a nasal tube — normally mad. I think he is on his way home and Guild says he now has complete faith in his recovery.

I am sending a bunch of flowers for you both as soon as he has sufficiently recovered, which I pray God may be very soon.

Dudy and the children are still in Philadelphia and will stay, if her fath remains well, until after Easter. Her father and mother have gotten as much joy and pleasure out of their visit, Dudy hates to leave.

Well now that winter has passed and the school season is about over those who live in the country can get sufficient gasoline to take their children to school. This applies t little Charlie who has been out of school the entire winter because Charlie, Sr. has not received sufficient gas to drive to town and it was an impossible journey for little Charlie to go with his father by train, especially when Charlie, Sr. had to leave him at seven A.M. It has been a lonely winter for the little fellow and I am glad he will have a couple months' contact with other children.

Glenn Martin is after me to have night office hours -- from eight to ten -- I took it under consideration but decided against it. I am working very hard and feel the extra might break me down and make me useless. As it is I am treating many of his night shift people in my day hours. If I were a young man I would try it for a while but un-fortunately I am not so blessed. I really think it will be wiser for me to stay home this summer and keep up my regular practice. Ma is a busy woman and I thank God for her mathematical brain when I see what it means for her to play her ration cards. Boys, I could never do it, I would rather not eat and just have it over. Every mouthful must be cal-culated weeks ahead because the loss of a few points will mean missing meals. She just takes it in her stride and never loses hope nor faith. She even makes a gallon and a half of gasoline a week look like the loaves and fishes. How she does it is a deep dark mystery.

I am enclosing the photo of our newest dive-bombers. Thought they might interest you. Swepson Earle who has been retired from the Navy after a bad heart following a frontal sinus, tells me the Navy is getting in super shape and will surprise our enemies. They have several new gadgets which have panned out very well for us. He believes we are getting the goat of the submarines with some new methods of attack. I hope so because they have recently been particularly destructive and many more in numbers. I take off my hat to the merchant marine. Those boys really are up against a difficult and dangerous job with never a squawk. One of those boys went out to the club to see whether he could get a job for a month driving a tractor. Said he wanted to get away from ships and water for a few weeks and get his nerves straightened out -- following three sinkings. Says he cant sleep on shipboard any longer and feels the need of a little rest and diversion of a peaceful nature but needs the money to live on. He is from the university of North Carolina and an old quarter back, about thirty I should say.

More later.   Love from Ma

and

153

Major John E. Bordley, M.C., O-405012

General Hospital No. 118

A.P.O. 927, c/o Postmaster

San Francisco, California, U.S.A.

Dr. James Bordley, Jr.

330 N. Charles St.,

Baltimore, Md., U.S.A.

April 7, 1943

Series II., No.49

Dear John and Jim,

We hold an election primary today, all City offices. I am betting that not more than 20% of the voters will go to the polls. If I am correct, it will be a tragedy. Out fighting a war to establish a democratic world, the fundamental of which is the peoples choice of their governors and only 20% go to the polls to vote for such officers! It seems hardly worth the sacrifice. No wonder we are building -- or having built for us -- a stronger and stronger central government, have about lost all the rights of the states, have Government encroachment on the private rights and business of the voters. Well the organization controls 10% of the voters by creating offices and this establishes a vicious circle which can be broken only through votes and we who are fighting for freedom will not take the trouble to insure that freedom by voting.

Since the above was wrotten, the election has taken place with the return of Jackson as Mayor. Less than 15% of the registered Democrats voted and less than 10% of the Republicans. Speaking of the freedoms for which we are fighting it seems to me that of choosing our Governor is far and away the most important, but, only 11% of the clamourers think so apparently.

I have been treating John's Mrs. Dr. Moses, thinking she was an unusual looking Jewess. In discussing the Jewish question today found out I had made a mistake -- almost a tragic one, but, recovered in time. People should be more careful about their sign posts, especially where they carry a name. Of course, I know her husband had somewhere a Jewish ancestor. The name never came over in the Ark and Dove, nor did it land at Jamestown or Plymouth, but what of it. I know some Jews who are nicer than some Christians.

Any spare time I get I work on your ancestors. My! how many you had. I am glad the records are lost beyond Adam and Eve. Such curious people you came from too, but that makes the study more interesting. I found one who was known as the great dueller. He challenged anybody for anything and when the stock grew low he advertised in the papers for more. Curious it was that when the British attacked Queenstown he was the first to arrive in Centreville from the battlefield and when a fellow traveler impuned his motive he shot him. Then another, challenged to fight, threw himself at the feet of the Legislature and demanded protection -- and got it. But when the Indians attacked his community he was the hero in its defense. And still another who slapped a man for insulting his wife left her defenseless when the other gentleman drew a gun. It takes a lot of people to make a world but your ancestors did their part in supplying the deficiencies. Fifteen to a family was just a few months' work. I sometimes wish birth control had been the practice in the past ages, but if so maybe I would not now be writing of your ancestors.

Everyone is planting a Victory Garden, especially those who never before had a garden. The Lord is not helping much. He has turned on the cold with a vengeance. Today it was 22° and more promised. This is disastrous to the oil stock. We were given 1500 gallons less than a year ago but we still have tickets for five hundred gallons. In other words, we have saved 2,000 gallons. I can see now how we have wasted heat in the past.

Sam Crowe is getting along very well. Had no recorrence of collapse or hemorrhage.

More later. Love from Ma

and

April 13, 1943.

Dear Boys,

Yesterday I went on a rampage: went out to Uncle Charlie's for dinner, then over to see little Charlie's wife and baby and Charlie of course.

Milton came home for dinner, he is in the Air Corps and trying to get to the ground Cadet School. He has been down in Florida and was transferred to Washington by mistake and will have to go back and start over again for some other place. He has worked out some sort of scheme for quick repairs which has attracted the attention of his superiors and with his training they think he should get officers training so as to give force to his plans. Little Charles is working on some new gadgets, I don't know what. He has had one promotion after another and has been assured a fine post war job.

Worthington isteaching at the Cavalry School and I heard indirectly he was given a first lientenant's commission.

Beale is in England with the Artillery. We heard he had gone to North Africa but it was a mistake. He is still a private.

With you boys in the Army the whole family are now engaged in Uncle Sam's job. I think that is a hundred percent. because Murray's step-sons -- two in the Army and one working here in the ship-yard -- completes our man adults of fighting age.

Dudy called me up on Saturday about her State income tax and was delighted to know she could deduct $5-1/3%. She says Jimmy is so big and developing so fast we will not recognize him. They are all well except her mother who is down in weight to 88 pounds. They carted her off to a hospital last week for a good rest and some forced feeding. She has had too much responsibility and I feel sure the rest will do her a lot of good.

My clerk, Ellen, and her two kids are fine. Father and Mother Fisher are going to California to see Bill who is located there temporarily. Just when and for how long Dr. Bill did not tell me and I have not asked Ellen.

We are preparing a vistory garden, not much of course, but, we have hopes that if our plants are not eaten up by the children of Hirohito we will be able to supply the table with some essential vitamins.

The President has clamped a ceiling on all essential foods, which should have been done months ago. Prices have been going up so fast and so high that it must be difficult for the poor to get enough to eat. We are down to a green vegetable, a meat, fish, eggs or chicken, potatoes or some similar thing and a simple dessert. Soups take too many points except for baby foods and canned juices are too expensive in points to use often. Don't get the impression we are hungry for we are far from actual want. We just no longer need a dining table twelve by fivefeet. Really I think it is grand because I have always insisted on not eating what I did not want, and this just eliminates the abusive criticism I have had to put up with.

Ma is a real provider, just a first class specialist. She never kicks and never complains except at those who patronize black markets. She looks at every ceiling price sheet and believe me no extra pennies are added.

It is really very interesting to watch the reaction of all this mess on our people. You seldom hear a kick and I am happy to say that those of our class are the most punctilious in observing the rules. It can never be said they used their money to the disadvantage of the poor. The honest merchants are up against real competition from the black market rats. As an example these skunks and polecats of New York have cleaned the Eastern Shore of poultry at a price above the market (Thank God most of the checks have been returned as no good). Of course the buyer had nothing on the seller, but Baltimore markets have been left with an empty basket.

Today has been a full one for me; Twenty patients in the office, a visit outside, a conference at the Hopkins, one at the Museum, and another at the Maryland Historical Society, to say nothing of getting up at six fifteen to fix the furnace and then having it to fix on my return home. And honestly I am not tired, no more so than I would have been twenty years ago. In lots of ways I am a joying myself, especially I think because I expected to be sort

Lt. Col. James Bordley, III., M.C.

General Hospital No. 118,

A.P.O. 927, c/o Postmaster

San Francisco, California, U.S.A.

April 17, 1943

Series II.. No. 51

Dear Boys,

We have had the damndest weather for the past two weeks. The temperature nearly every day in the 20s and flurries of snow most any time. The oil ration board on March has left a lot of people cold. We were more economical than some and have not been cold but it gives me a shiver to see how low the tanks are getting. It has been too cold to plant our Victory garden, those less experienced than Ma put theirs in and now it must be done all over again. The early peaches in our State are gone as they were in full bloom when the cold struck. It is a funny thing though, the peaches are killed every Spring but there is always an abundance in the summer. We have gotten so far ahead in our tank and heavy car production that two of such plants have closed down and it was stated over the radio that in three months some 600,000 workers in such plants -- including some types of air planes -- will be out of jobs. The trouble is we have not adopted an over all manpower plan which results in an unequal distribution of manpower. The Baltimore papers for instance carry large front page advertisements for workers but in New York they are a glut on the market. There is some light however as stronger men replace college professors and parlor reds in the running of the war efforts. Such foolish things were done -- such as a ceiling on retail meat and no ceiling on cattle on the hoof and which kept the cattle dealers selling at higher prices in a black market where the hungry and selfish went for more than ration tickets called for. Recently a first class man was put in charge and his first move was to remove all ceilings on meat. This has left the black boys holding a very full bag which cost a lot of money. It is a hard job without full public support. If they insist on breaking rules no sort of management will succeed. During the Revolution all beef cattle and hogs were commandeered by the State Governments and paid for at a fixed price. It cost a little more but it immediately stabilized prices at the Government's own figure. Of course, that is now ancient history and we never regard the lessons of history. While we actually have more beef cattle on the hoof than ever before we have had a serious shortage of meat. It is getting better now.

It was announced over the radio that a new glass is being made which sheds both snow and rain. It means no more windshield wipers and no more frosting. At present, the Government takes the entire output. I cannot begin to enumerate the wonderful discoveries that have been made, they are legion. They hold out wonderful hopes for the post war years as means of employment. For instance, there is a new plastic used as a substitute for wire screens. It costs less than half of the present copper screen and will outlast it by years. It is being used on planes, in homes and even for fencing.

Crowe is well on the way to complete recovery. He had a right sharp time for a few days but pulled out O.K.

We are well and looking forward to the return of Dudy and the children which will be delayed a couple of weeks by Mrs. Ross' stay in the hospital where she needed very much to go. Ellen and her kids are O.K.

Love from Ma and

Your

Major John E. Bordley, M.C. O-403012

General Hospital No.118

A.P.O. 927, c/o Postmaster

San Francisco, California, U.S.A.

Dr. James Bordley, Jr.

330 N. Charles St.,

Baltimore, Md., U.S.A.

April 21, 1943.

Series II., No. 52

Dear Boys,

The snow has changed to rain and the west wind to the north east. This has been a poor season for the new gardeners. I hope they will not be too much discouraged because the way things are going in food supplies they may need a few fresh vegetables before another season comes around.

I have a new farmer with a German name -- Wessel -- but the family has been here since before the Revolution so I suppose he will try to make profitable crops. Wheat is selling around $1.40 but most of the farmers got rid of their crops at a dollar or less and the speculators will get the cream. The Government has just advanced the price of corn five cents but much of that had to be left in the fields because of no labor. Mine has just been husked but the quality is so poor it will bring next to nothing, not enough I am sure to pay for the taxes. The new farmer is a young man of progressive inclinations -- is thirty-one and has five children. He also owns a combine, tractor, truck and car and is looking at the market to see what is going to be short so he can plant just that. I like his looks and will help him. His two boys, 11 and 12, can handle his plows behind the tractor and do the odd jobs around the barn and as he can hire no labor they are a great help and he has had them excused from school for the balance of the year.

We have added a new cook to our household. She came last Wednesday at eleven, Thursday was her day off, Friday she had to leave to report to Glenn Martin as a riveter. As she did not bring her birth certificate they would not accept her so she is back. While she was away her mother came out to work. She said her daughter was 26 and she herself was 36. When your mother questioned her, she said "I suppose I did get married right young". Well there seems some difficulty about the birth certificate and I suppose the mother has not been able to definitely name the father.

I am invited to eat terrapin at the Fishers Thursday. Sox Elting sent Bill some and Bill and his wife have gone to see Billy. Ellen decided to give us a party.

We have had a curious disease among the children and all of ours have had it. Just nausea and abdominal pains with a bit of temperature. It lasts for about forty-eight hours and is gone leaving no aftermath. It has attacked few adults and is I think on its way out.

More later. Love from Ma and

Your

Dear Boys,

I got sort of tired out so pulled away for two or three days' rest and did not have time to write because I was too busy. Vacations mean harder work than working days for me. There was so much to be done at home and nobody to do it that I put in a good many hours.

I suppose you know Mrs. Ross was operated on on the 26th. She had gained three pounds prior to her operation and was very much more cheerful. The operation I can only report as finished and the lady in good shape. I confess I was a bit uneasy about her but apparently with little foundation for worry.

Griff Davis died last week at seventy-six. He worked in his Victory Garden one afternoon and greatly exhausted himself, went in and to bed. His housekeeper to his room to call him some hours afterwards and found him dead. Thus ends a life of great usefulness and I lose one of my old time friends, one with whom I worked for forty-three years. My first operation was just forty-three years ago when I went out to help Ridge Trimble to remove a large fatty tumor from a man's back. Griff gave the anaesthetic. It was in the days when most operations were performed at home. Ever since then Griff has given anaesthetics for me, first chloroform and then ether. I shall miss his grouch which was his outstanding characteristic.

There was a nice write-up of your Unit on the first page of the Sun this morning. I would send it but understand it makes too much weight for mail and packages are not allowed. It did not go into much detail, was more a birdseye view. Mrs. Fox (Henry's wife) called mother up this morning and told her the New York Times of last Tuesday carried a page of the pictures of your new hospital with a pretty full description. I have ordered several copies so I could send them around to the wives.

We have had out first real Spring and the trees and flowers tell us of coming summer. This makes me wonder when the gods will dispense in the way of war. It looks better and Germany seems to be in for a real fight on the West. Of course, we are told nothing, as it should be, but it keeps everyone on edge with expectation and anxiety, especially now with so many families represented in the fighting forces. I am one of those Americans who believes that we cannot be licked when we set our minds on winning.

All the families are well and send love with Mother

and

Lt. Col. James Bordley, III., M.C.

General Hospital No. 118

A.P.O. 927, c/o Postmaster

San Francisco, California, U.S.A.

Dr. James Bordley, Jr.

330 N. Charles St.,

Baltimore, Maryland, U.S.A.

May 3rd, 1943.

Series II., No. 54

Dear Boys,

Another of the President's poor choices has bit the hand that fed him.   John L. Lewis who took a half million dollars from "the poor starving miners" and gave it to the President in exchange for labor power has struck against his old chum, because, he failed to be named President by the last Democratic Convention.   That is all, nothing more and nothing less.   It may not be treason to scuttle the Ship of State in the midst of war, but if it is not it is certainly coming damned close.   If I were President I would let twelve is Lewis' peers(and they would not be hard to find) say what they think.   It is bunk to talk about his being persecuted. Any man living under our Government who declines to abide by the laws and recognize the constituted government is a revolutionist and as a revolutionist he should be subjected to the punishment prescribed for such offense, or, the Government itself becomes a menace to the people.

There is too much loose talk about liberty and its infringement.   There can be no liberty without laws and any man who stands above the law, especially one made at the personal behest -- as was the Labor Board -- is a menace to the security of liberty.   In this one instance the people will have the final say and make no mistake where they stand, they want coal mined and it will be.   It does seem odd that the President's dream should be shattered by his bed fellow.

The weather is still playing pranks with the victory gardeners.   In the past week we have had two frosts and a terrific lot of wind.   I hope those who have worked so hard to help in the food shortage will not be too discouraged.

Mrs. Ross was getting along well at last report and Jimmy weighs sixteen pounds, so things are looking up with Dudy.

All the families are well.

Sometime drop Ma and me a note.   It has been weeks since we heard direct.   Everyone is delighted with your new Hospital as depicted by the New York Times. Winford Smith says he is afraid you will like it so well that you may not want to come back to the Hopkins.

Well I must run as I have a lot to do.

With love from Ma and

Your

Major John E. Bordley, M.C., O-403012   Dr. James Bordley, Jr.

General Hospital No. 118
                                               330 N. Charles St.,
A.P.O. 927, c/o Postmaster
                                               Baltimore, Maryland, U.S.A.
San Francisco, California, U.S.A.

                                               May 4th, 1943

Dear Boys,
                                               Series II., No. 55
        A nice quiet day ahead, only 12 patients in the office, one hospital to go to and
one visit in the country. This is a let down but it is limited to today for tomorrow I have a
full house including a difficult operation put off by the Major, in fact a very difficult one
it would have been for a novice.

        The sun is shining and the wind is blowing a gale. Every day a howling wind keeps
the ground dry in spite of repeated rains. It is good for golf (when you can find time
which is seldom) but hard on the farmer who wants to plant his corn and tomatoes.

        The coal strike has been settled for 15 days. A "truce" John Lewis calls it. Think
of a truce between the Government and a private citizen! If the President sticks to his
guns the coal strike is over but as he seldom arrives at a logical conclusion we may have
more of it.

        We have an election today: Jackson vs. McKeldin. I suppose Jackson will win as
he has a strong organization. I wish he would lose because I feel no politician should
hold office too long. The job then becomes a money making institution instead of a government for the people. The Republican has at least put a me daylight into the private activities of Jackson's Insurance Co., the people at least know what a money making proposition
he hasmade of the Mayor's office.

        The Governor has done one of the most constructive things yet advanced to set
straight the medical tangle. A survey is being made of the medical needs of the poor in the
City and counties. The proposition resulting at least tentatively is that two county hospitals be constructed after the war is over and be so placed geographically as to best serve
the counties' poor sick needs. These hospitals are to be staffed under the advice of a
committee appointed by the State Faculty and application for treatment will be made through
the County Health Officer. The State to pay Hospital expenses and medical fees on a scale
arranged by the State Faculty. Where hospitalisation is unnecessary the Health Officer is
to see that a list of local physicians is given the patient for selection and the resulting
medical fee is to be paid by the State. The whole scheme is to be conducted by a Board on
which there is adequate medical representation.

        It looks to me as the most sane plan presented and if it goes through, which seems
probable, it will end State medicine as proposed by the Surgeon General of Public Health as
far as Maryland is concerned and will set up a model for other States to copy. It is so
rational and simple and so unpolitical that it may not be agreed to by those who want to make
chambermaids of doctors. At least it forces the medical profession to come to life which
is quite a trick.

        We are all jubilant over the success of our Army in Africa! I never doubted its
ability to lick the Germans if given a real opportunity. God bless every man of them is
my earnest prayer. What a thing! A lot of farmer boys and clerks in one year of training
beat Hitler's professional soldiers at their own game.

        More later. Love from Ma and

P.S.--Mrs. Ross goes home today much improved. I thought she would probably die from the
operation.

160

Lt. Col. James Bordley, III., M.C.   Dr. James Bordley, Jr.,

General Hospital No. 118   330 N. Charles St.,

A.P.O. 927, c/o Postmaster,   Baltimore, Maryland,U.S.A.

San Francisco, California, U.S.A.

                                May 10th, 1943

Series II., No. 56

Dear Boys?

Well Mayor Jackson was defeated which leaves me a poor prophet. Some sixty thousands less votes than were cast at the last election is probably the answer. McKeldin -- the "South Baltimore Boy" won by 20,000.

Most of the business men, except the Insurance crowd, are disturbed. Why I shall never know because this city is in a deplorable condition. Dirty, filled with rats and pavements about as bad as possible, still the Mayor found money enough to hire twenty-two secretaries, buy a park so far out that without an automobile it cannot be reached. We have had strike after strike among the City employees and needless expenses one on the other just to keep alive a political machine.

They tell me that McKeldin has real ability and sound judgment. He ran against O'Connor for Governor and reduced his majority for a hundred to eight thousand. He says he is going to run the City as a business enterprise and disregard politics; he will retain all competent City employees who are needed and fill the jobs of the inefficient with efficient persons regardless of their politics. It is the proper approach but whether his political friends will back him up I doubt. The entire Democratic ticket won with Jackson the exception. This does not keep McKeldin from having a majority on the Public Works Board which is the plans making outfit.

(Several days later). I just heard, in fact was told by Mr. Crook (appropriate name for a politician -- but Mr. Crook is not a politician?) that the cause of Jackson's defeat was a woman's campaign started several months ago to get the City cleaned up and the rats exterminated. Right or wrong they pinned the failure to accomplish this much and benefit on Jackson.

Tunisia has definitely brought the civilian population into the war. I know because Frank Chew is buying Government Bonds. Of course, they are two percents because he does not expect to live long enough to cash the War Bonds. There is the first evidence of excitement since Pearl Harbor, the first time people have button-holed each other. The rapidity of the changes in the battle and our overwhelming strength is an eye-opener to everyone. Of course, Africa and continental Europe are two distinct problems, but no one can convince me that Germany is not on a rapid down grade. How could it be otherwise; she is not superhuman; she cannot grow good without fertilizer and man-power and she has neither. It was quite a job to feed their eighty or ninety millions in peace time and no matter how large their storage space, three and a half years is a long time to provide for so many hungry mouths. Then they must have exhausted their stored gas. A Standard Oil man said they were working on their stored gas a year ago. The British and Americans have been knocking hell into their industries and they have no extra materials to waste. It may take more than this year to complete the destruction so successfully carried on by Russia but I doubt it.

Dudy brought her little family home yesterday. Either Jimmy or I should go in a circus. Everytime he looks at me he laughs until he gets hysterics. He is as big as his daddy. Pay looks her lovely self and is brimming over with mischief. Dudy looks very well and says her mother looks better than for years.

More later. With love from Ma

                  and

                      Your

Major John E. Bordley, M.C., 0-403012   Dr. James Bordley, Jr.

General Hospital No. 118   330 N. Charles St.,

A.P.O. 927, c/o Postmaster   Baltimore, Md., U.S.A.

San Francisco, California, U.S.A.

                                           May 13th, 1943

                                           Series II., No. 57

Dear Boys,
        Your father is distressed to have you know that he is in the clutches of the law.
A parking ticket, the first one in thirty-two years. What a bad example for my sons. I am
offering no excuse, though I can think of scores, am just paying my fine and charging it
against expenses. I do hate to have my record broken and it really was not my fault and
I will charge the fine to those who detained me, but my good name has a smear on it.   Of
course you cannot appreciate this feeling, neither could your mother who has had far more
experience with the legal workings of the traffic court than I, and, who in a sense, is a
hardened criminal! She denies but one summons but pleads guilty to several warrants.
        We are all enthusiastic over the complete victory in Africa.   Our part was rela-
tively small but done in a first class manner and it leaves no doubt that our clerks and
farmer boys make just as good soldiers now as in the times of Washington and Lee.   We are
proud of them and should be. The boosted professional German soldiers (with a little g)
are not after all supermen. They just had a super training in everything but humanity
and civilization which our boys possess without training.   In the end it counts for more
because no matter how much you learn hot to fight if you have not confidence in your own
soul you can't get far when you are cornered.   I hope this fight is emblematic of our
qualities and intentions and I believe it is.
        We received John's letter last night and mother and I enjoyed it very much.
Nothing like a direct communication.
        We are producing better than seven thousand planes a month and with a large
proportion of heavy bombers and long range fighters.   They are being flown to England in
six and a quarter hours. The best time is six hours and twelve minutes and they are going
in flocks.
        Churchill is here again with Wavell and the top ranking Army and Navy men of
both Great Britain and U.S. It is expected here that a meeting between Churchill, Stalin and
the President is in for the near future. This will delight all of us, it means a concentration of power for the near future against Germany. It is rumored that Italy is seeking
a separate peace but I find no real foundation for the rumor. I hope I am wrong provided
it means a complete surrender. This Germany may prevent with its troops, but even if it
attempts it provides a new front if the Italians decide to fight.
        More later.
                        Love from Mother
                                and
                                    Your

Lt. Col. James Bordley, III., M.C.

General Hospital No. 118,

A. .O. 927, c/o Postmaster,

San Francisco, California, U.S.A.

Dr. James Bordley, Jr.

330 N. Charles St.,

Baltimor 1, Md., U.S.A.

May 17, 1943.

Dear Boys,   Series II., No. 58
        Another week has come and I wonder what it will have in store for us. Things are
moving fast, nothing faster than rumors of things to come.   Yesterday we were told the King
of Italy had abdicated, that Italy was now in the hands of friends of the Allies; today we
hea the Germans are pulling out as far as the Brenner Pass and have told Italy to take care
of itself. If you believe the stories it would be fine but I know if Hitler is proposing a
defense of Germany he wants as much land as possible between the llied forces and that God-
forsaken land.   The King may have abdicated but Hitler's concenience may have beenserved
as the King has always been a friend of England. Well a few days may tell us.
        Things in this country mull along and by the grace of God we are steadily making
progress in spite of the John L. Lewises. All the business men with whom I talk tell me that
in spite of the vaccilation of Government and the departmental jealousies production is
steadily on the increase and that we will not want for material when the crucial test comes --
which it will in the not distant future.
        I would like to tell you of some of the ingenious investions which have reduced
certain essential production activities from days to minutes; how obsolete materials have been
brought back to positions of great importance by changes in chemical reactions; how vibra-
tions are taking the place of power. It is marvelous and our ingenuity is bounded only by
necessity. When the war is over and the story is told it will astound the world. If we
exhibit the same political ingenuity in the peace we may live in a better world, but, my
lack of faith in our political leaders is as weak as my faith in our industrial leaders is
strong. Christ said he came not upon earth to give peace but to show the way. All I have
to say on that is that He left the job to a poor bunch when politics supplanted statesman-
ship.   When I think of my grand kids and those of others I wish He had taken the job in His
own hands and endowed it with His great philosophy.
        There is n t much change in the ways of life of our social set. A change in
transportation and in menu but not much otherwise. Those who have earned their food by their
sweat are booming. The stores cannot supply their needs. They are for once saving some
money by having ten percent. takenout of their wages for the purchase of war bonds. Those
who live on income from invested capital are now obliged to use their capital because the
increase in the costs of living are based on war and not the peace when their incomes were
created. Interest rates goes down while vegetables and meat and clothes go up.
        Jimmy is some boy, he grows like a weed (but blossoms like a flower). He is full
of fun and laughs. Apparently appreciates a good story and likes a bottle. I predict great
things for him. Pat is the smartest thing you know and is etting worldly wise rapidly. Her
particular penchant is trying to grab match boxes, bu always gives sufficient notice by saying "Pat don't touch that match box" and then proceeds to make a rush for it. As soon as she
gets it she says "Mammy says no, Pat". She has the darndest vocabulary you ever heard and she
is very cute, correcting herself when she uses a wrong word.
        Anne and Brucie were down to have me go over their eyes last week because the
school wanted it done. Anne was a hundred percent. but Brucie had a slight near-sightedness.
Not much but enough to correct Her her studies and school work. The both look very husky ,
in fact Brucie is putting on some weight which will be a help to her.
        Well, more later.   Love from Ma

                                                and

163

Major John E. Bordley, M.C., 0-403012

General Hospital No. 118

A.P.O. 927, c/o Postmaster

San Francisco, California, U.S.A.

Mr. James Bordley, Jr.

330 N. Charles St.,

Baltimore 1, Maryland, U.S.A.

May 21st, 1943

Dear Boys,   Series II., No. 59

I can see a real change in this division of our nation. It has taken place in the past sixty days. To get a good back ground to have to visualize about 50% of the people without servants or at the least very inadequate help; then there is no one to cut 80% of the lawns; then everyone who owns or rents a lot is or has planted a garden, in many cases plowing up their lawns. The city is dirty and the streets should be turned over to the fish commissioner; whenever it rains there are more than sufficient pounds to raise the fish to supply the city. Of course that means no help and a limitation on effort demanded by the Unions. Persons with whom you discuss the situation show the first real worry, a sort of indefinable uneasiness not so much over the military as the civil. It is remarkable that it has taken a year for the populace to get wise to what they would have to contribute. They have found it out when they are called upon to pay two years' taxes in one, when they can't buy butter and meat and vegetables as they expected. It is a great strain but have no fear, there is an increasing desire to get the Germans and the Japs, this country will not tolerate any let down in the effort. We have a venomous snake to deal with, the Black Market. I am far from satisfied over Washington's attitude towards it, a bit suspicious of the remedies proposed by the Professors and the New Dealers. I would either put on a ceiling from consumer to producer or limit the food tickets to production. Both can be watched and the Black Market man will find a market beyond his competition.

I heard a great debate last night by a labor leader and a congressman. A bill has been introduced in Congress to prevent strikes again the Government -- think of having to introduce such legislation at this time. In the end it became a debate on John L. Lewis and at the close the labor leader castigated John Lewis. The applause was so strong in every attack made on John by the Congressman that I believe it unnerved the labor man. There is no doubt that any restrictive legislation against labor would meet with a hearty and an overwhelming reception by the nation. I am a believer in the union of labor and I fear the assininity of its leaders will set it back a generation. They are making the same mistakes made by industrial leaders -- trying to hog everything and entirely without an eye single to the common welfare. The public is slow to wrath but with overwhelming power when aroused.

We have an acute gasoline shortage on the Atlantic Seaboard. Not a drop for distribution in Maryland even for essential purposes. The management of the whole fuel problem has been rotten from start to finish. One day they say drive at your pleasure, the next day no gasoline. It is believed generally that gasoline is now being conserved for war purposes soon in continental Europe. This is speculation and not I think well founded although precisely lit it was before the North African campaign. Today the streets are almost free from automobiles.

We had a streak of luck yesterday when a very nice colored woman dropped in and took the job as maid. I may marry her!!

Fulton Leser was driven home by a taxi driver last night and Fulton asked him, for some reason to spend the night. When he left in the morning he carried away $8,000 worth of the Leser property.

More later. Love from Ma who thoroughly enjoyed John's cable for Mother's day.

Love

from

Lt. Col.James Bordley, III., M.C.

General Hospital No. 118

A.P.O. 927, c/o Postmaster

San Francisco, California, U.S.A.

Dr. James Bordley, Jr.

330 N. Charles St.,

Baltimore 1,Md., U.S.A.

May 24th, 1943

Dear Boys,   Series II., No. 60

Well little Jimmy is now legimately James Bordley, IV. The preacher fixed it up
yesterday in spite of a gasoline shortage that seriously reduced the numbers present.   It is
against the rules to use cars for any pleasure driving and while regular church services are
not on the ban, special church exercises are. The family could go but not the outside friends.
Think of the U.S. without gasoline for cars! Well that is exactly where we are. Mary Goodwin has been unable to practice medicine for several days and I suppose there are many others.
Doctors are given sufficient tickets for gas but there is none for sale in Baltimore sotickets
are of no use. I have made a habit of keeping my car filled up so I have enough for about a
week more. You should see the street car station at the bottom of our alley. Usually one or
two persons, now it looks like a New York subway station at 5 p.m. Many people drive from
the country and park near and walk to the station and the whole of Guilford is riding by
trolley. One first class hot dog stand and the whole complexion of our dignified suburb would
be altered.

Peggy, Chandler and Mr. Ross' nurse were down for the function yesterday. Pat needed
about four keepers. Her natural enthusiasm knows no bounds and we were a bit afraid she might
decide to drink the water before the baptismal service or make some suggestions to Mr. Baker.
She did very well however, nothing worse than roam around and make a few pertinent remarks.
All the grandchildren were there except Carroll. Ellen thought her duties as Godmother might
be interfered with too much, to my disappointment she was left at home. She is Pat plus when
it comes to human energy and force of personal decisions. Brucie was there with her dignity
and Anne with her cheerful smile. Charlie too, who suggested to Anne he would like to kiss
her and, she accepting, did. Altogether it was a very happy occasion for me and I am sure for
the balance of the family. The only blot was your absence. After the function all the cars
were left at the Church except those required to take the little party including the children
home. They all had to take the bus and go back for their cars after drinking the health and
happiness of Jimmy and his father.

The middle west is in the throes of a terrible flood, the worst in thirty years. It has
inundated about a million and a half acres of producing land which is the worst damage. A
few war plants have had to suspend but without material stoppage to the war effort.

We have an international food conference going on. The Government has bought the Hotel
at Hot Springs and it is there the conference is being held. There is too much secrecy
concerning its meetings including exclusion of the press and radio commentators. This is
poor stuff as it is this country which must carry the burden. Its people should know in
advance of our Government's commitments and decide whether they approve. It is too much like
the last peace treaty which they promptly upset. If we are to participate we should know in
advance of our responsibilities. We are believers in Democracy which means a voice in our
commitments.

More later. With love from Ma

and

Your

Major John E. Bordley, M.C., O-403012

General Hospital No. 118

A.P.O. 927, c/o Postmaster

San Francisco, California, U.S.A.

Dr. James Bordley, Jr.,

330 N. Charles St.,

Baltimore, Md., U.S.A.

May 26th, 1943

Dear Boys,   Series II., No. 61
        No gasoline for automobiles, no buses and only an occasional street-car. A strike
on the United Railways brought about by a fight between two rival unions and the refusal of
the Company to restore seven drivers who were caught driving busses and street cars while
drunk.   This strike is causing the loss of thousands of man hours work in all the war plants
and is one of the most outrageous and unpatriotic acts which have occurred in Baltimore since
the war started. It has greatly aroused the average citizen and is a blow to the ultimate aims
of organized labor. It has lost them thousands of friends who will take the first opportunity
to get even.   Already they are flooding their representatives in Congress with demands to
pass represive legislation and to rescind portions of the Wagner Act.   This move is getting
nation wide as one community after the other is subjected to the deviltry of the leaders.
At present half of the Chrysler Corporation's war work has stopped because the Union is dissatisfied with a Government ruling, 46,000 rubber workers have closed the three largest
rubber companies because, the Government would not permit a rise in the wage scale.   All
over the country similar outrages are taking place.   I stand now, as always, for a decent
wage and I stand as ever against the stinking, rotten, low-type leaders who have infiltrated
through the ranks of labor to fill their pockets with the hard earned wages of laboring men.
They are each and almost everyone small type Hitlers who are out for their own personal
advancement and to Hell with the toilers and with their nation!
        The President has coined: "No man has a right to strike against the Government in
time of war".   He should broaden it to: "No man has a right to strike against his country's
safety at any time".   Labor is the spoiled shild of the U.S. and a first class spanking is
right in order.
        The floods still take their toll and even here we are having extraordinary rains.
The weather man promises us to stop it this afternoon and with so many people walking it will
be very nice.
        Pat had a birthday party yesterday and was a very nice host, eating the choice
tit-bits of her guests and always insisting they have more.   A birthday cake was provided and
when she finished cutting and helping the only place not covered with icing and cake was the
seat of her britches. If anyone ever enjoyed a party she was the person.   They let Jimmy
in on it to the extent of lying on his belly on the floor and having his toes pulled by the
guests. He was in a gale and you might suppose he knew just what was going on.   His admira-
tion of pat is complete. If she is around you just waste your time trying to make him pay
attention to your feeble efforts to entertain him. He smiles or laughs at everything she
does.   In fact he is far more attentive to the little girls than the boys.   A sort of
early natural selection.
        The Kennels has requested its members not to come to the club in automobiles
and to obey the orders to conserve gasoline.   In Monday's paper there was quite an article
on the number of cars at Country Clubs, naming the Clubs. I suppose this is a reaction but
as there were only two cars at the Kennels I see no reason for reminding its members to
conserve. There were 87 at the Baltimore but as a great many people take their meals there
I think it probably not a very large number in fact.
        Well more later. Love from Ma
                            and
                    Your

Lt. Col. James Bordley, III.,M.C.

General Hospital No. 118

A.P.O. 927, c/o Postmaster

San Francisco, California, U.S.A.

Dr. James Bordley, Jr.,

330 N. Charles St.,

Baltimore, Md., U.S.A.

May 31, 1945

Series II., No. 62

Dear Boys,

Another minor triumph over in the Aleutians. Just a straw to show which way the war is going. There is a rapidly increasing expectation of collapse in Germany. I am not convinced how much the impression has gained from German propaganda and how much solid truth there is behind it. It ispoor policy not to try and counteract the impression because there may be a let down among our workers. I still believe that Germany is taking punishment that is desperately hard to stand but with nothing to lose and much to gain personally I am sure Hitler has no intention of stopping until he has shot his last cartridge which is some months away.

We still are in the throes of a street car and busstrike but only three hundred and fifty out of three thousand have struck. The vagabond three hundred and fifty are amusing themselves throwing bricks through car and bus windows and todate only one arrest. If the authorities really wished to catch more of course they could but it is the old story of votes and politicians and the spoiled child of Congress.

They published a decree today denying the right of automobilists to drive to the cemeteries on Decoration day. This gives you a good idea of the shortage which is apparently growing worse rapidly. So long as essentials are met I think it is a good lesson for our free and easy compatriots. It at last emphasises the war.

We just eceived Jim's letter telling us about the Hospital. It is evidently not the hospital as depicted in the New York Times, that was a ten story building built on lend lease by the Australians to be returned to them at the end of the war. It was full brick with what we judged an adminstration building, in the front, and a beautiful layout of help cottages in the rear. If you get a picture I would love to have it so I can show it to the doctors interested in the Unit. They all get a kick out of the activities of the Unit.

It is nice to know that we have taken another island away from the Japs. It may not be large bu its capture is helpful and its location bades no good for the Japs. England and the U.S. are certainly making life uncomfortable in Germany and Italy and they must have seriously interfered with war production. The rumor still persists that Italy wants to get out but I am sure it will only come through unconditional surrender. We made a mistake of that kind in 1918 and I don't believe we will repeat.

Our street car strike has not yet seriously interfered with production and from the looks of it I don't believe it will. The local A.F. of L. is trying to precipitate a general sympathetic strike but its suggestion has been turned down by the National Organization.

Our gasoline situat on is still pretty bad but getting alittle better. The food situation offers more obstacles and is very unsatisfactory. The President has just created another bureau of coordinate war and civil food problems. Bureaus are multiplying so fast that it is beyond an ordinary individual to fathom their functions. They interlock and duplicate so much that they create real confusion.

Well, I must run. It is a legal holiday today for everyone but war-workers and doctors.

Love from Mother and

Your

Major John E. Bordley, M.C. O-403012

General Hospital No. 118

A.P.O. 927, c/o Postmaster

San Francisco, California, U.S.A.

Dr. James Bordley, Jr.

330 N. Charles St.,

Baltimore, Md., U&S.A.

June 3, 1943.

SeriesII., No. 63

Dear Boys,

The summer has arrived. Following days and days of rain, we have suddenly dipped into a heat wave but it almost feels good after the bad humid time.

Well John L. Lewis has called another coal strike and if any man ever received a castigating in this land he is getting it deservedly so. Well it is just the cat coming back, this stage was prepared by the President years ago and while he now blames Lewis for the less the public has not forgotten his past.

There is a strange lack of real news to write you outside the war stories. This results from the enforced stay at home of most people after working hours and the dread of starting any kind of function not connected with war. People are critical, some from inability to follow Jones, others because they dread criticism. It is a good state of affairs because it tends to a greater concentration on the war in both thought and effort. Slowly we are becoming steeped in war and the reaction is helpful to production and personal economy both of which are essential if we are to be delivered whole out of this awful mess.

They are sticking poor Jimmy so full of stuff -- diptheria, whooping-cough, small-pox, etc. that I am afraid his blood may get mixed up when he contracts anything. He is a good sport though and takes it as it comes without complaint. He is getting better looking by the hour and if Pat does not watch out he will be just as good looking. He and I remain on excellent terms. Pat calls him "Jiminnee" and is very fond of him in fact a bit too affectionate at times to suit Jimmy's desires. Pat is the greatest talker you ever listened to. She never says Pat is going to fo thus and so, she always "You" are going to do, etc. It gets quite confusing at times because you are not sure whether it is a statement of facts or a request for action. If she uses a wrong word or pronounces it incorrectly she repeats it correctly. It really is very odd that she can realise the difference.

Brusie had a birthday the other day and was tickled pink to receive a cable from her father. She too is very careful. If you send her a little present she sits right down and writes you a very nice note and supplements that with a telephone call. I think it fine and it reminds me so much of her father.

More later. Love from Ma and

Your

P.S.Carn.amble,Sr. went over the Styx day before yesterday at 80 years.

Lt. Col. James Bordley, III., M.C.   Dr. James Bordley, Jr.

General Hospital No. 118   330 N. Charles St

A.P.O. 927, c/o Postmaster   Baltimore, Md., U.S.A.

San Francisco, California, U.S.A.
                                                       June 5, 1943.

Dear Boys,   Series II., No. 64
        The on again, off again coal strike is off again with no settlement of any dis-
puted point. Congress took a hand and both Senate and House have passed anti-strike legislature making it a $5,000 and one year in jail penalty for any labor leader to provoke a
strike against any industrial plant under Government control.   It also requires every
union to make a public declaration of its assets and income.   There are four other less
important provisions but it has teeth.   Personally, I do not believe the President will
sign it. Congress has the votes to override a veto but I don't believe it will, so as far
as I can see it is a major political bluff in a pre-election year.
        The President's social security plan has been introduced into Congress.   It istoo
long and too complicated to write about but it is just the resident's old whim of making
the industrious carry the lazy, preventing iniative, penalizing the smart and trying to bring
to a common level -- a lower average level. He says it does away with the necessity for
socialized medicine but it supplies the treatment and hospitilization under Government direction and if that is not socialized medicine it is its twin brother.   The worst feature of
the bill is that it was written and introduced by Senator Wagner whose labor bill is a curse
to the country, including labor and is largely responsible for our war labor difficulties.
I don't expect the Senator to be fair and just and long sighted.
        The four freedoms are to be the basis of our peace efforts as representative of wh
what we are told is the best in Democracy.   Freedom from fear and freedom from hunger by
Government direction and support are as far away from my idea of the American way as the
North Pole from the South Pole. It is fundamental that this country has prospered not from
Government help but by the energy and ambition of its people, from an opportunity to advance
their material welfare through their own foresight and energy.   Let the Government start out
on a campaign of freedom from want and we will merely duplicate the iniquities of the New
 eal when whole families of able bodied people laid down on the job and let the thrifty
support them.   If there had been a ew in each City or County it would not have been so bad
but in truth there were thousands, many of whom still hold out their hands in spite of the
greatest opportunity for profitable employment this nation has ever enjoyed.
        Jimmy and I are getting closer and closer and he is beginning to realize the
superior treatment he can expect at my hand.   This morning he was lying out in his cart
under the trees, theoretically to sleep and you never saw a wilder animal in a cage. I went
over to inquire for his health and he started doing stunts for my delectation and was so
pleased with his efforts that now and then he would stop and have a good laugh at himself.
If he had a long tail he could pose as a kitten.
            Well more later.   Love from Ma and
                        Your

Major John E. Bordley, M.C., 0-403012

General Hospital No. 118

A.P.O. 927, c/o Postmaster

San Francisco, California, U.S.A.

Dr. James Bordley, Jr.,

330 N. Charles St.,

Baltimore, Md, U.S.A.

June 7, 1943

Series II., No. 65

Dear Boys,

War is a darned inconvenient way to spend your time. The civilian population has to give up its golf. It is really funny to see the boys going out to the Club on the street car -- and that included me once a week or less. It is gratifying though never to hear a kick. Most of the men playing are engaged in war work and go out either Saturday or Sunday and there are not more than fifteen or twenty. The course is mowed by a pair of first class mules and a pretty good negro farm hand. The greens are taken care of by a one-eyed man and a super annuated gentleman. George Bennett, Richardson and a few others have volunteered for three hours a week to use a scythe on the rough. Our caddies are most the young sons and daughters of members who live close enough to ride on bicycles. It is increasingly hard to get balls and other necessaries. A nice patient of mine gave me two dozen balls -- not the best but perfectly serviceable. I really miss the exercise but if it is a contribution toward winning the war I am all for it. The grill is closed and the Club house is running with about four old men for help. There is not even a night watchman and the other day somebody broke in and carried off some hundreds of dollars worth of liquor which does not bother me as I never take a drink. The old digestion is not as good as it used to be.

It was announced in the press that Baltimore will be used as a port of debarkation for wounded troops as soon as we get busy in Europe. In fact it is being used for North Africa. Plans are made for taking over some of the larger hotels and everything is ready in the way of equipment. It is to be run by civilian doctors largely. I feel a keen intrest in doing my part so it makes a vacation doubtful. If we involved in a European drive and the casualities are coming in before August 1st I shall stay here and serve on a team, if not I will go away until I am needed I would not go at all but I feel for one of my age it would be folly not to stop completely and rest. I have worked very hard for a year (10 months) and while I feel fine I know what another year added on would do to me and I am convinced I will be needed even more the next twelve than the past twelve months.

Saturday was the mildest day professionally that I have had for many, many years. I thought travel difficulties and gasoline shortage had permanently slowed me down but today has convinced me it was only a pleasant dream.

Ellen Fisher is going off for a few days with the family. She needs the vacation and I am glad to see her go. She is not used to routine life and she hasbeen 100% faithful and I can realize that a break will help her.

Sis has had mumps in her house. None of her immediate family but her sister-in-law. The incubation period has passed and nothing wrong with her children. There has been very little mumms this year. I had one to drop in here for something else and one case of chicken-pox which was supposed to be a mild skin irritation following a cold. Except for our visiting population and the unsanitary conditions under which they live we would have had a season pretty free from contagion. We did have a burst of virus pneumonia, whether that resulted from more virus or from a better acquaintance with the disease I am not sure.

Well I am called away, so good-bye until the next time.

Love from Mother and

Your

Lt. Col. James Bordley,III.,MC.,O-396822

General Hospital 118,

A.P.O. 927, c/o Postmaster,

San Francisco, California, U.S.A.

Dr. James Bordley,Jr.

330 N. Charles St.,

Baltimore, Md., U.S.A.

June 12, 1943.

Dear Boys,   Series II., No. 66
        People in general have been making money so fast that it is disturbing the financial
balance of the country. A commentary on having everybody rich.
        Well one of the results is to increase real estate values, including Guilford. A
year ago you could not give away houses in Guilford now they are snapped up and the prices are
from twenty-five to fifty percent. higher than for the past ten years. Two people are after
our home and if either one meets my terms they can have it. I have no certainty either one
will take it as I am holding for a larger price than any property has sold since the depression. I am willing to sell because the house is too large for just mother and me, the taxes
are too high and the servant question too acute. Mother and I will take life more comfortably. I am having no dreams about our prospects, except a night-mare about where we will
place our wonderful collection of treasures. No apartment would hold a tenth.
        Well we are making mo. progress in Mr. Mussolini's lake. The pounding given that
little island must have been terrible. I wish we could do the same thing to the whole of
Germany and Japan. It would rid us of lots of parasites. The funny thing is that England
has gone soft on the bombing of German cities and there is a strong feeling I understand in
this country. To me it means the saving of thousands of allied lives and the destruction of
a group of people who for centuries have been in the middle of every great war in Europe. How
can anyone give birth to the idea that Germany should be treated with less severity than she
has dealt out to her enemies. We cantoo well remember how lack of punishment of that nation
started this war. The only language the Germans understand is brute force, their philosophy
of life is predicated on that assumption so why argue morals with such wild beasts. Christ
said he came into this world not to bring peace but to show us how to get it and if we cannot
read His handwriting on the wall it is just too bad, if we really want no more wars. Maybe
we have over-developed our humanity. When I think how we lavished money on the Japs after
their earthquake and loaned billions to Germany to rebuild her war machine I am pretty sure
we have. We are starting out with our four freedoms as a basis for peace, we should add
another one: freedom to work out your own salvation, financial political and social. It is
the basis of our democracy and the reason we are great. I have little sympathy for the senti-
mentality of our Vice-President who would have us put a quart of milk in every door-way. It
smacks too much of the paternalism we are fighting to destroy and calls back the unpleasant
picture of our P.W.A. Let every man sail his own ship and every nation work out its own
destiny. If we start otherwise we will find ourselves surrounded with ingrates and enemies.
Giving is a dangerous procedure among individuals, it is worse among nations.
        Dudy took Pat to Philadelphia for a long week end. Her father and mother go to
the Adirondacks next week and Dudy follows the second week of July, Jimmy stayed home to keep
me company. He is getting bossy with me and is due for a real shake down. His teeth are
coming and his mouth is pretty uncomfortable but not as bad as his stomach about meal times.
He eats like a horse.
            Well more later. Love from Mother and
                            Your

Major John E. Bordley, M.C., 0-403012

General Hospital No. 118

A.P.O. 927, c/o Postmaster

San Francisco, California, U.S.A.

Dr. James Bordley, Jr.,

330 N. Charles St.,

Baltimore, Md., U.S.A.

June 14, 1943.

Series II., No. 67

Dear Boys,

    Good old summertime has arrived and it is now the custom to discuss the comparative heat of this and the last war and I know no one in a better position to discuss it than the Italian Duce (short for Jackass). We are certainly putting the screws on him. One of the best informed men I know says the Italian will soon give up. I hope so but I afraid the Germans will have too much to say about it. What I have been afraid of has happened; Congress was driven to passing repressive legislation against the labor unions. It is all the fault of such leaders as John L. Lewis. Until they purge themselves of such tripe they can expect nothing better. It is debatable whether the President will sign the law but it is generally believed he will be unable to find a way out. In the end it may show labor its proper position and responsibility. I hope so. I am sure the leaders will try and make them do some foolish things because the legislation is directed at the leaders and it will be their defense. The Government is getting properly tough on the politicians who have flagrantly disobeyed the rules in gasoline conservation. Our State Comptroller of the Treasury has had his tickets taken away for a year for going off on a joy ride to Georgia and our Governor's wife has been asked to explain a trip she took (for her health) to South Carolina, to the Gardens in Charleston. Her modest request was for 2,700 gallons a month (mine and most other doctors is for 450). The Board cut it down to 1,200 and there is such a public protest she may lose it entirely. I hope so. If I cannot drive two miles to the gold club for much needed diversion, why should she joy ride to South Carolina?

    I am still very busy. Operations, office and house visits leave me little time for recreation and rest. I have not been in bed later than six thirty for weeks and seldom get to bed before eleven. I ordered reservations today for Rye Beach the last of July and if the Government lets me travel I am going. I am too tired to argue against going.

    The Hospitals are rushed to death. To get a room is about as hard as getting the King's suite in Buckingham Palace. The U.M.H. has only six internes and when I operated there on Friday six operating rooms were going full tilt. Thismorning four. At the end of this month it is doubtful whether there will be any internes or residents. This is very bad but the ManPower Board of the Government Can8t be made to see it.

    It is interesting to see the gardens of the Victory Army. They are literally all over the City and will, weather permitting, go a long way toward supplying needed food. Indeed we might have been up against a serious problem and may still be. The Government's Handling of foods has been extremely poor. Like in most of the civilian activities nothing was done until trouble was so apparent it could not be avoided. Just the good old way of politicians and believe me this country is filled with such lice.

    Nothing to write about home, we are well and send love.

                      Your

Lt. Col. James Bordley,III.,M.C.O-396822   Dr. James Bordley,Jr.

General Hospital No. 118   330 N. Charles St.,

A.P.O. 927, c/o Postmaster   Baltimore, Md., U.S.A.

San Francisco, California, U.S.A.

                                              June 18, 1943

Dear Boys,   Series II., No.68

        Things are moving along at a rapid pace. The food conservation, gas saving, troop
movements and our home life changes keep every one on the job.   Some dissatisfaction but
this is over-balanced by a real desire to help promote the war plans. Of course the labor
situation is far from satisfactory and just what will result from the new labor laws is hard
to determine.   The President has not yet signed them but it is currently believed he cannot
resist the public clamor. I am sorry labor has given the President small choice and how
ungrateful for the stupendous service he has rendered.   I have always felt that he has not
placed sufficient safe-guards against ambition labor leaders.
        There is a probability that I may get a purchaser for our home.   Tentatively
mother and I have decided if we do and can get Dr. Gamble's apartment we will take it. I have
some yet undeveloped plans about the use of his offices which I will know more about later.
If I sell I shall re-organize our lives and take things easy for the balance of my short span.
I shall always have some serious occupation but it will be measured by my own desires.   I
always intended to retire at sixty-five but circumstances prevented that.   I think seventy
none too soon.   Dr. Osler told me years ago that the time would surely come and to prepare
for it by developing some congenial hobby. I always took his advice seriously.
        The hospitals are having a bad time and making as many rules as the Food Administra-
tion. They are really essential. Such as: Nose and throat operations must be performed and
without interne assistance after one-thirty; no operation can be posted before 8.00 a.m.;
a complete physical must come in with the patient, including laboratory tests or the patient
must enter before 10.00 a.m. the day before operation and eventhen no special examination
can be made such as X-rays, blood, etc. These are only samples of a very long list.   In our
work this means more expense to the patient because physicals must be done by outside in-
ternists and laboratories.   The hospitals have been so depleted of man and woman power --
a most unnecessary thing -- that conservation is essential.
        The Food Administration is working out a five-year plan for food conservation.
In my judgment the day war ends the hue and cry of the public will be for lifting of all
bans on restrictions without a far better scheme is presented than anything yet suggested.
I don't believe the American public has the slightest intention of supplying world deficiencies.   Our war debt and taxes plus the essential restructions required will be a large
burden and it will take a genius to sell it to the public and I know no geniuses in American
politics.
                    More later.   Love from Ma and
                                        Your

173

Lt. Col. James Bordley,III.,M.C.O-396822   Dr. James Bordley,Jr.

General Hospital No. 118   330 N. Charles St.,

A.P.O. 927, c/o Postmaster   Baltimore, Md., U.S.A.

San Francisco, California, U.S.A.

                                             June 18, 1943

Dear Boys,   Series II., No.68

    Things are moving along at a rapid pace. The food conservation, gas saving, troop movements and our home life changes keep every one on the job. Some dissatisfaction but this is over-balanced by a real desire to help promote the war plans. Of course the labor situation is far from satisfactory and just what will result from the new labor laws is hard to determine. The President has not yet signed them but it is currently believed he cannot resist the public clamor. I am sorry labor has given the President small choice and how ungrateful for the stupendous service he has rendered. I have always felt that he has not placed sufficient safe-guards against ambition labor leaders.

    There is a probability that I may get a purchaser for our home. Tentatively mother and I have decided if we do and can get Dr. Gamble's apartment we will take it. I have some yet undeveloped plans about the use of his offices which I will know more about later. If I sell I shall re-organize our lives and take things easy for the balance of my short span. I shall always have some serious occupation but it will be measured by my own desires. I always intended to retire at sixty-five but circumstances prevented that. I think seventy none too soon. Dr. Osler told me years ago that the time would surely come and to prepare for it by developing some congenial hobby. I always took his advice seriously.

    The hospitals are having a bad time and making as many rules as the Food Administration. They are really essential. Such as: Nose and throat operations must be performed and without interne assistance after one-thirty; no operation can be posted before 8.00 a.m.; a complete physical must come in with the patient, including laboratory tests, or the patient must enter before 10.00 a.m. the day before operation and eventhen no special examination can be made such as X-rays, blood, etc. These are only samples of a very long list. In our work this means more expense to the patient because physicals must be done by outside internists and laboratories. The hospitals have been so depleted of man and woman power -- a most unnecessary thing -- that conservation is essential.

    The Food Administration is working out a five-year plan for food conservation. In my judgment the day war ends the hue and cry of the public will be for lifting of all bans on restrictions without a far better scheme is presented than anything yet suggested. I don't believe the American public has the slightest intention of supplying world deficiencies. Our war debt and taxes plus the essential restructions required will be a large burden and it will take a genius to sell it to the public and I know no geniuses in American politics.

    More later.   Love from Ma and

                Your

174

Lt. Col. James Bordley,III.,M.C.,O-396822

General Hospital No.118

A.P.O. 927, c/o Postmaster

San Francisco, Californiam U.S.A.

Dr. James Bordley, Jr.

330 N. Charles St.,

Baltimore - 1, Md.,U.S.A.

June 28, 1943.

Dear Boys,

Series II., No. 72

Hoot Mon!!! For some 17 days the weather man has treated us rough. Temperrture every day 95° or over. This is June's record breaker. The kids are thriving in it and Dudy is picking up weight. I confess I have had to pant a couple of times but have not really suffered much. We had a sort of family reunion yesterday, with our home crowd was Charles,Jr. Catherine and Ann. We sat out under the trees in the back yard and in spite of the heat we had a fairbreeze and in the end a very small shower. The girls all had a mint julep but Pop drank ginger ale (and kept cooler).

Jimmy grows more and more cute end big. He is a good natured fellow and was captivated by Charlie, as was Pat. I had to go out in the country to see a patient in the morning so stuck two small seats on back of the regular seat and took Pat and Charlie. It is a real treat for them to get in an automobile and they sang songs and had a high old time -- and so did I. My grandchildren are my real joy now-a-days and they make me one of them -- mostly the burden bearing ass.

Ellen and the children are due back today. I am afraid they had an uncomfortable time but probably not as bad as I think. When I was their age I lived on the Eastern Shore but if it was hot I was seldom aware of it except when a parent thought it a good excuse to make me stay home when I had something on hand.

I operated again in the office on a crossed eye. It is hopeless to try and get in a hospital. More hopeless still to get an anaesthetist.

I went out to the Club Saturday to play a few holes of golf. From the second tee I was called to see the Chef. Fortunately I declined, thereby saving his life. It was a hot day and the man passed out supposedly from heat. As a matter of fact in lifting something in the morning he brought on a supture which he did not appreciate -- because it did not hurt, in three hours it was strangulated and that was why hepassed out. Lay Martin was there insisting on making a careful examination,he discovered the hernia and the man was sent to the U.M.H. for immediate operation. For once it paid me not to stick my nose into somebody else's business and it also saved me much future embarrassment.

The propaganda man says we should not write our sons any of the complications and difficulties of the home government. What do you think? It strikes me you have a greater strength in this country than ever before and that you experience a vital interest you never before felt. If I am correct I am glad I have written you thestory of the successes and failures as I have observed them. Of course I have no inside information to divulge, what I write is common knowledge, so, why should I try to paint a false picture and why should the facts be hidden from the men who fight our battles. It doesn't make sense. He probably doesn't want the armed forces to know an American citizen who harbored a German soldier is to be hanged while John L. Lewis who has almost completely upset our war plans is strutting around the country laughing at the weakness of our Government for not hanging him. That does not make sense either, so the Government has been told by am overwhelming majority of our people. Write me your ideas.

Love from Mother and

Your

Major John E. Bordley, M.C., O-403012

General Hospital No. 118

A.P.O. 927, c/o Postmaster

San Francisco, California, U.S.A.

Dr. James Bordley, Jr.

330 N. Charles St.,

Baltimore -1, Md., U.S.A.

July 1, 1943

Series II., No. 73

Dear Boys,

Well Ellen is back on the job and says she had a nice vacation and the kids had a good time. No complaint against the heat.

Today is positively cold. A rain yesterday and a drop of forty degrees in in temperature. We can really do weather stunts in and about here. What a day for a golf game, even by street-car, but I will not need such conveyance as I have a patient that carries me by the gate which makes the use of my car legitimate. Unfortunately I cannot find anyone to play with.

The Barkers are looking for an increase in their family in September. Polly has had not a single person to help her for months but she keeps on producing just the same. The twins are so wild that no help will stay. They have put in and done all the work on a lovely Victory garden. How they can find the time I cannot understand. I understand his father is in a desperate way with a face cancer and he has to go there twice a week.

Johnnie will not know his Papa Fisher when he gets back. He is developing a new paid of ears. I had him get a hearing device but his hearing started to improve before it came, not only in his voice bearing low voices at 25 ft. with his back turned, but his audiomster test shows a uniform improvement of about 20 decibels. He is delighted and seldom uses his hearing device. I have outfitted his brother also with the audiear with some success. I am trying to get the family straightened out, coming your return.

The political pot is boiling: now a fight between Wallace and Jesse Jones. The Vice-President spoke out of turn and the repercussions are loud and many. It is rumored that the President and Voce-President are manouvering for position for the next election and the attack on Jones was to discourage the President. It is disgraceful.

Dudy is packing to go to the Adirondacks on Monday. We will miss them very much. Ma and I are going away ourselves on the 27th. I am tired especially of the difficulties attending operations and hospital practice. Of course, the operative side of my work is booming now it is difficult to get in hospitals. I believe the U.N.H. will have to partially close before long. The Army is taking three more internes it promised not to disturb. This almost completes a clean up, in my judgment it is unnecessary and very harmful. It has been functioning with only six for sometime. The hospital aides have done much to save our hospitals but of course they can help only in the non-technical branches. They are faithful and work long and hard.

More later.   Love from Ma and

Your

176

Lt.Col. James Bordley,III.,M.C.,0-396822

General Hospital No. 118

A.P.O. 927, c/o Postmaster

San Francisco, California,U.S.A.

Dr. James Bordley, Jr.,

330 N. Charles St.,

Baltimore -1, Md., U.S.A.

July 7, 1943

Series II., No. 74

Dear Boys,

Well the Fourth has come and gone and I got two days' rest, the longest period since last September. I really needed the stop.

This week I operate practically every day and already we are booking operations for next week. Boy they are certainly coming in and Pop loses some enthusiasm each day. I guess I am getting lazy.

Dudy and the kids left yesterday for New York. We are going to miss them very much but are sure the mountains will be fine for them. Pat was as anxious for a train ride as a child twelve years old. She is in fact a wise old lady. Jimmy is as cute as possible and growing like corn after a warm rain.

The weather has been wonderful for July but the rain deficient. The combination never suits mortal man. I had my car parked in front of the home of a patient yesterday and the cops took my number for pleasure driving. Well it was a charity patient who cost me about a dollar in gas, oil and tires. I told him if he thought that was pleasure he should follow me around for a couple of days. So far nothing has happened and I don't think will. I drove out Charles St. and not a single car did I see either in front of, or, behind me the whole way to Lake Ave. They arrested a woman for having her car parked near a movie house. Two of the tires and the battery were stolen out of it last November and it was parked on her property. The only penalty is taking away her gasoline ration tickets. She can buy neither tires nor battery so the penalty is not particularly severe.

The Jap beetles are back with us but they were two weeks later and have not been as numerous or destructive as last year. A new poison has been developed to destroy them. The work has been carried out by one of the entomologists at the Maryland University and the experiments are being tried out at Elkridge. They capture the worm from the soil before it breaks through, grind it up and infect it with a certain type of bacteria and it is then injected into live Jap beetles and they are sent out to infect their friends. They also make a sort of mulch of the same stuff which is spread on the ground and it kills the little devils by the thousands. The idea is to destroy them in large numbers before they go back into the soil for winter sports. They hope this will eradicate them in a few years. The only trouble I see with the scheme is that the beetles are in every field, woods and garden. It will take an immense quantity of the poison and an army of workers. It is claimed they will never reappear in the area treated.

Since I started this we have had a wonderful rain which I hope will augment our rapidly dwindling water supply. We have some 320,000 strangers here and using vast quantities of water (some of them show little signs of that use) and the voters authorized a new compound and filtration plant, taking the water from the upper Patapsco river. It is to cost $12,000,000 but will not be completed for a couple of years so it will be of little help for this emergency. I think there is a lot of bunco in the continual talk about a water shortage. A few years ago we had not a drop of rain from April to Sept. and always enough water for ordinary needs, this year we had abundant early rains and all the wells, springs and streams are full. The trouble now is that we had 19 days of temperature over 94° and there was tremendous evaporation as well as extra use. Since then it has been too cold even to take a bath (for many).

More later. Love from Ma and

Your

Major John E. Bordley, M.C. 0-403012

General Hospital 118

A.P.O. 927, c/o Postmaster

San Francisco, California, U.S.A.

Dr. James Bordley, Jr.

330 N. Charles St.,

Baltimore, 18,Md.,,U.S.A.

July 9, 1943

Series II., No. 75

Dear Boys,

Well, Congress has adjourned for a vacation, the first in three years. It voted some hundred and fifty billions of dollars, most of it for the war and most of the balance for the New Deal tricks. It showed, toward the end, an independence not before exhibited since the establishment of the Roosevelt dynasty, even had the nerve to override a veto.

Most of the present administration seems to have lost sight of the fact that Democracy is only a partnership and that every man and woman should pull his weight or not enjoy the blessings incident to Democracy -- making allowances for the mentally and physically incapable. The New Deal has set apart a portion of the population to support the balance. This does a two-fold damage: It makes bums and loafers out of a huge mass of people and it discourages individual enterprise. Of course, the foundation of the New Deal is politics and uncontrolled politicians are mainly to blame for the present world chaos, the New Deal adding its bit. My fear of the coming peace is the division in this country brought about by two parties. I believe in two parties but in their union on foreign policy. As I view the present sutuation, no matter what policy is advocated by the Government it will be opposed willy nilly by the Republican party. There has been no evidence of a meeting of minds on post war questions. The Administration has never been candid with the country and today in spite of persistent urgings by the most able men we have no indication has been given of its post war aims. Wendell Wilkie is correct when he says to the Government "Define your aims and lets argue them out before we go to the peace table so we can know what our Nation wants." If this is not done we will be impotent as a final factor. We have t ings rolling now and the end while not in sight is not so far away that we should not begin to think of the implications of peace upon our body politic. I was opposed to the injection of peace before our war machine was ready. It is now ready and for what do we wish it to fight? To destroy Hitler and Hirohito is a small part of what should be our program. World order, honor among nations, a willingness to sacrifice for the sake of the well being of mankind are more important.

I have just heard a most interesting story about our new plane with only wings, and double the load capacity of the Mars. A bomber being built for a special purpose. Gen.Wilson told over the radio last night about a new fighter which is just coming off the assembly line. It must be a wonderful fighter. The wingless bomber is an entirely new thing in aeronautical engineering and has its power plant so distributed that it will be almost impossible to seriously cripple it. Donald Nelson told us last night that by Fall this country and Canada together will be making a new airplane every $4\frac{1}{2}$ minutes. If they can find the boys to fly them what a sensation is in store for Germany and Japan. Remember the planes coming off the line now are much greater in weight, fighting power and engine capacity than those of even two months ago. The new gasoline has made much of this possible.

We have had too much loafing but at the same time we have done a tremendous job the size of which I had no realization until I heard the facts from Donald Nelson.

There has been a sharp let down in the office in the last few days but an increase in outside work. I am glad for the change.

More later. Love from Ma and

Your

Lt.COl. James Bordley,III.,M.C. O-396822

General Hospital 118

A.P.O. 927, c/o Postmaster

San Francisco, California, U.S.A.

Dr. James Bordley, Jr.

350 N. Charles St.,

Baltimore - 1, Md.,U.S.A.

July 12, 1943

Series II., No. 76

Dear Boys,

We are all excited over the attack on Sicily. It must have been a remarkable picture: The two thousand ships and hundreds of planes, the tremendous bombardment and the paratroopers landing everywhere. My, I hope it all goes well, it means so much to the whole world.

What a different picture from last year when the Axis was sweeping all before it,when we were taking it and they were giving it. What a fool -- to say nothing of his being a scoundrel -- Hitler has been. He could have won the war long ago if he had gone to England but now the last chapter in his career is being written by those for whom he expressed the greatest contempt. We will have a hard fight but we are prepared for it.

The Curtiss-Wright Company is in Dutch. An investigation shows they have been using defective materials and installing defective engines and worse they have been protected by the Army Inspection which tried first to block the investigation and then falsified reports. It is a dirty stink. Glenn Martin'e B-26 is not to be manufactured as a result of the necessity for super training of pilots. Its high speed landing has taken too large a toll of pilots. Martin has been commissioned to make the largest bombers yet produced --p the one with wings only. He will continue to make the Baltimore for England and the Navy plane (rated the best plane yet built). Plane manufacture has had a great over all success and is going ahead by leaps and bounds.

Perrin Long has been put at the head of Army Medicine in Africa. Got his appointment a few days ago and the papers are full of praise. I was very glad to hear he is appreciated.

Staige Davis' boy (in the Navy) got a submarine the other day and the Navy sent the pictures to the Sun. I heard last night that since then he has discovered and destroyed another. He is on "Navy Patrol off the South Atlantic Coast". I called Staige up to congratulate him and you could hear him smile over the phone. He comes from an Army ancestry and I think he wanted Howland in the Army but is now perfectly satisfie.

Had a card from Dudy saying she and the kids arrived after a very comfo table trip and that everything is going along very well.

We had a full day of rain yesterday and the Gunpowder dam is about full again. We need the rain for the crops and it was sufficient.

Ma and I were sitting in the Library last night and at 10.29 we heard a sharp crack and the Library light almost went out. This morning an earthquake was reported by the Fordham Observatory and the exact time. There is no mention of it otherwise.

More later. Love from Ma and

Your

9 β ..

July 16, 1943

Dear Boys,

Dr. Barker died day before yesterday, I have none of the particulars so can tell you little. He was a very unusual man, or more correctly he had a very unusual mind. I had the opportunity to watch his career from his first appointment. He started a real scientist with tremendous application. He was not very original but amassed a large stock of knowledge. He was on his way fast when he suddenly found himself in big money. You know what happens to most men who are bitten by that bug and he had no immunity. The Baltimore Sun said editorially that he had the instincts of a fine family doctor with an unusually broad knowledge of medicine in all of its specialities which made him a wise advisor. He was not my idea of a family doctor. I sort of never forgave him for giving up what promised to be a brilliant medical career, a constructive career, but, maybe, he realized his lack for original research.

One by one my contemporaries are departing but most of them could have little regret because their lives were filled with usefulness, most of them made the most of their abilities and opportunities.

We are still having a cat and dog time over in Washington. The President yesterday fired the Vice-President and Jesse Jones from the Commodities Corporation for calling each other slackers and liars. That is only a sample. The day before the deputy director of OPA, the retail sales crowd, resigned because he claims that body has prepared and is now putting in action a plan for the Government to siege and run all business and that none of his protests has in any way changed their policy. He had just been asked by the President to become General Manager of OPA and is probably one of the ablest men in Washington. It has caused a stink.

I got a ticket for stopping at the Elkridge in my car on July 5th. The case has not been settled. I had asked the Rationing Board whether if I were called to see a patient beyond the Club whether it would be permissable for me to stop at the Club and play golf. I was informed that I could. I had a patient beyond so stopped and was reported by the police. The punishment is to take away all or a portion of gasoline ration tickets. The joke is that I was given a book to expire on Feb. 2nd and on July 12th I used the last ticket. I have traveled on street cars more in the past ten months than in the preceding sixteen years just to save gasoline, not because I had to but because I wanted to. Tom, Dick and Harry are given "C" books, the highest rating, because they are war workers. Most of this gas is used for pleasure. I hear many of these tickets are sold at $1. a piece and that you can buy all the bootleg gas you want at 30¢ a gallon. Then they come along and cite me for doing what they gave me permission to do. It just does not make sense.

Ned Broyles' family have gone to Rye Beach for the summer. Ned is going away and will get two weeks the first of August and expects to go up. He has been home off and on all summer. His sister-in-law, Miss Whitely has a beautiful Victory Garden on her front lawn and as she has gone away and Ned's family have gone only Menges, their driver, is left and boy will he have a lot of nice cheap food. Miss Whitely has sold her house to one of the Wickes' girls and vacates in September.

Ames' death leaves his home vacant and I understand it is to be sold. Mrs. McPhail, our neighbor, has sold her home to a person whom they say is not --- but he certainly looks like he is and so do his children. You see our neighborhood is due for a real shake up. Same Crowe spends a very large portion of his time on our preserve -- at a neighbors.

Well we have a new kind of Income Tax. You are certainly lucky to be down in Australia and I may join you. Life has grown so complicated with the rules and regulations that I bet when you fellows come home you will insist on a thorough house cleaning. Maybe we will never be free again from dictation but I hope its authors will be made to see our difficulties. I am not kicking, I am only regretting.

Wendell Wilkie announced yesterday he will be a candidate. Thank God. He is the one man with both feet on the ground. He will take his contest to the Illinois primary and has invited that old varmint McCormick of Chicago Tribune to come in the fight

9 B̄ᵗ̄ʰ

Dear Boys,

Dr. Barker died day before yesterday, I have none of the particulars so can tell
you little. He was a very unusual man, or more correctly he had a very unusual mind.
I had the opportunity to watch his career from his first appointment. He started a real
scientist with tremendous application. He was not very original but amassed a large stock of
knowledge. He was on his way fast when he suddenly found himself in big money. You know
what happens to most men who are bitten by that bug and he had no immunity. The Baltimore
Sun said editorially that he had the instincts of a fine family doctor with an unusually
broad knowledge of medicine in all of its specialities which made him a wise advisor. He was
not my idea of a family doctor. I sort of never forgave him for giving up what promised to
be a brilliant medical career, a constructive career, but, maybe, he realized his lack for
original research.

One by one my contemporaries are departing but most of them could have little
regret because their lives were filled with usefulness, most of them made the most of their
abilities and opportunities.

We are still having a cat and dog time over in Washington. The President yesterday
fired the Vice-President and Jesse Jones from the Commodities Corporation for calling each
other slackers and liars. That is only a sample. The day before the deputy director of
OPA, the retail sales crowd, resigned because he claims that body has prepared and is now
putting in action a plan for the Government to siege and run all business and that none of
his protests has in any way changed their policy. He had just been asked by the President
to become General Manager of OPA and is probably one of the ablest men in Washington.
It has caused a stink.

I got a ticket for stopping at the Elkridge in my car on July 5th. The case
has not been settled. I had asked the Rationing Board whether if I were called to see a
patient beyond the Club whether it would be permissable for me to stop at the Club and play
golf. I was informed that I could. I had a patient beyond so stopped and was reported
by the police. The punishment is to take away all or a portion of gasoline ration tickets.
The joke is that I was given a book to expire on Feb. 2nd and on July 12th I used the
last ticket. I have traveled on street cars more in the past ten months than in the preceding sixteen years just to save gasoline, not because I had to but because I wanted to.
Tom, Dick and Harry are given "C" books, the highest rating, because they are war workers.
Most of this gas is used for pleasure. I hear many of these tickets are sold at $1. a piece
and that you can buy all the bootleg gas you want at 30¢ a gallon. Then they come along and
cite me for doing what they gave me permission to do. It just does not make sense.

Ned Broyles' family have gone to Rye Beach for the summer. Ned is going away
and will get two weeks the first of August and expects to go up. He has been home off and on
all summer. His sister-in-law, Miss Whitely has a beautiful Victory Garden on her front
lawn and as she has gone away and Ned's family have gone only Menges, their driver, is left
and boy will he have a lot of nice cheap food. Miss Whitely has sold her house to one of
the Wickes' girls and vacates in September.

Ames' death leaves his home vacant and I understand it is to be sold. Mrs.
McPhail, our neighbor, has sold her home to a person whom they say is not --- but he
certainly looks like he is and so do his children. You see our neighborhood is due for a
real shake up. Same Crowe spends a very large portion of his time on our preserve --
at a neighbors.

Well we have a new kind of Income Tax. You are certainly lucky to be down in
Australia and I may join you. Life has grown so complicated with the rules and regulations
that I bet when you fellows come home you will insist on a thorough house cleaning. Maybe
we will never be free again from dictation but I hope its authors will be made to see our
difficulties. I am not kicking, I am only regretting.

Wendell Wilkie announced yesterday he will be a candidate. Thank God. He
is the one man with both feet on the ground. He will take his contest to the Illinois
primary and has invited that old varmint McCormick of Chicago Tribune to come in the fight

as a means of determining whether the people of that State are willing to follow the Tribune's lead of isolation. The old fox (or rattle snake) will never accept the invitation.

I am enclosing a letter from the Hopkins to Jim. I suppose I am correct in forwarding it.

More later.   Love from Ma and
Your

Major John E. Bordley, .C. O-403012

General Hospital 118

A.P.O. 927, c/o Postmaster

San Francisco, California, U.S.A.

Dr. James Bordley, Jr.

330 N. Charles St.,

Baltimore -1, Md., U.S.A.

July 17, 1943.

Dear Boys,   Series II., No.78

The war do move!   It is wonderful how how that things are moving that we can win
all the major contests.   The great victories in the Solomons, the Mediterranean cleared of
Nazis, Russia slugging hell out of Hitler, the air pounding of the continent and most important the end of the Submarine menace by the baby air-plane carriers. Of course, there will
be hard fighting ahead and only too many casualties but we are out to win and nothing else
counts.   The advice given the Italians to quit before they are annihilated was the most
sound advice given anyone by the President.   I suppose it will not have any open signifi-
cance but I do believe under the ground it will inspire effort I hope and that will be
revolutionary and helpful. Yesterday the baby air-plane carrier B met a pack of eleven
submarines and destroyed them   There is a rumor coming from Norway that many of the submarine crews have struck, officers and men, and that many more are coming in for "repairs"
and find it impossible to get conditioned for weeks. This sounds like the end of the last
war but it may be only inspired rumor.

Worthington will see you before long he writes. He has not been able to get
leave yet to visit your hospital but expects it soon.   So far as we know Beale is still in
England and Madison in Boston, or, perhaps on the Pacific Coast.

Had quite an experience yesterday. Ellen brought Carroll to spend the afternoon
with Ma.   She took a nap in our room and locked herself in.   Ma went to get her up and
could not get in the room.   I came in about that time and went up to help her.   Carroll
is bright or she would still be there. We explained to her how to turn the key but she could
not do it. So she took the key out of the lock and started it under the door. I hammered a
wedge under the door and dragged the key through only to find she had bolted herself in and I
knew how tight the bolt was. I asked her to look for the bolt and press it back. She found
it and said"I can't move it and I ain't going to try any more because it hurts my finger."   I
persuaded her to go in my bath-room and get my wash cloth and tie it around her hand. She
was smart enough to do it and worked hard until she slid the bolt. It was a relief because I
was just getting ready to send for the fire company and have them get in the window.   When
she came out I told her what a dreadful thing she had done and asked her what would have
happened to her if she could not have gotten out for food. Her reply was on the moment;
"I guess I would have grown thin".   I thought that was pretty smart. She was not frightened
one bit.

More later.   Love from Ma and
                          Your

Lt.Col.James Bordley,III.,M.C. 0-396822   Dr. James Bordley,Jr.

General Hospital 118

A.P.O. 927, c/o Postmaster   330 N. Charles St

SanFrancisco, California, U.S.A.   Baltimore -1, Md.,U.S.A.

                                                July 27, 1943.

Dear Boys,   Series II., No. 79
        I was derelict in my duty last week but to tell you the truth some Jackass announced
in the society column that mother and I were leaving for the balance of the summer and then the
rush was on. I am glad to go tomorrow because I am mentally tired out. This has been a strenuous year both in and out of the office. Mr. Ross, of course you know died last week. Ellen
saw Chandler and he told her that his father had a terrific attack of angina and died in it.
I think Dudy was not told of his intense suffering. He was buried from Philadelphia Saturday
but I could not go up because of the large number of out of town patients whom I had to see.
I wrote Mrs. Ross and Ellen Fisher took it to her and brought me back word from Dudy not to
think of going up as they had no conveyance for meeting us and the house would be full of relatives. Maybe Mrs. Ross relieved of her work and anxiety will pick up in health and strength.
She has had too much responsibility.   Old Sawdust Ceasar has at last been thrown
in the ash can. What an end for the Emperor of Africa and the Mediterranean. After all he
was just another man playing the old con game, the same old stunt to enrich the insiders at
the expense of the populace. The trouble with him was that he started believing his own lies.
Well he will stain any page of history where he appears and he thought he would be the golden
edge of all. He did and could have continued doing fine things for the physical aspects of his
country if he had not forgott n the souls of his people. He should have known that no political
scheme was ever successful without it came from the hearts and souls of th people incolved. It
is a breake for our side and a blow to Hitler's. The Germans w ll not be far behind. An un-
willing mass of them are taking terrific punishment and they are not supermen, in fact damn puny.
I am anxious to see what the reaction of Mussolini's downfall will have upon Hirohito's monkeys.
I don't know them well enough to form an estimate. They must realise that it brings them much
nearer to the centre of our might.   We were disturbed by certain remors that 118 was losing
medical personnel. On inuiry of the Surgeon General we were assured the base was to be expanded
to 1,000 beds andthat the personnel withdrawal was temporary I am wondering how much he actually
has to do with it. In the last war his office only supplied medical assistance abroad on General
Pershing's requisition. Maybe now it will be the same with General MacArthur. That was my job
in the last war so I know.   Wilkie is gaining by leaps and bounds in all the recent polls
some 65% in the last one. He was out with some observations on the negro question yesterday.
They were quite correct and fair. Summed up it amounted to inadequate housing and no political
status.   I ventured to write another letter for the Sun -- Sunday. I wrote about the
necessity for viewing the peace as both political and economical. That no plan could be adequately formulated nor carried into execution without proper men were given th task. I proposed that the people have their platform for the coming election and that platform to be one
plank -- whom they wished to represent them at the peace negotiations. I called to mind the
entire fulfillment of butone peace after any war in which we were involved and that plan represented years of study by a great group of statemen and out of their deliberations came our
nation and liberties. I gently suggested that the coming peace was foredoomed to failure if
negotiated by those springing from the root of our present partisan politics. I am afraid of
the New Dealers, th y have added to the complexity of our lives but nothing to the joy of living.
We are a hand fed people and I fear for its effec upon our initiative which has beenour principal glory. Their toats is: "Here's to Hell and may it be as pleasant as the paths that lead to
it!" But will it be?   More later. Love from Mother and
                                                Your

Major John E. Bordley, M.C. O-403012   Dr. James Bordley, Jr.

General Hospital 118,   330 N. Charles St.,

A.P.O. 927, c/o Postmaster,

San Francisco, California, U.S.A.   Baltimore -1, Md., U.S.A.

                                             July 27, 1943

Dear Boys,   Series II, No. 80
          It will probably be several days before I will have an opportunity to write again as
I sail by railroad tonight at the ungodly hour of twelve.   Things are moving fast both here
and abroad.   There is a rumor that negotiations are being carried on in the Vatican for the
retirement of Italy from the war and that already the Italian troops have been ordered out of
Albania and the Balkans, also from Germany.   Of course, these latter moves might be the
defense of Italy -- if so, I am betting it is defense against the Germans.   Already they are
kicking the Germans around and the people are rioting for peace.   Graham Swing says it will
take a while to get the Germans out and before that it would be bad policy to lay down their
arms to the Allies.   It is intriguing to think what will happen soon in the Balkans if the
Italians withdraw because they have twenty-two divisions there and their withdrawl will give
the native bands an opportunity to consolidate for help to the Allies when they start through
which is not far away -- another guess.   On the home front -- the Pittsburgh U.S. grand
jury had indicted about twenty labor leaders and laborers for starting a strike in one of the
steel companies. This is under the new conspiracy law and the penalties are very severe. It
is high time and should have been done months ago.   There is to be some relaxation of
the gasoline use by Sept. 1st   The present rules are farcical, not that it bothers me. You
can get a permit to take a trip as far as your coupons permit, if for a vacation, but I could
not, for instance, stay in at home, drive a half mile to any place of amusement.   It puts a
premium on vacations and adds a hardship to those who stay at home.   On Sunday over 30,000
cars were in Ocean City, the largest number on any day since 1940, but a half a dozen of us
had to ride two miles on a street car to get to play golf.   Typical New Deal Stuff.

          We have a black market comparable to old Prohibition days. You can buy anything
rationed from butter to gasoline, if you want to pay the price.   To me this is as unpatriotic
as giving aid to the enemy.   I would no more buy a rationed article against regulations than
violate the laws against murder, but with some it is the same game we played during prohibi-
tion-- beat the Government and laugh at it.   Of course, there is one section of our population
which cannot resist making the extra money and a lot of them are getting very rich.   They and
their friends are never in want but they are piling up antagonism and when this war is over
someone may get very rough with them. They never think that far beyond the dollar.

          I sometimes would like to look into the minds of many of our fellow travelers just
to see their thoughts on why we are fighting this terrible war. I think most people -- or a
very substantial minority -- look upon our efforts as just a fight to lick the Germans and
Japs, a sort of prize ring affair.   They seem to have no comprehension of the stakes involved
and less idea that liberty is a thing which springs from man's soul, and if he wishes to safe-
guard it he must be willing to risk his body.   I hear intelligent (?) people say "I wish the
damn war was over, it interferes with everything I want to do."   But if it had never been
fought by liberty loving men what could they do then?   Most people are stupidly selfish.
          More later.   Love from Ma and
                              Your

                                                                                        185

Vol. #III

Notes on Letters to Jim and John 1942-1945

Sept. 17, 1943 "Ellen is home…" refers to Ellen Webb.

Sept. 30 and Oct. 4 are both letters are called Vol. III, No. 4. At the start of the war he owned two farms, one on the Eastern Shore and one west of Baltimore in Howard County.

Oct. 27 "Mrs. Roosevelt at museum…" probably means Balto. Museum of Art.

She had been his patient in early 1030s.

Jan 21 and 29, 1944 letters are both numbered "30". To avoid confusion between the originals and the scanned copies, this has been continued.

Mar 20, #039- Homer Saint-Gaudens (1880-1953) was the son of sculptor August. His mother was first cousin of John Singer Sargent. August did a sculpture of Sargent's sister. Returning the favor Sargent painted Homer age 10 with his mother. Homer became director of the Carnegie Inst. of Art in 1922, and the portrait hangs there. We do not know why JB jr. knew him. This info. is easily found by 'Googling' Homer.

April 24 and 27 are both labeled Vol. III No.46. Again, we keep this numbering to avoid confusion.

April 27 No. 46 He had owned one of the row houses on Mc Elderry St. just east of Hopkins Hospital for some time. Jim and John had lived in it as medical students and or residents. He continued to rent it and in April 1944 he had not rented it for the coming academic year.

May 4 No. 47 John Gibbs was John Sears Gibbs, President of the Hopkins Hospital.

May 8 No. 48 I believe he bought 2630 Guilford Ave, a row house, for his brother Worthington, who had financial problems. They did eventually move there, remodeled, and stayed several years before moving to an apartment. I recall him shoveling coal into the furnace, so he did not get the oil furnace, at least initially.

June 30 No.59 Beale Bordley, Worthington's son, (nephew of JB jr.)

July 5 No. 60 Tyrothricin was a new antibiotic. It is tryocidine and gramicidin, used as a topical antibiotic in treating infections caused by gram-positive bacteria.

July 13 No. 62 UMH is Union Memorial Hospital.

Dear Boys, Well here I am home, the place I love best in the world in spite of the destruction
by unprecedented drought and heat.   It looks a bit cheerless on the outside but the spirit is
still alive on the inside and I am glad to be here.   The war is moving steadily towards its
final phage and Germany just as rapidly toward utter destruction - to satisfy the pathologic
ambition of one man. It is all toog and too tragic but there was no other way to solve our
fast declining civilization. Or, is this just a phase of its advance toward a higher and better
plane? It seems tough to have to walk through a fiery furnace just to convince ourselves we can
survive the heat. Italy gone, soon it will be the Balkans and before long Germany. Then for
your old friend Hirohito, then home to your wives and children. We have enjoyed every minute
with them and they have been splendid actors in this drama but they want you and I pray God that
in a little while their hopes and prayers will be answered. Then when you get home you must
work even harder to set out National house in order.   It needs a good house-cleaning before
you come but it will never get it because the conflicting interests of politics, business,
agriculture and labor can eb composed only by those whose will it is to settle them and that
will does not now exist.   The old plant needs new blood and a revived determination and you
are the only Americans who can supply both needs.
        Within the past few days we have had three tragic railroad accidents on the three
crack trains of three roads. The Congressional on the Pennsylvania, the Century on the New
York Central and The Flier on the Lackawanna. Scores of people killed. There ismuch talk of
sabotage but I believe it is just overwork of men and material. The Railroads have been and
are doing a grand job but their roadbeds and rolling stock are taking a terrible beating. You
can never visualize the millions of passengers and their mountains of baggage, nor, the endless
train loads of freight. Everybody is making money and trying to spend it and travel is an
outlet and, since the limiting of gasoline, a necessity. There are a few patrons of the gasoline
bootlegger but only a fraction of those who own cars.
        It was a wonderful and remarkable sight coming down from Boston. Every factory
was in full operation and their lights made it like daylight nearly all the way down.   I had
no idea that so many industrial plants existed, thousand there were. It made my heart leap
with joy to think that in spite of the bungling, the strikes, the shortages and the incompetents
we were really living up to our greatest dream of industrial power. And now all of this building is nearly complete and the fruits of our struggle are coming to full flower. What a grand
thought: we have realized our dream and made the best of our great opportunity, have overcome
seemingly impossible impossible obstacles and risen to the highest point of our material possibilities. We are a great people, both in retrospect and prospect and, what an honor to be one
of them. Democracy may be crazy but its works give life and liberty and they are the greatest
conceptions of God and man.
        Dr. John Dorsey died yesterday. Had a frontal lobe tumor -- malignant.
                        More later. Love from Ma and
                                        Your

Series III., No. 1

Sept. 16, 1943

J.B. III.

Major John E. Bordley, M.C. 0-403012

General Hospital 118

A.P.O. 927, c/o Postmaster

San Francisco, California, U.S.A.

Dr. James Bordley, Jr.

330 N. Charles St.,

Baltimore, -1, Md., U.S.A.

Sept. 17, 1943.

Dear Boys,   Series III., No. 2

This is a wonderful country. Up North and down South the rains have been more
abundant than for years, along the coast from Massachusetts to North Carolina hardly a rain
in two months. Up at Rye it was cool enough to require two blankets, down here they had
52 consecutive days of temperature above ninety. The crops here were killed by the heat
and drought and those in the north were more abundant than for several years. So we
evened up pretty well in production but we are away above the average costs in food.
Peaches six dollars a basket, soft crabs four and five dollars a dozen, oranges (2nd grade
a dollar a dozen, bananas five cents a piece, apples and pears five cents, small lemons
ninety cents a dozen and garden vegetables out of sight. You have to buy butter -- when
you can find it -- in quarter pound lots. Everything pretty nearly is rationed and some
things with ceiling prices which are far above normal. You hear much and read much about
the control of inflation but if you go out to spend a dollar you see it is not much
controlled. Still few of us would be willing to change places with the boys who are
fighting on the Italian coast or those killing Japanese in the jungles. -

Dudy is back in Philadelphia and telephoned last night that the kinds were so well
and fat that it was difficult to get food enough to keep them filled up. Jimmy has developed
splendidly and if full of pep.

John's children are fine and are now getting ready to go back to school.

Ellen is home with her family from a three weeks' stay in Rehoboth. Ellen needed
the rest as she has not had a servant for a year and has been doing all of her own work
even the laundry.

More later. With love from Ma and
Your

James III

Dear Boys,   Series III., No. 4

More changes in gasoline rationing have taken place than there are stars in the
Milky Way. Honestly it is a hard job to keep abreast the latest. There is one ration for
the West, one for the middle West and another for the Eastern Seaboard. Yesterday a ration
coupon was worth three gallons -- a week's supply -- today it is worth two -- still a week's
supply. I thought it was due to drain brought about by the African campaign but I was mistaken. Of course it does not affect me except it means more riding because people who live
in the county cannot waste their precious gas coming to a doctor, they need it more to go to
the grocer.

Since I wrote the above on Saturday, the ration value has changed again to two
and a half gallons (Monday). We are to get new books in a few weeks rationing everything
from food to clothes. This covers everything except some perishable foods. This should
have been done months ago but it was put off until we were face to face with serious shortages
all along the line. We are getting a new tax bill on luxuries sufficient to collect ten
billions. A drink of liquir will be taxed 12½ cents and a package of cigarettes 10 cents.
I am all in favor of paying for as much of this war as possible as it goes along and I feel
the pressure for the sale of bonds could have been made much lighter if an adequate tax had
been placed on everybody for everything. A man in my position cannot save a cent. Fellows
making fifty dollars a week in a war factory are better off than professional men who have to
maintain an organization and whose fees are pretty generally ftozen. Money counts for very
little in our reckoning of the war but in civilian life it is still worth what it will buy of
the necessities of life. Most of the men to whom I have talked discount all savings and
profits but there is growing up in this country a new aristocracy of wealth. It is becoming
quite manifest in Guilford. It is unfortunate that no educational qualifications are required and no background of national service. How they get the money and how they keep it
I have no idea but it is clear that these items are no obstructions. Dick tells me that the
contractor for whom he works saved above his taxes, last year, a half million dollars.
Before that the banks owned him body and soul. We have a new neighbor who was a cappenter a
short time ago. He bought an expensive home and keeps three cars and made his money since
Pearl Harbor in general contracts. This is all very interesting sociologically and it will
be interesting to watch the results. These people will, as all people with wealth, have a
definite influence on our social trends. I would have no anxiety if these people had sound
educational and cultural support. It is not bad in a democracy to have one crowd pass the
crowd ahead, it gives democracy its necessary life blood.

The war news is inspiring. I have felt the Germans were drawing the Russians on to
turn on them in due course and knock the stuffing out of them but the war wise say it cannot
be done that way and that the loss of territory and war materials mean a tremendous handicap
to the Nazi and that in no sense was their withdrawal voluntary. I hope so.

The kids are well along with their mothers from last reports.

Love from Ma and

Your

Major John E. Bordley, M.C. 0-403012

General Hospital No. 118

A.P.O. 927, c/o Postmaster

San Francisco, California, U.S.A.

DMajor James Bordley, Jr.

330 N. Charles St.,

Baltimore -1, Md., U.S.A.

September 30, 1943.

Series III., No. 4

Dear Boys,

The old grind is on again, but guided by more enthusiasm since I had a nice long rest. Every moment is filled for days and weeks ahead both consultations and operations. When 1943 end I will have done more cataract operations than in the preceding five years put together. I thought I would be carefree by this time, both from choice and the advent of a group of better qualified doctors, and here I am working as hard as ever and with zest.

At least in being in Australia you get away from a hell of a mess. It is not only discouraging but disgusting to see what goes on around you from high Government officials to caddies. There isan utter indifference to all real responsibilities, it is a veritable scramble for self and nothing, not even war, intervenes to change the trend. I once thought that this dreadful holocast would change people and make them more serious in their outlook on life. I was mistaken and badly.

We had a little rainthis morning, nothing to brag about. We need rain for the Fall planting. I understand this is local but when you own a farm and have the taxes to pay it is a considerable item when you cannot raise crops. I have a new farmer.

I have just had an offer for my land out in Howard County and I only hope the fellow lives long enough to take it off my hands.

Jimmy weighs twenty-two pounds and Pat is flourishing. Dudy comes down on Tuesday to pack her belongings for transportation to Philadelphia. It will be a sad day for Ma and me.

Anne and Brucie have started school again and Ellen Webb's kids are in college also. They are all growing up too fast.

Love from Ma and
Your

John

Dear Boys,   Well the Wagner bill for the political control of medicine has been sent to a
Committee in the Senate.   It provides for the expenditure of three billion dollars a year and
the full control over all hospitals and medical schools.   As an attraction it offers any doctor joining up a salary of $5,000 a year. It pays $5 a day for every bed in all private hospitals, $2.50 for Government hospitals.   One hundred and sixty-eight millions for drugs, forty
eight millions for education and research giving every student $700.   Individuals will be
submitted lists of doctors in their district with the right of choice and physicians retain
the right to reject those they do not care to treat.   We had a full meeting of the Medical
and Chirurgical Society and unanimously voted to fight the bill which very clearly shows that
any doctor not joining will have no standing or opportunity to practice, teach or advise in
any hospital or medical school.   The appointments will be political although this phase is
beautifully camouflaged. The New Dealers are trying to rush the bill so as to get it over
before the 45,000 doctors serving in the military forces get home and have a voice. The sop
is that many of these doctors will have lost their practices and this provides an immediate
wage of $5,000 a year if they join up.   I don't know whether it will pass but it is solidly
supported by rganized labor which is making a real fight.   The only stimbling block is an
emphatic no by the medical fraternity and a unanimous decision not to join up.   What the
attitude of the hospitals will be I do not know, but they always look out for their own interests first.   Of course there is much dissatisfaction at the present time with hospitals, or,
rather there is much room for dissatisfaction. This is being pointed out as one of the shortcomings of medical practice which is absurd as it is no more a shortcoming than is the employment agency of Martin's because it pplies an insufficient number of workmen. The rank and
file of our people have a superabundance of money and they are demanding luxuries in mediciane
as well as in cosmetics. I fired a man from the U.M.H. yesterday who was in for a cataract
operation because he was insulted because the resident and head nurse had failed to drop in to
say "Good morning". He said it was insulting not to have such courtesies shown him. Two years
ago he would have been happy to accept a free bed in the ward. I told him to get out and get
another doctor as he was too frivolous to understand the serious reason for his being in a
hospital and I was too busy to waste my time in silly chatter. Mr. Baldwin of Congressional
Representative told us last night that he had canvassed Congress and the medical bill would
not pass. People are getting fed up on Government intervention in their civilian activies and
are loudly protesting to their Congressmen and Senators. He thinks most of the Ne Deal stuff
will be done away with and there is no prospect of Congress passing additional. The President
is gradually eliminating his professors and professional social workers and replacing them
with men of reputation and experience. Whether this is just a bid for the 1944 election,or,
whether he has seen the light I don't know but as he has been in some eleven years I imagine
the light is beginning by now to trickle through. There is a persistent rumor that he will not
runagain. I never tried to take a bone away from a dog but once and he bit me. I feel that
betting on the President's declining the nomination is about as silly.   Dudy has been down
to pack her winter necessities for transportation to Phila., she looks very well and says never
felt better. If she carts Jimmy around she will soon wilt away, he is almost round and never
fails to anticipate his meals, he learned to crawl up the steps and the hour of food without
notice, the alarm clock insidehas perfect adjustment. Pat grows more lovely, hope she does not
find it out. The John Bordleys are busy ladies now that College is in season.

Love from Ma and

Your

191

Jim

Dear Boys,

The great national discussion now is what is going to happen at the Interallied Conference in Moscow with the Anglo Americans supporting one crowd in the Balkans and the Russians the other. Mr. Hull is going to undertake to care for our interests. Unfortunately the State Department is under attack by a rather powerful opposition which may embarrass him in his efforts. It is trying to place him as anti-Russian and he deemed it necessary to go on the radio and explain his position to the country and he has issued a "white paper" to show the efforts of the State Department prior to the war. Fortunately, he has done a first class job and I implicitly believe in his judgment even though he is a rather old man and muchset in his ways. My faith is pinned on him because he can still cuss when the occasion demands. Of course Russia will present yerritorial demands and will want to establish a sphere of influence in the Balkans and I don't blame them after the tragedy that has hit their country. They want to know whether our pledge for help in the future will be based on a treaty which the Senate will not upset. This constitutional restriction is hampering Mr. Hull's plans and the two major political parties are formulation two foreign policies which does not help. If they could put country before party just once it would help much. Wilkie is right; "This is no tim for arty politics, ra her it is the time for party discipline and cooperation on a matter vital to the entire world."

I am really weary. Every minute crowded, four or five new patients a day and hospitals to go to and operations without end. When this war is over I am going to quit, if not for good, for a very long vacation. Last year was tough, but this year is tougher and then some. It seems to me the whole City is ailing. When I finished up last year I had saved about two thousand dollars in Victory bonds which I distributed among my grandchildren. That was the sum total out of a tremendous practice. This year I will be fortunate if I can make ends meet out of a still larger practice. Still I would not change places with any corporal on the fighting front and what he gets of hat I make he is more tham welcome to.

My old friend, Mrs. Requardt, died a few days ago. Many people will miss her charities. She was always objective in her help, seeking the individual rather than giving promiscuously. She was always generous to my causes.

Cousin Zeke Forman — some ninety-two or three — passed over the line last week. You see we have our casualties in civil life. The old fellow is getting around quite frequently among my contemporaries.

Honestly you would not recognize the old home town. The only things which have not changed are the buildings and the ward politicians. You never see anyone you know and the streets are filled with Hill-Billies. It sometimes looks like a mountain village. All we needed before were the moonshine stills and now they are working at top speed. Horse and carriages and wagons, double teams, single teams but not yet tandems(or new rich have not yet thought that out).

Love from Mother and
Your

Jim

October 19, 1943.

Series III., No. 8

Dear Boys,

Last year was a corker medically but this year is a killer. Every fifteen
minutes another patient, operations morning and afternoon. Where the devil they all come
from I don't know but they flow in streams. I am only helping to pay for the war which I
can't help to fight because I keep precious little, no more than living expenses. Then
the work is made doubly hard by the fact it is impossible to get some medicines and all
instruments. You have no assistants in the operating rooms and the nurses with the exception of the head nurses are as green as grass. I have requisitioned Warren Buckler and
this week he is giving four or five anaesthetics. It is impossible to get anyone else as
there are only two others left. Take it altogether, the Woman's Hospital is in better
shape and crowded and their head nurse is splendid and most helpful. This really is no
time to get sick but the town is full of it. The word is more doctors are to be taken.
I think it will be a near tragedy and terrible on home morale. We are down to bed rock
and every doctor is working his heart out. Now they have the spectre of socialized medicine
for the defeat of which we have raised three hundred and fifty thousand dollars. I will
send you a copy of the Bill as soon as I can get hold of one for you.

The news still looks good. Evidently from General Arnold's report the air plane
trouble Germany is having will give us many advantages. Hirohito seems to be taking a
fine lacing every time his planes venture out, but we have got to finish this job and do
it well enough to discourage another war in your generation. There is a great difference
between Germany and Japan as expressed by the public, it hates Germany but loathes Japan.
I see precious little difference except in the treatment of war prisoners. In Germany
apparently they are not cruel but in Japan they are murderers.

You cannot visualize the change in this country. While we still live well,
we live in a different atmosphere. You can sense it but not describe it.

More later.   Love from Ma
                              and
                         Your

Dear Boys,

The weather is too perfect. Fortunately we had one day of tremendous rain which has now made it possible to plow and plant wheat. We farmers are asked to raise ten percent. more Just how it is to be accomplished with no farm labor we are not told. My farmer is a young progressive fellow with an abundant faith in his wisdom and strength. More, he has all the mechanical devices necessary but he is the rare exception here. Most of them still plow with horses and mules and cut and thresh their wheat with hired threshers and have to take their place in line.

There is a very interesting show going on behind the War drop. The President, ever anxious to spend money, has conceived the idea of a subsidy for all food products and dropping the retail price by an equal amount. Butter, for instance, at present price of forty-five cents will be sold at forty and the creamery re-imbursed the five cents. Congress is definitely opposed. It says the Treasury is only robbing Peter to pay Paul. As a matter of fact the scheme is definitely inflationary leaving as it will much more money to be spent as food bills are the largest single item of domestic expense. It really does not rob Peter to pay Paul but robs both to pay both, because what is paid in subsidies must be raised in taxes. Personally, I am opposed to any and all Government subsidies, called by any name and for every purpose, but, this controversy with the President on one side and Congress on the other is unfortunate not only because of the war, but also it lines up the President as the friend of labor, in keeping his food costs down, and it lines up Congress in favor of Agriculture in that it demands that the law of supply and demand be not tampered with. I believe Congress will win. The truth is labor has demanded more money or a drop in living costs and the President, always politically afraid of labor, is trying to dodge a show down, -- the country on the other hand is fed up on labor's selfishness and extravagant demands and is supporting Congress. There are thousands of laborers on strike, some very serious -- coal, for instance, which has closed some of our large steel furnaces. The people are sick of the whole labor defection and blame all labor and are insisting that Congress get busy about it. As a matter of common knowledge labor is trying hard to get the predominant political voice both domestically and internationally which is bad because no group should ever gain political control. We saw the evil effects of industrial control.

Wendell Wilkie made a powerful speech the other night and included this phase in his argument.

Love from Ma and

Your

194

Dear Boys?

Their geologist think it possible there is a substantial pool. They will not move, however, until some action on the price of oil is taken by the Government. To complicate the fuel situation we have a coalstrike on.   Damn the people responsible for our intrnal troubles. Instead of using a feather duster, it is time to use a club.

Mrs. Roosevelt was at the Museum last night to dispense her wares. It cost a hundred dollar War Bond, to hear her. I have bought enough bonds to do my part so I dispensed with the agony and stayed at home. The Museum sold fifty-two thousand dollars worth so everybody has not my objection.   It was a worthy cause.

The Sun carried a long story about Base 18 So far they have not carried your Hospital but as they are taking one after the other of the various outfits I suppose yours will come along. You should have as good a press agent as the University of Maryland Unit, they get something every few days.

I must run to the U.M.H. where I have two operations this afternoon.

Love from Ma and
Your

John

Dear Boys,
        The Evening Sun busted loose with about two columns on the use of Sulfa drugs in common colds and sore throats. The solution referred to was Pickering. A long list of studies was out lined and many men mentioned but neither John nor Perrin Long. A very comprehensive study was published in both the A.M.A. Journal and the newspapers of experiments carried on by the University of California men on common colds -- preventive -- in the Lockhead factory. They used a new Sulfa.

        I have done a number of eye operations in which I opened the globe. I have been washing out the eye after the operation with our regular Sulfadiazine nose solution. It is remarkable in that the eye shows hardly any reaction to the operation, pain ceases in six to ten hours, there is no discharge to seal off the lids. I had one cataract operation and several hours after the operation the patient had an acute gastritis with extension of the iris the result of vomiting. A beautiful way to pick up an infection. I kept the Sulfa going and no infection has shown up. The solution is more easy to use in the eye than a powder and finds its way into the anterior chamber.

        If we do not have a social scandal around here it will not be because a certain chief's automobile is not parked at a neighbor's house day and night, day after day. I am afraid something will blow up. Her husband is in the Army Intelligence (God only knows how he made the grade).

        Dudy was coming down next week but has had to postpone her visit as our cook has just had a uterine tumor removed and will not be back for two or three weeks -- if ever -- Ma has been unable to find a substitute. The servant problem is complicated by the wages in the war plants. We have to pay twenty dollars a week now for fourth grade help -- when you can find it. I am going to a hotel if we cannot secure a cook. The work is too much for Ma to be doing.

        Since writing the above, we have decided to go to Mrs. Tilghman Davidson's over in Roland Park for dinner and have breakfast at home and lunch down town. It is tough but better than having Ma doing all the cooking.

        I am just in from an operating campaign. Boy, I am getting fed up with so much work but I should not kick because it takes a lot of work to meet expenses and at least I am doing that. Fortunately Congress will not agree to increase income taxes but rather increase taxes on luxuries. Income taxes are driving people on fixed incomes crazy. They have great difficulty making ends meet especially those with children to support. It costs now about five dollars a week per child. Think of a bookkeeper with four or five and drawing a hundred dollars a month. He must take 19% out of his wages for taxes. If the increase asked by the Treasury had gone through he would have had 33% taken out and then what of his rent, food, clothes and children? He can do away with luxuries. The boobs drawing a hundred and fifty dollars a week for eight hours a day working in a war factory are the ones who should be made to go to the captain's office but as they belong to labor unions there is not a chance. Labor is pretty rotten, not only does it get killing wages but all sorts of special government protection and then if its every wish is not gratified it goes on strikes -- such as the coal strike with every miner out and plant after plant doing war work having to shut its doors. These get a minimum of $7. a day, some making as much as $400 or $500. a month and kicking because they were just granted a raise of $1.12 instead of $1.50 asked. They have not sense of responsibility and even less patriotism.

We have a strike among the crane drivers at the Fairfield Ship-yard.   Three hundred men putting thirty-thousand men out of work in that plant to say nothing of the thousands at subsidiary plants.

I guess I am too old to get the proper point of view so I had better stop.

                    With love from Ma
                                    and
                                         Your

November 3, 1943.

Series III., No. 12

Dear Jim,

I am primarily writing this to make inquiry about Bill Guerin, former Secretary to Hugh Young. His mother is much upset -- very much -- because no word has reached her about him for eight months. She has written, cabled, several times, and made effort through the Hopkins to find out about him. Her daughter told your mother that Mrs. Guerin's condition is a matter of serious import to them as the result of her anxiety. If he is not inclined to cable or write you let me know about his health so I can see his mother and tell her he is all right. You know so many rumors fly about, planted rumors, that many people are getting jittery and that is just what Hitler and hirohito want. One of the commentators told in detail about his supposed statement about the boys on the Aleutians, it reached the boys on that far away Island group and very greatly upset them. He was unable to trace the lie down but its intent was perfectly clear. We hear such things every day. I am sure this boy's mother has heard some such tale about him and it should be corrected at once. You have no idea of the tragic stories we have heard about the Hopkins Units. We have been sufficiently informed to spike them but even then they are further circulated.

The Government's attitude is silence but that is not always helpful when so many thoughtless, ignorant, people are concerned.

You might send me one of the short cables, at my expense, and if it contains no negative I will know he is with you and well (one of the sixty cent kind). Say a birthday greeting, which will be taken as positive proof.

          Love from Ma
                and
                     Your

John

November 12, 1943
Series III., No.13

Dear Boys,

What a hectic week.   One day a regular thunder storm for an hour o so, the next morning a snow storm and now as cold as winter weather.   The rain during the thunder and wind storm washed out roads, flooded cellars and farms, washed out bridges and the wind knocked the stuffings out of things.   We seldom have a summer storm of such violence.

I have been very busy both in and out of the office and to add to my worries I have a law suit to defend.   A contractor who was employed to build the barn and stable on my farm used green wood which was split into about a thousand pieces and exposed the interiors to the elements so that they cannot be used.   I declined to pay the bill until the work was made good and he entered suit against me.   Mr. Constable was consulted and he advised me not to pay and does not believe the contractor can win his suit.   It is a damn nuisance but as the work must be done again, I am going to make him pay if possible.

Dudy was to have beendown with the kids this week but was unable to make it so she will come next week.   She says the kids are fine.

Anne took part in a show at school.   She insisted her mother come to see her. Ellen went and said Anne's part was a walk across the stage and nothing to say but she was happy because Ellen was there, so that is all that counts.

Dr. Holt has discovered that Vitamin Bl is formed in the intestines by bacteria, in some individuals in those treated with the Sulfa drugs the formation ceases.   The report of his experiments is out in this weeks Journal of the American Medical Association.   The work was done at Harriet Lane on about fifty volunteers.

The Hospitals are all having a hectic time except the Womans.   Stout has managed to keep a pretty full staff -- except internes.   How is a mystery, or, he is a genius.   It is far the best place to have patients.

There have been several full page pictures of both of the University Units and General 18.   Nothing is said about 118.   You had better get a better press agent.   Every day there is a story of one or more of these Units and this has kept up for weeks.   Yesterday General 18 was pictured and the photo of Bruno and his brother were excellent.   Doctors and nurses shared the space.

Whiskey is now five bucks a pint if you can find any.   It has disappeared from the market.   Less than a year ago when the distillers wantedto make alcohol for smokeless powder they said they had more than the necessary quantity of liquor for six years.   A banker told me a year ago that they were lending no more money on whiskey certificates because the volume in bond meant a heavy loss to the producer.   As whiskey is not sold until it has been in bond four years somebody must be lying about the present shortage.   Most people believe it is artificial and for the purpose of greatest profit.   The boot-legger cannot flourish this time because he cannot procure the sugar.   We have out little mix-ups, but, what the Hell!

Love from Ma and

Your

Series III., No. 14

Dear Boys,, I went to Swepson Earle's funeral yesterday and met most of my old white-haired, bent over contemporaries. My, they were an old looking lot, and the truth is they are holding on to life by their finger tips. I am glad I can look with sympathy and feel none of the pangs of age.   Swep spent Saturday afternoon with us and was in high good humor.   Sunday morning before I got up Georgia called to say she had found him dead in bed.   I am not surprised. Last winter he was forced to sleep in a barracks filled with plaster dust for over a week. He got his lungs full and, his nose, resulting in a serious bronchitis and a very bad frontal sinus.   Was kept in a Naval Hospital for three weeks with temperature and no diagnosis. During a violent fit of coughing had a coronary thrombosis. Pulled out of it but left his heart crippled. He came to me and I opened his frontal which was filled, sent him to an internist who found his bronchi filled up.   We put him in a hospital and the Navy ordered him back to its hospital near Washington.   In a few weeks they discharged him from the Navy without pension rights and said his trouble was only an exacerbation of an old trouble in his bronchii and that, in spite of the fact he had never before had a bronchitis, to say nothing of no coronary and an acute frontal sinus and a crippled heart which their own records on five different occasions withint the year had found normal.   Well, he is dead now and only his widow is left without his support as his children are married. Rotten treatment, both medical and Navy.

Well poor old Dudy had to postpone her trip again and we were much disappointed but agreed she was correct. I want Jimmy to know us and grow up with some knowledge of his grandparents.   Candidly I also want to spoil him just a little bit so he will particularly care for me. I am conservative in my spoilings and know when the kids have jad enough.

The Evening Sun has carried three stories of your Unit in the last three days. The City Editor called up and said the censored stories had arrived with photographs but the pictures were too small and asked if I could find him a picture of Jim. We sent the only two we had and he selected the one with both of you -- taken I think in Australia.   Like most of such stories they deal with personalities and only a brief description of the place. We were all astounded to know the size of the Hospital and the population. The Editor's note was that it was the largest Army Hospital outside of the States.   The pictures used were those taken before you left.   I imagine the pictures received were the very small photos for enlargement but not glazed and the newspaper will not use them because they do not reproduce well on print paper. We were all glad to get the stories because the doctors and nurses were nearly all mentioned in some way and each family could collect some direct information from official sources. I am collecting them and will keep them for you. The next time the reporter comes along have Wink give him some nice glazed pictures of the Hospital and personnel. This to n looks like a gypsy village. Where the women don't wear bandannas they have on pajamas. The faces are those of hill-billies and hundreds of them.   Congress and the President are fight ing over food bonuses. The President wants to keep prices down by paying so much at the production sources and Congress wants the law of supply and demand to determine prices.   God knows which is right, I don't but I do know that prices are rising and labor is asking for more wages. If something does not happen we will have a runaway market and inflation of a serious proportion.   Love from Ma

                                and

                          Your

John

November 23, 1943

Series III., No. 15

Dear Boys, Well you have been making the headlines on front and back pages of all the Sun-papers. Group stories and individualstories. Telling your life histories and special attractions. In fact, the reporter is doing a very good job in covering the whole south and southwest Pacific area -- in medicine. I have heard many complimentary things said about the make up of the articles and the choice of material. He lacks illustrations for your hospital group but the Sun has called on us to help supply them which we have done as far as possible. The article which I have heard most about came out only yesterday morning -- "The Re-union of the Bordleys in Australia". We supplied the three pictures and the reporter wrote an interesting article, it appeared on the back page of the morning Sun. Today, an article giving the names and A.P.O. address of all the Maryland doctors outside of General Hospital Units appeared in the morning Sun. It told their assignments (which surprised me much). It supplied a real need because so many friends want to write and have no idea where their letters should go. People at home want direct information from men in the Army and Navy, official, authentic news. So many wild rumors float around and articles like these bring great satisfaction to family and friends. Just a word is all they ask. Well, your Dad has really sunk lower than he ever expected. He wipes dishes, helps "house clean" and plays parcel boy. We have had no servants for weeks except a woman to clean up twice a week and a laundress. Most of our friends are in the same boat but we get along pretty well. In fact I have the best cook in Baltimore. Most of us give our cooks time off on Thursdays and Sundays and take them out to the Club for dinner, then once or twice in between my cook and I go over to the Poplars for dinner, but I am not much smitten with boarding house living. A man and woman are thinking of buying our home. Neither one knows the difference between algebra and grammar and oh, boy how I would hate to see them living in our real gem of a home. That particular class is rapidly becoming the rich one, some of them have made fabulous fortunes and are trying to live up to their money. They are buying Guilford by leaps and bounds. We have two such families as neighbors. There is much disturbance over the whiskey situation. You see a certain class owns all the distilleries and supplies all the whiskey. Suddenly it is announced there is no whiskey and it goes to $5. a pint. Then the high-jacker and the boot-legger suddenly come into being again and grab the market. Well it is the same whiskey that is supposed to have been exhausted. The Government has gone after them and finds whiskey stored away by thousands of cases. In other words, it is being sold in the black market at tremendous in - crease over the ceiling prices which would b impossible in legitimate channels. Fortunes, oh boy! Work still keeps getting more and more, but I am holding my own. I confess however a few days off would be a help but there are no prospects. You see now an interne can only stay on your service for 18 mos. and residents 27 mos. They must then serve in the Army. This makes things rather bad because knowing their services will be automatically terminated there is a distinct drop in interest. The internes - a fair proportion - tell the residents where to get off. In truth this spirit prevails among all. It is shocking but under the circumstances there is no defense against such attitude and practice. If you lose an interne, orderly, nurse, maid or cook you cannot get another and it is wiser to be insulted than to fight back. This lack of responsibility and dignity is the worst feature of the war and will make for serious trouble bye and bye.

More later.   Love from Ma

and Your

Lt.Col. James Bordley,III.,M.C. O-396822

General Hospital No. 118

A.P.O. 927, c/o Postmaster

San Francisco, California, U.S.A.

Dr. James Bordley,Jr.,

330 N. Charles St.,

Baltimore,Md.,U.S.A.

November 26, 1943

Series III., No.16

Dear Boys,   Well, Thanksgiving 1943 is a thing of the past and what a beautiful day. It was like late Spring, just enough frost in the air to make it delightful and not too cool for the children to play in the yard.   We had the full dining-table for the first time for two years with twelve people seated. We got a turkey only the afternoon previous and that because a patient and his wife were invited out. You have no idea how hard it is to get certain foods. We had a cook for the occasion and the girls -- Ellen Fisher, Ellen Webb, Katherine and Ann (big Ann) all helped.   Mother, of course, worked like there was no one else around and her table was lovely, except she had no flowers which no one ever buys except for funerals.   I made the wine jelly -- believe it or not -- help set the table, did the marketing and bought the birthday cake -- it was Charlie Webb's birthday.   The kids had a wonderful time and we all missed Dudy and her kids.

Dudy wants Ma and me to spend Sunday in Philadelphia but I have no one to look after my patients, either in the hospitals or outside and I decided it unwise to be away. Ma is going some day soon.   Mrs. Ross istaking a rest in the hospital and Dudy thought it opportune to have us.   I am sorry not to see her and the kids, I so enjoyed them last winter and have so missed them this winter. Indeed, the old house sounds like a cave when Ma and I call each other.

Congress and the President are at daggers points.   The fight grows stronger and stronger. It looks to me like a coalition to defeat the re-election of the President -- even his renomination.   The present fight is on taxes -- subsidies to producers.   The Secretary of the Treasury asked for ten billions in taxes and Congress has cut him in two by more than a two-thirds vote.   The President says the ten billions was to take purchasing power out of the hands of the public. Congress says that forty million people hold sufficient money to pay the extra and that ninety millions -- not helped by war wages and profits are now nearing destitution and cannot pay.   Then came along subsidies to the farmers. This the President says was to lower prices of foods to the consumer and make it profitable for thefarmer to produce by jacking his anti.   It gets my goat: Taxes to take away consumers money to keep down prices and their subsidies to increase the incomes of farmers -- one-third of our population.   Organized labor is backing the President and the farm bureaus are supporting the Congress. One wants cheaper foods although making more money than in the world's history and the farmer with double his usual income wants subsidies for all he raises. Well take your choice: The whole trouble lies in the fact that in order to make this the Chief Executor's war he for months has boycotted Congress only using it as a place to get more money. It he had followed wise advice and asked for a working Committee from Congress to sit in as advisors on all war plans none of these storms would have come to plague the country. The President, was to say the least, very unwise, and surely he did not observe the soundest of democracy in excluding the representatives of the people.

More later.   Love from Ma

and

Your

Major John E. Bordley, M.C., 0-403012   Dr. James Bordley, Jr.

General Hospital 118   330 N. Charles St.,

A.P.O. 927, c/o Postmaster   -1
                                                                Baltimore, Md., U.S.A.
San Francisco, California, U.S.A.
                        Series III.,No. 19   December 8, 1943.

Dear Boys,

The Democratic party is split wide open on the soldier vote. The whole thing hinges around the negro vote. The President wants all soldiers to vote (which I think should be a right as well as a privilege) and a bill was introduced into Congress to permit the same, but, a coalition of Northern Republicans and Southern Democrats (according to our "friend and patient", Senator ------) defeated it. The Republicans were afraid to turn the machinery over to the administration and the dissenting Democrats were afraid of the negro vote. The opposition wants the States to handle the whole show, although some states by Constitutional provision do not permit absentee voting. Well, it is a hell of a mess and may definitely split the Democratic party. I really think the party opposition to Roosevelt and another term is directly responsible, the opposition is looking for ways and means of heading the President off. The trend is strongly in favor of the Republican party and many informed men are convinced that the opposition to Roosevelt is at the bottom of the trouble. Personally, I see the fine hand of the defeated isolationists at the bottom of most of the stew, it is their real chance to gain control before the peace settlement. Led by Senator Wheeler they are a shrewd lot and a serious menace to our well being. To me all the bickering and fighting isoutrageous and it shows the caliber of our rulers -- little men in important places, asses trying to hold down intelectual jobs. The war should be first but with many of this gang it is last.

Well my life has been so changed that I thought I might as well change my habits. I have after some sixty years given up cigarettes and taken cigars, I have also given up cocktails for hot water. Of course, this is the interest of longevity and present comfo t but nevertheless it is sort of a strain after sixtyyears' indulgence.

John W. Owens has resigned as Editor-in-Chief of the Sunpapers. He will continue to write occasional editorials and will have a voice in editorial policy but as an active agent he is through. This followed a serious illness and his physicians' advice.

The kids are fine and all send love, and so do Ma

                                                    and
                                                        Your

203

John

Series III., No. 17

Dear Boys,

Yesterday, I sat down to write you a long letter and right in the middle of it Colonel Dawson called me up and mother and I spent the balance of the afternoon withhim. He had seen some of the articles published in this country about the Unit so I carried them over for him to read and will get copies for his personal files as he was much interested in both the text and pictures. He told us the story from Melbourne to the finished Hospital, told us much about your work and above all how gratified he was at the opportunity of commanding such an outfit. When he left you he went to Moresby and from there back to this country and is now assigned to a hospital in Mississippi -- Camp Van Dorn -- with a bed capacity of twelve hundred. He hopes some of you will write him. Until he told me I did not know that your Unit is supposed to be one of five constituting a Medical Center. So far as he knows yours is still the only outfit there and that you are over your quota -- or what we all supposed was your quota.

The new Surgeon General is one of our Eastern Shore boys. I don't know whether he is still a member of our Society. He is a fine man of real ability. If we can be helpful in your plans it will give us much pleasure to talk with him.

Col. Dawson says Wink has taken some fine pictures. Why not send some along, I will gladly stand any necessary expense. Most of the wiveslike portraits and I will see that they get a look at them. If it is O.K. to let us look at some of the hospital views we will all enjoy them.

We are all well.   Love from Mother
                            and
                                Your

LT.COl. James Bordley,III., M.C. O-396822

General Hospital 118

A.P.O. c/o Postmaster,

San Francisco, California,U.S.A.

Dr. James Bordley, Jr.

330 N. Charles St.,

Baltimore, Md.

December 6, 1943

Series III., No. 18

Dear Boys,   Life grows more strenuous: I have not only fallen to dish-washing but even cooking.   Ma has a touch of intestinal flu and as we have no servant, certain duties fall to my lot.   Oh, boy! What a war,even worse than Sherman thought it could be.   Well, we are only following the rule and are not exceptions and while it is bad it will be nothing after we win the war and establish lasting peace.   We sent Jim a cable last night and signed it Jiminie Bordley so it would carry both names. It was more fun trying to make the operator understand the name.   She made me spell it a half dozen times, left the phone (I suppose for consultation) and when she came back, she said "you are sure about the name because I never heard such a name".   I said, "Miss if there is any mistake my mother and the preacher made it and I am only a reflection of their ignorance." Her apologies then came thick and fast.

The papers and radio are making a long and loud protest over the fact the British News Agency (Reuters) beat them to the story of the Cairo meeting and the Russians to the Teheran Conference.   It was agreed to break the story together and when details were available.I I hope this is not a sample of what the post war cooperation is to be.   After all the layman got the news and that is all that interests him.   Unfortunately the anti British and the anti Russian members of our Congress have fallen on the incident like turkey buzzards on a dead mule.   The Baltimore Sun thinks the same spirit is developing which destroyed the last peace; partisan and factional.   I wish the boys in the armed forces would take the stand that they are fighting not only to preserve their way of life now but to save their children from the horrors of another war and they will brook no political traffic in their objectives.   Some of them have clearly and emphatically expressed themselves and if more would join the chorus it would have a salutory effect.   All politicians are selfish but all are damned cowards. The inner circle of the Republican party are trying to destroy Wilkie but the mass of the party wants him.   He cannot be used,therefore the professionals don't want him. In my judgment he is the outstanding American stateman and his only real opponent is the President whose net has developed many holes, so many in fact that there is serious doubt it will hold the voters. The President's mistakes are not in his handling of the war but along domestic lines. He has appointed too many fools to direct the home economy, too many untried to important jobs who have tantilized and irritated the public.

I had a note from the President of the Zenith Radio Corporation in which he told me that Bill Jack is located in Chicago and has a tremendous practice, is on the staff of the Henrotin Hospital and has been elected to its Board of Directors. I thought when Kilmer died he was probably through. His life there was not conducive to the development of energy. He did not mention his field of operation.

It is said by informed persons that when this war is over we will be terribly short of metals and oil.   We have accumulated sufficient for the completion of the war but we will have nothing to spare for the upbuilding in the devastated countries after the peace. This is remarkable in view of the often repeated statements that we have sufficient iron and copper for four hundred years. It may be that somebody is building up an alibi for higher prices later on.

I wish Jim many happy returns of his birthday and for both a Merry Xmas.
      Love from Ma
            and
                  Your

Lt.Col. James Bordley,III., M.C. O-396822

General Hospital 118

A.P.O. 927, c/o Postmaster

San Francisco, California, U.S.A.

Dr. James Bordley, Jr.

350 N. Charles St

Baltimore -1, Md., U.S.A.

December 11, 1943

Series III., No. 20

Dear Boys, A cold windy day, the first for December which has really been ideal. The golf course and greens are still beautiful, and green but not given to much wear and tear. It is seldom you see anybody there except on Saturday and Sunday and then seldom more than a dozen persons. I get out there now and then but have not played eighteen holes for weeks. Now and then I would blow up if I could not get away. Not only is medicine pressing but finances even more so as the result of steadily rising prices and taxes and, to add no servants at home and you have a faint picture of the effects of war on those at home.

We are in the midst of an influenza epidemic. Most of the hospitals are curtailing because illness of such a large proportion of their nurses and help and there is hardly a house without someone sick. The cases are mild, temperature from 100 to 102, many with painful abdominal symptoms, headache and prolonged cough. It is markedly affecting industry. Very few deaths, most from virus type pneumonia. From Washington last night 90,000 cases were reported. The poor general practitioners are rushed to death. A patient of mine from New York called up from the Lord Baltimore Hotel and asked me to get her a physician. We called eight or ten before we could even get the promise of a visit, all were booked up and declining calls. The Health Department expects it to be over quickly, I hope so.

Dudy was down yesterday. She looks like a million dollars. She surprised me when she told me she had gained two pounds, she looked ten pounds heavier. Says the kids are fine and she is coming down for a short visit after the holidays and bring the kids. My assistant Ellen is looking fine and her kids the same. I don't know what I would have done without her. If I can arrange a couple of divorces I may take her on permanently.

The damned politicians are still playing with the war. You know I think with all the interference industry has done a remarkable job. Congress started out by giving labor anything and everything it wanted, then it put a ninety-five percent. tax on profits, which prevented the accumulation of any capital, then advanced money for expansion (when the war is over the Government will virtually own as well as control business). In spite of all the handicaps industry in some war lines is so far ahead of requirements that plants are closing to release workers for new requirements, some of the steel furnaces have been banked because the steel production is above requirements.

The Mars made a trip to Brazil and back in fifty-five hours, carrying a freight load of 35,000 pounds. Her gross weight when loaded has about 150,000 pounds. She made two stops on her return with a 15,000 pound load. She made 161 miles an hour and traveled 5,900 miles. This was not her maximum speed. This time she took off from deep, broad water without a flutter. More of her kind are to be made at once and to be used as heavy transports for long flights with essential freight for the front. She carries a crew of 16.

Love from Ma

and

Your

Major John E. Bordley, M.C.04003012

General Hospital 118

A.P.O. 927, c/o Postmaster

San Francisco, California, U.S.A.

Dr. James Bordley, Jr.,

330 N. Charles St.,

Baltimore -1, Md., U.S.A.

December 14, 1943.

Series II., No. 21

Dear Boys,   Well, Congress has decided to let you vote but cannot make up its mind just how.
It has defeated the Administration's bill to have the National Government engineer it and substituted a state supervision which the Army and Navy have virtually declined to carry out as
impractical and unwieldy. The question has resolved itself into one of constitutionality. The
states lone have the right to determine the eligibility of voters and if the National Government distributes the ballots it opens the way to a legal contest after the votes are counted.
Old Senator Carter Glass says "to hell with the constitutionality, just let the boys vote and no
court will upset their privilege."   I have sold my Ellicott City farm. Got a good
price as land is going up. Indeed there is a good deal of worry about the rise in farm values,
it may help along the inflationary tendency and invite such wild laced speculation as we had
during World War I.   I have another farm down on the Eastern Shore and if prices go much
higher I will certainly sell it.   I believe farms should be owned by people who live on them.
They are always insured then against want.   As an investment they bring more trouble than
financial return.   Many of our industrial plants are taking up civilian work.   This is fine
because the more that can get back on that basis before peace will greatly help the re-adjust-
ment from war to peace and the more workers who are freed from non-essential to essential war
work the less the strain on our man power problem.   it is interesting that most plants in
transferring have not dropped wages. Whether this is the industrial policy of the future I
don't know. I do not believe that peace time profits will justify such a stand.   I hope I am
wrong.   The flu is all invading, hardly anybody has missed a touch.   It has been like
a prarie fire, extending the length and breadth of the country and all in about two weeks.   It
still remains quite free from serious consequences.   This morning's paper quotes the
Public Health as saying the epidemic we have is not influenza but a mild upper respiratory infection.   This is poor dope; In many of the patients I have seen, the thing started with
acute pain in the abdomen, temperature from 101 - 4, then intense sore throat associated with
very severe headache.   Then came acute ears, acute sinuses, a severe cough, extreme lassitude
and pains in all the joints.   It is true there has been but little lung involvement but except
for that the symptoms are the same as in 1918.   The Public Health has certainly missed the
majority around here if it calls the disease a mild upper respiratory disease.   The Army
through the cooperation of LIFE has just had printed the story of the 8th Army Air Corps.   It
is intensely interesting and is being dramatized for the Radio.   If I can secure a copy I will
send it to you as I am sure it will prove worth while reading.   I have been surprised at the
intricacy of the whole business and the tremendous amount of work required to keep the planes
flying. You may know more about it than we know and it may be old stuff.   I am taking
off a couple of days to get a little rest as I am very tired. I am going to the Eastern Shore
to see my new farmer and I hope to bring home some food.   It looks and feels like snow now
and if it materializes I will not go.   Bill Fisher is down there now looking for ducks. He
has had lots of wind and much severe cold and I suppose will come home with a full bag.
The papers are full of the returning soldiers not receiving any financial help, not enough to
buy a ticket for home.   In the last war I anticipated this and had a fund to pay their compensation and advance needed funds.   I loaned about a hundred thousand dollars to my boys
and lost only eighty dollars.   This time nobody thought about it.
                    Love from Ma
                         and   Your

Lt. Col. James Bordley,III.,M.C. 0-396822

General Hospital 118,

A.P:O. 927, c/o Postmaster

San Francisco, California,U.S.A.

Dr. James Bordley,Jr.

330 N. Charles St.,

Baltimor -1, Md., U.S.A.

December 18, 1943

Series III., No. 22

Dear Boys, We are in the midst of the coldest spell we have had in these diggins for many a year. Fortunately, it has been clear and beautiful while north and south of us there ha been much snow and wind. Yesterday the extreme weather resulted in the worst train wreck in many years. A rail broke on the Atlantic Coast Line in North Carolina and derailed their crack flier coming north and 40 minutes later their other crack train going south plowed thru the overturned cars. Somewhere around 100 persons were killed and another hundred injured, most of them military men. We have had more railroad deaths in the past 6 months than in the preceding 10 years.   Pop was not feeling up to the mark so went to Charlie Austrian for a complete overhauling. I have more wounds now than most of the boys from a South Sea Island. The whole force looked for some vulnerable spot and struck a hole in it.   In the end it was resolved that I was only a bit tired and a rest was ordered. I feel so much better as the result of th battle that I am begging for commutation of the sentence. Indeed it is next to impossible for me to go anywhere until this damnable pandemic is over. very doctor here is crushed with work and I hesitate to throw an additional burden on them.   I am willing to work for 4 hours -- in which I can see 15 or 20 patients -- and rest the balance of the day.   I sought help because I have lost about 10 pounds and my old pump was not working smoothly. I am assured my heart disturbance is only an extra systole or two and is in no sense serious and my loss of weight is the result of too much work and responsibility. This knowledge really makes me feel better because when my heart kept me awake at night I thought some piston or other was leaking and maybe the old machine would stop.   Things are getting in a mess in the country, a mess which bodes no good for the future.   There are two serious conditions: First, labor. It has come to pass that it openly tells the Government to get to hell out. It defies all rules and regulations. The Railroad Brotherhoods have notified the Government of their intention to strike after Xmas because extra pay of $3. a day was not granted them by the War Labor Board which thought 4¢ an hour would compensate for the increase in their living cost. Then foolishly Congress came along and granted them 10¢ an hour raise, but, it is not believed the President will sign the bill.   The steel workers demand a raise but have not threatened to strike. Forty or fifty other organizations say if Congress doesnot pass a bill to subsidize foods and thus hold the price down, they intend to quit. Then Green and the head of the C.I.O. have served notice they do not intend wages shall be reduced after the war and they intend also to demand adequate housing,etc.,etc. The whole trouble with labor is that it is the spoiled child of the President, and if I am not mistaken th people of this country are going to register their protest at the next election.   I am sorry because I am for decent wages for decent workmen but I am only for that and I am forced to believe that the leaders of labor are a bunch of hogs and as unpatriotic as Benedict Arnold.   There was a good bunch of pictures in the Evenin Sun a day or so ago of your Unit personnel. I think it fine as it creates a good impression among those who have boys fighting down your way. I was at the Hopkins yesterday and dropped in on Winford Smith. He has some nice pictures and promised to have them copied for me. He is very proud of General Hospitals 118 and 18.   John's Anne had the flu and a bad ea I watched it for several days as all of the other children with similar middle ears have gotten well without surgical interference. As it did not clear up I opened the drum and her temperature is now normal and the drum in good shape and discharge lasted only a day and disappeared. (Good old Sulphadiazine 3%). I tell you this because I promised her if she would be very good and let me do it without an anaesthetic I would tell you about it. She was a good as gold,although surrounded by agonizing relativ s. Be sure to write and congratulate her on her heroism. She is all right now and eating like a horse.   Love from Ma and your

Major John E. Bordley, M.C. O-403012

General Hospital 118

A.P.O. 927, c/o Postmaster

San Francisco, California, U.S.A.

Dr. James Bordley, Jr.

330 N. Charles St.,

Baltimore -1, Md., U.S.A.

December 20, 1943.

Series III., No. 23

Dear Boys,   Well Xmas is nearly here and what a hot spot old Santa Claus will find whenhe starts climbing down chimneys. In not a single se-called civilized country will he be able to drive his reindeers without bumping into a war vehicle either in his aerial flights or on the ground. How lonely this old fellow, who specialized in good cheer,will feel.   Wehumans can certainly make an awful mess of things when we are left unescorted.   When the history of this gene ation is writ, to be appropriate, it should be on black paper.   We have mortgaged our souls to make material progress, have forgotten our duty to our neighbors, have sent our sons out to be slaughtered, and some have even defied God for gain.   Still the sun shines and the rains fall and I guess when the chickens are counted in the future they will all be there.

I have not sent you the book I promised -- about the 8th Air Division -- because I have not yet got it.   I am going to send you another one also -- "The Ten Commandments". The latter book is said to be the finest of the war time literature and is a compilation of short essays by Thomas Mann, Erskine and eight others. Each essay deals with one commandment, and the reviewer for the New York Times says they are their finest short stories.   Each is an expose of the acts of the German Government in its attack on Christianity. ~~The~~

The flu runs merrily on and our death rate is on the increase but as such a large proportion of our people had their attacks when it was mild I hope we will escape a debacle. There is a great discussion as to whether it is of the same type as that of 1918.   As I saw hundreds of cases then I feel competent to compare at least the symptoms and I feel sure it is the same but less fatal.

You would be surprised to know how few of the common presents of the usual Xmas you are able to buy now.   Not only are they fewer in numbers but even intypes.   Even childrens' toys are limited to wooden ones.   Such things as doll babies with clothes are impossible to find, as a matter of fact childrens' clothes are hard to get. Ellen Webb had to go to New York for her children's and then found but little more there than her .

The President is home safe and sound thank God (I never expected to express such a sentiment but I really feel it). I hope he will stay home for a long time as it would be disastrous for us to be without a head for the Government.   He tells us that the meeting of Churchill, Stalin and himself has eliminated the possibility of another war "inthisgener- ation". It is sort of letting us down to use such arithmetic. We want no future wars. And what is the present generation: me, you or your children?

Anne is well and up and ready for school. Her drum has healed and her cold is well. Pop Fisher went down ducking last week and ran into a four day temperature around 10° coupled with high wind. He got his ducks but says it was his worst experience as a hunter.   He gave me a pair of canvas backs.

More later.   Love from Ma and

Your

Lt.Col. James Bordley,III.,M.C. O-396822

General Hospital 118

A.P.O. 927, c/o Postmaster

San Francisco, California, U.S.A.

Dr. James Bordley,Jr.,

330 N. Charles St.,

Baltimore -1, Md.,U.S.A.

December 23, 1943

Series III., No. 24

Dear Boys, Christmas is just around the corner and I am in the same dillema I have been in for some 40 odd years; no present and no ideas for a present for Ma. Being a rational being I can never understand why women are so secretive as to what they want on birthdays and Xmas, if you buy them a wrap they neak away and change it, if you buy them jewelry they think you are grossly extravagant and what other things can you get a woman? Oh, hell I have survived before and probably will in spite of my mortification this time. I was glad to get Jim's letter telling us about the progress of the hospital and about the Colonel. Both were very interest-ing. The F.B.I. has just unearthed a million dollar syndicate dealing in bootleg whiskey They had thousands of bottle all of which will be confiscated and put on the market as it is bonded whiskey. Their loss will be a million bucks and sometime in jail. You know who they were. The usual tribe that specializes in doing their friends, customers and Government.They had thousands hidden in Baltimore which is one of the driest places in the nation. You cannot buy whiskey of any kind at any price except in the black market. I blame this on Ritchie who had a chance to have the State handle theproduction of all the distilleries. I urged him to do it but good old politics was more important. The first thing we know prohibition will be back. Since I wrote the above yesterday, the Public Health has reversed itself and declares in screaming headlines that there isno difference between the flu now and in 1918 except in fatalities and warns that it may assume the same proportions. It took them two months to find it out and now it is, in this State, on the decline. We have a big strike on at all the plants of the Western Electric. It is too damn silly to believe. A question of separate toilets for whites and blacks. The Government to prevent "a show of partiality has decreed that both races use the same toilets". The whites struck and the Government has taken over the plant and the white strikers will not return to work and the Government will not permit them to go into any other jobs. It is an outrage for the Government to interfere with out war effort just to carry out the theories of a bunch of Yankee New Dealers. I don't blame the whites for striking and I would have joined them. It is at least not making votes in this State for Roosevelt and that was its intention. We are promised a major railroad strike on Dec.30th and I was just told by the Manager of a large ship-building plant that at the bottom of this is also based on the attempt of the Government to equalize whites and blacks and to force the latter into skilled trades of the railroads. On the durface it is a strike for higher wages - three dollars a day for one and all. Yesterday they offered to compromise on 64¢ and overtime beyond 40 hrs.a week. The steel workers are asking a raise of 25¢ an hour but have not mentioned strike. I personally believe if the President had used the big s ick on John L.Lewis and his coal strike instead of giving them all they asked we would have had none of this trouble. It all leads up to infla-tion and the Administration is largely responsible. It is in for a real crack next November as the public is fed up and is convinced that our war effort is being seriously hampered. What a condition we will be in when peace comes. The most gigantic national debt of any country in the history of the world; wages which can never be s pported; a race question of serious import; food at its greatest price and a much disturbed general economy. If we had a two fisted President we would all be happier and the country safer. It is no time for a jelly fish with whims.

More later. Love from Ma and

Your

Major John E. Bordley, M.C. 0-400012   Dr. James Bordley, Jr.

General Hospital 118   330 N. Charles St.,

A.P.O. 927, c/o Postmaster

San Francisco, California, U.S.A.   Baltimore, Md.,(1) U.S.A.

                               December 27, 1943.

Series III., No. 25

Dear Boys,

Xmas has come and gone and except that you were not here, our Xmas was very nice. Ma and I had two celebrations, on the 25th at Ellen Webb's and on the 26th at our home. We had the children and a Xmas tree with all the day's trimmings. Our presents were many and very nice and best of all we secured a cook for the whole day, put out the silver and drank wine to celebrate. The 25th was a beautiful day, the 26th a sleet storm which lasted the whole day. Everybody was well but Ellen Webb who had the flu in mild form but with temperature and a vicious headache. We missed her very much. Thank God the flu is rapidly on the decrease. Sulfadiazine has been a Godsend and we have in it a wonderful agent to prevent the secondary features. I will give you a pointer. It is most important to shrink the nasal tissue so the solution reaches the vault of the nose. I use a 1% cocaine solution but give my patients a Neosynephrin solution to use at home. Spray the nose, throat and mouth and have the patient swallow the Sulfa spray. The spray does not reach the trachea but that swallowed does the trick. I have given none by the mouth. If you get in within the first twelve hours you can prevent sinus complications. In fact I have not had a single sinus except those which developed before I saw the patient. I have had two cases allergic to Sulfa. Their noses looked like extreme hay fever and they sneezed for hours. Inhalations of steam stopped both. The pediatricians are using Sulfamerizne in quarter gram doses for kids with flu. Mary Lee Carroll's baby was cured in forty-eight hours of a nasty attack. We have had none of the penicillin to try, nor the English penicillin, both are retained for seriously ill patients. Dunning tells me that all the scientists in his laboratory are working on the synthetic production of penicillin and they are making satisfactory progress.

It is funny to look back and see things. When I was a youngster the niggers used to scrape mold off of stones to put on sores and cuts. Father would raise the devil with them and tell them of the danger of blood poisoning but they always made a speedy recovery. They were always careful to get a mold of a certain color. I wonder whether they were using penicillin fifty years or more ahead of schedule? They also drank "catnip" tea for malaria and when I was a kid I used to collect the catnip from the fields and sell it to our servants for ginger cakes and cookies. Maybe we had better look that up too.

Congress has adjourned until after the New Year. Probably help the war along -- certainly it has done nothing to stop strikes as today we have a paralyzing steel strike and a threat of a railroad shut down on Dec. 30th. A fine bunch of patriots who are out for all they can get and to hell with the country. This is democracy as translated by our ardent patriots, they are willing to have the soldiers go to war to save their bacon but have not sufficient sense or gratitude to support them. But just look the average fellow in the face and you can understand.

       More later. Love from Ma and

               Your

Major John E. Bordley, M.C. 0-40612

Dr. James Bordley, Jr.

General Hospital 118

330 N. Charles St.,

A.P.O. 927, c/o Postmaster

Baltimore, Md. -1, U.S.A.

San Francisco, California, U.S.A.

January 8, 1945

Series III., No. 27

Dear Boys,   Well prohibition is back again and well informed men in Washington are very uneasy about the passage of a bill to be introduced. It is a vote getter, therefore both parties are afraid to shy away from it.   It is the same old story -- "A war measure to keep people at work by reducing the alcoholis content to one half percent."   The pressure for the bill is from the south and the central west. The damn fools can't realize that the iniquities of enforcement are worse than an occasional drunk. I don't believe the President will sign such a bill but he is unpredictable and with a neck to neck run for this election he may try to get his portion of the votes.   When it comes to a show down I believe the pressure against the bill will lick it.   It is inconceivable that we want to breed more Al Capones. Somebody said -- it is supposed to be General Marshall -- that the agitation for strikes and the Army having to take over the railroads will add months to the war and hundreds of thousands of lives.   Well, boys, you have never experienced such a din and I truly believe it has sa scared the labor leaders very badly. They are trying to wriggle out but the radio commentators and newspapers are making it stick.   I am convinced it has done more to awake the fathers and mothers than anything so far. They say Congress isbeing bombarded to curb labor and put it in its place. Just for sixty cents a day extra the safety of armed forces and the country have been jeopardized. It sounds bad and is bad.

We have a new plane propelled like a rocket. It is said the substitution of this force for propellers is going to give us the greatest fighting plane in the world. It was invented in England and perfected by General Electric and constitutes a great advance in aviation it is said.   It will use less than half of the gas used in present planes. It is now in full production at Bells. We have furnished Russia with seven thousand planes and a million and three quarters motor vehicles to say nothing of five millions pairs of boots and billions of dollars in clothing and food. I believe we have been very helpful to the "bear who walks like a man". Of course that is not more than ten percent, but it is a good and useful present and has saved thousands of American lives.

Well I have sold the Ellicott City property I offered it to a man for fifteen hundred dollars and he turnedtit down . In a few days another fellow came along and offered metwo thousand -- which I promptly took. If God ever made a wilderness when he first constructed the world, I am sure that piece of property could be used as a likeness for it. People are buying real estate as investment fearing inflation but if we can inflate faster thanthat property neither cash nor real estate will be worth having.

George Bennett is trying to make me sell the little house over by the Hopkins as a permanent home for his residents. It is too good an investment for me to sell. I wish I had bought a dozen like it.   .

Everybody in the family is well. Mother had a nasty attack of intestinal flu but she is now back on the job and really looking better than before she was sick.

I have been invited to take part in a symposium of Maryland Art and to speak on the characteristics of early Maryland furniture.   I am going to do it as it will be a diversion from medicine.

                    Love for Ma
                              and
                         Your

Lt.Col.James Bordley,III.,M.C. 0-396822 Dr. James Bordley, Jr.,

General Hospital 118   330 N. Charles St.,

A.P.O. 927, c/o Postmaster   Baltimore -1, Md., U.S.A.

San Francisco, California, U.S.A.

                                                                      March 13, 1944

Dear Boys, Politically things grow more tangled. The really serious part of the story is that in every by-election that has been held this year for Congressmen the Republicans have won and today the great Democratic majority has been reduced to just one. In the Senate the Democrats have about sixteen majority with thirty-two seats to be filled at the November elections. This does not mean that the President has sixteen majority because nine of the Southern Senators are opposed to him, so a change of five seats at most will leave him without Senate support. Now this will mean after November a Republican Congress beyond doubt and a possible Democratic President. Of course, this will seriously interfere with both our war and peace aims because by the nature of politics they will never pull together. The only way to stop the Republican trend is for the Democratic party to nominate a man like Byrd (and there is no chance) in whom the people have faith. The personal strength of Roosevelt may re-elect him but he cannot carry Congress along with him. His strong stand will be on war issues, his weakness on domestic policies and it is the latter which will bring in a Republican Congress. One after another his domestic policies are being exposed as totally fallacious or inadequate and his coupling up with the C.I.O. has a mess of Democrats worried. It is a fact that this branch of labor today dictates the domestic policies of the Administration and carries them from bad to worse.   I am branching out as a photographer with John's camera. I regret to say that his two rolls of films were dated for Oct.1,1942 which necessitated my buying others. My old tripod camera really takes beautiful pictures but is unhandy to carry around. I am taking pictures of furniture details and propose writing a complete story of the Maryland product. The trouble is I have to practice medicine and it interferes a great deal, in fact, leaves me little time, but, by systematically plugging I will finish in due time. Ellen Webb is going to help me as my pictures are in colors which requires a bit more skill than I have.

Our cook has a cold (so she says) and has been home and visiting friends for a week, so I am back at dish-washing and bed making. The damned niggers are the most shiftless, unreliable bunch that God ever made. Wages and living conditions play no part in their philosophy of life. The great trouble now is that there is a concerted drive from a great many directions to help them and the would be helpers do not take sufficient account of their nature. They are by and large dirty and shiftless and no matter what habitations are built for them they will never adequately care for them. Demand is being made to have Southern Colleges receive them as students, that business open its offices to them as secretaries and stenographers and that industrial plants take them on equal terms with whites. They are too utterly unreliable to be trusted with business responsibilities. I mean the rank and file for whom the Roosevelts are demanding social equality.

            More later. Love from Ma and

                        Your

Lt.Col.James Bordley,III.,M&C. 6-396822

General Hospital 118

A.P.O&. 927, c/o Postmaster

San Francisco,California, U.S.A.

Series III., No. 28

Dr. James Bordley,Jr.

330 N. Charles St.,

Baltimore -1, Md.U.S.A.

January 10, 1944

Dear Boys, Just a picture of my schedule for a single day. Up at five-thirty, three fires to build because oil truckmen are on strike and we have no oil, operated at eight, office at nine fifteen to see a score of patients, out about two to go to the Maryland Historical for half hour, back to the hospital, then tosee outside patients, home in time to get the market list and dash over to do the marketing, home in time to do a few odd jobs before a cocktail and a mother-cooked dinner, then washed the dishes, then sat down to hear a little over the radio while I wrote the thesis I am to deliver on the furniture of Marylanders, interrupted a thousand or more times to answer the telephone. Well, war is hell! but we are better off than the fellows in the fox-holes and I am not complaining. I am quite sure that these things are good for us because through them we realize the uselessness and folly of much that we haveconsidered essential. We find that we are more resourceful and less helpless then we believed ourselves and we are learning more about the habits and customs of those less fortunate than ourselves. Not a bad thing to take stock of one's life now and then so as to find out just how it may be restocked with usefulness. The worst feeling brought by age is the dread that you may have to live after you are useless, so a little turning up os such things as we are getting now give the elders an opportunity to observe certain essential facts of helpfulness, really makes them sure of their ability to carry on. I know it is that way with me. I have gotten a great stimulation out of our so-called "trials". They have been but good omens of things to come. Our brothers in Russia are the most wonderful fighters of all time. It was said in the last war whentheylicked Hindenburg in a battle that their only weapons were shot guns and staves. Boy, how they can fight now with modern weapons and how fast they can make those weapons. I really think their industrial triumph is equal to their battle skill. How many good American boys they are saving and still there is on foot a scheme for using their politics as a slogan in our coming election. The Governor of Maine came out with a blast against the pin heads of his Republican party and stressed the advantage to us of Russia's efforts and damned those - by name - who were trying to stir this country up against a sound foreign policy based upon friendship for our allies. He extolled Wilkie as the outstanding American who could see afar as well as near and, brought out the fact that his approach to Roosevelt's policy was an honest attempt to unite th nation in the time of trial. It has electrified the country and is one more evidence that some statesmen are left to guide us. The Republicans have the foolish notion that anyone they nominate can be elected. I don't believe it. If they fail to nominate Wilkie it will swing millions to Roosevelt, including me. If we cannot get a great man, why change? We had John's letter telling about Xmas party. It must have been great for the boys down under and I am so glad everybody pitched in with so much enthusiasm. You have no idea of the effect of such things on the home folk. I heard a young lieutenant from your area last night tell of his experience in a hospital. he mentioned no names but his observations and praise were very appealing and reassuring to mothers and fathers with injured sons. I hope it was your hospital.

With love from Ma and

Your

Major John E. Bordley, M.C. 0-403012

General Hospital 118

A.P.O. 927, c/o Postmaster

San Francsco, California, U.S.A.

Dr. James Bordley, Jr.,

330 N. Charles St

Baltimore, Md. -18, U.S.A.

January 12, 1944

Series III., No. 29

Dear Boys,   At last the President has seen the light and asked for an all inclusive draft
of man and woman power. It was two years before th light penetrated and now only partly.
We are ridden by strikes, worried for fear of serious inflation, anxious about an adequate
labor supply and now he asks for a draft which will permit the same wages, the same control
by lab r leaders over labor, the same opportunity to strike. What a farce! The President
has lost the confidence of not only Congress but the country by its many and foolish shifts
He exhibits no backbone, he creates official bodies and then intrigues with labor and farm
and what not to dissolve their decisions. This draft business is to placate those who oppose
him on the g ound that we are not making an all out effort in an all out war. More politics
than clear executive thinking I am afraid.   The United St tes Court of Appeals has
just struck States ights in the solar plexes. It has declared the Baltimore Transit Company
an interstate Co poration and ordered dissolution of its locally created labor union and makes
it amenable to all nati nal regulations. This is directly contrary to the spirit of our
constitution and is a blow to the States Rights equal to any effort of the Federalist party.
I am not su prised because I know the composition of the Court but I am nevertheless shocked
because I believe our greatest security as individuals lies in our dual form of government and
I am convinced that to give the national Government license to attack our States Rights is a
body blow to individual liberty. Becuase the Railroad Company buys power, street cars and
buses out side the State of Maryland it becomes involved in interstate trade makes it therefore an interstate corporation. If you buy your hat in New York and your coat in Richmond you
have not the right of security provided by your State, you become immediately a ward of the
National Government. That is as clear as mud, or, the philosophy of Hitler. We must be
vigilant if w wish to keep our rights and to me it seems too foolish to expend our blood
and treasure to free the French and Dutch and lose our perspective while we are doing it.
I could write a full dissertation on patriotic duty but why to two fellows who have amply
demonstrated their knowledge and feeling. The thing that tickles me most is to watch the
rats trying to get off the sinking ship of State -- the one with the Arms of the Roosevelts.
The same rats that took everything they could get, who led the country astray at election
time, th ones who followed the lead and never attempted to discriminate between right and
wrong, good or bad, so long as Roosevelt fed them fat meat.   Now one and all are rushing to
the attack, or sneaking to the attack on the obstacles to good government they helped to
create.   They are as loathsome as the Japs and not half as resourceful.
          We had an air raid alarm last night, a practice one of course. We were in the
kitchen, Ma cooking and I preparing a Manhattan, and both listening to the radio. An air
raid warden had to notify us to put out our lights. I felt sort of crestfallen because it
was our first mistake but as we were not reported it was not as bad as it might have been.
          More later. Love from Ma and
                              Your

215

Lt. Col. James Bordley,lll., M.C. O-396822

General Hospital 118

A.P.O. 927, c/o Postmaster

San Francisco, California, U.S.A.

Dr. James Bordley,Jr.

330 N. Charles St.,

Baltimore -l, Md.U.S.A.

January 21, 1944.

Series lll., No. 30

Dear Boys,   Your old Pop don't feel as lively as usual.   Had a touch of the flu intestinal and otherwise and had to be in bed a couple of days.   I know the value of Sulfadiazine.   It broke up a nasty little secondary in my nose in 48 hours.   If I had the nerve I would inject the stuff in the antra of allpatients.   It works wonders when you do.   I had 3 cases last week who were quite sick with enough cloudiness in the antra to justify puncture and a washout with Sulfadiazine solution.   All were entirely well in 36 hours.   I think it slowly feeds out into the nose and into the other sinuses by capillary attraction, some of course goes down and some is absorbed.   Try it if you get the infernal disease in your hospital.   We had a snow storm Saturday and the countryside is still covered and the streets very slippery.   I started this two days ago but have had so much on hand that I have had no time to finish.   It seems to me the older I get the more trouble I get in.   Walter Robinson called up last night and had a talk with us.   Said a lot of nice things about you both and the work of your hospital It was very nice to get first hand information and we all appreciated his thoughtfulness.   He is evidently impressed with your layout and your work.   Had John's note yesterday of the receipt of his boxes and we are glad to know that he enjoyed the food which Ma worked so hard to find.   She is a food sleuth when it comes to finding rare tit-bits and boy, things to eat are really getting scarce.   If you have a beefsteak of the most common variety you brag among your friends for a couple of weeks.   It is not that beef is really short but the required points are so high that it takes a week's allowance to get a couple pounds of beef.   And when they add butter to meat allowance and charge 16 points per pound you have to cook your beef in oleomargarine.   The distribution system is very faulty but that is not to be wondered at when bank clerks and lawyers instead of food experts make the rules.   Then such bureaus are presided over by college professors in economics instead of trained executives which adds an additional burden on the system.   Allen Woods is theSurgeon General's advisor on Ophthalmology. I have received some caustic letters on that subject from some of our leading Ophthalmologists who are much dissatisfied over the present and future Ophthalmology.   Allen seems to be playing the game with the administration since he started treating one of the President's close advisors.   He has had me out to discuss some of the phases of the work with which I was familiar during the last war but characteristically disagreed with our rather successful attacks on the problems.   I am through!   The Public Health has started another scheme to control medicine as their original bill has been successfully pigeon-holed in the Senate.   They propose to set the fees for services and have themguaranteed by the Government.   All desirous of free treatment must apply to the Public Health.   This means medical control and is being vigorously opposed.   Our State is fully organized - the Medical profession - to fight the proposition and is taking a very active part in its defeat.   Dr. Wharton is heading our activities.   The snow has gone and now we have slush and fog.   It is warm and we have had little sunlight for several days.   We were spoiled by a wonder December, clear cold and dry.   Our neighbor who bought Joe Ames' house has cut down most of the trees.   I often wondered why Dr.Ames did not thin them out but now that they are gone the place looks like the toothless mouth of a six year older. I am trying to prepare a talk on ancient Maryland furniture but my real duties come s thick and fast I am making no headway.   I want some lantern slides but the material is unobtainable, the Museum has had it on order for 3 mos.   You have no idea how many things of that kind you can't get but I will forego my part with a smile if they are putting the time and material into planes and ships.

More later.   Love from Ma   and   Your

Major John E. Bordley, M.C. O-403012

Dr. James Bordley, Jr.,

General Hospital 118

330 N. Charles St.,

A.P.O. 927, c/o Postmaster

Baltimore, Md., 1,U.S.A.

San Francisco, California, U.S.A.

January 29, 1944.

Series III., No. 30

Dear Boys, A week of summer. The longest warm spell for this time of year on record. Even the plants are showing leaves and the grass has turned green. I was out yesterday with no overcoat and hot. The temperature was up to 80°. It has saved us a lot of oil and as we have passed 52% of the cold weather and we still have 56% of our oil left we should get through O.K. Winifred Smith has just beenappointed the American representative on the Board for the manufacture and distribution of hospital supplies which includes instruments. He will not have to leave the hospital. I hope he unfreezes some instruments. I have had an order in for some since last June, just common things like scissors and forceps. Every American concern is booked to capacity and I hear the Army has stored enormous supplies so as to be able to meet any emergency. I think I told you we have a cook. Well instead of being in her forties she is near her eighties. But she knows how to cook and wash dishes and lives in the house so we are not kicking. Miss Rusk has gone to St. Louis for a wedding -- her nephew. It is the first time in about thirty years I have failed to have her at my side. Ellen is substituting and I keep her on the jump. She is a grand gal and most helpful. When John comes home he may have to look up another wife as we have decided to keep her down here. Of course he can see her fromtime to time if he decides to come back to the old stand. Miss Willets has lost her job and has little to do. She knew too much for her own good, she thinks. I have no place for her and what she will eventually do I have no idea. The country got a bad shock yesterday when the Jap atrocities were let out officially. It is the greatest sensation since Pearl Harbor and if it succeeds in increased efforts the publicity was timely. We had over two thousand strikes last year involving millions of days lost and we have had and still have too much common politics. Every radio announcer yesterday played a tune. The families are all well.

There is much agitation -- politics of course -- to bring the boys home for a rest. To me it is too dumb to agitate such a question which belongs strictly to military. Honestly some people have not the slightest conception that e are in a desperate war with the liberty of mankind hanging in the balance. The Congress and the President are still fighting like a pair of tom cats over every questionraised byt the Democratic National Committee has just unanimously endorsed the President for a fourthterm. It does not make sense. Now the people have come to life on the soldier vote and demand it be immediately settled which it should be. Whether it helps Roosevelt or the Repunlicans the soldiers have a right to express their choice and I am enough of a Democrat to be willing to accept the voice of the majority.

More later.

Love from Ma

and

Your

Lt.Col. James Bordley,III.,M.C. O-396822

General Hospital 118

A.P.O. 927, c/o Postmaster

San Francisco, California, U.S.A.

Series III., No. 31

Dr. James Bordley, Jr.,

330 N. Charles St.,

Baltimore -1, Md., U.S.A.

February 1, 1944

Dear Boys,

I think your determination to stay on is a wise one in spite of the fact the temptation to come home is very great and our desire to see you is no less esthusiastic. I can see nothing in swapping the devil for a witch which is precisely what it will mean. A month home and then to some other foreign shore. Keep your unit together and continue, what we are all led to believe by outside sources, your fine contribution to the war effort.

Of course the whole question of furloughs is a politically stirred up mess. Instead of leaving the whole question for the settlement of the General Staff just to make political capital the politicians in Congress are keeping the whole question stirred up. It is the worst moral buster the politicians have invented and they are legions. General Marshall made a telling speech last night over th radio and reminded the American people that the war is a long way from won and that the demands being made on the Army are poorly conceived. I like him and his quiet but perfectly firm manner. He is much like Gen. Robert E. Lee and just as sound.

I will make a search and let yo know what I can find out about the reasons behind the furloughs. I know if the Army is not in favor of the proposition and just driven to it and men take advantage of the opportunity they will be marked for something not so pleasant. It is a little way they have.

Ellen just had a wind-fall. One of John's patients from Australia is sending her a box of mylon stockings.   You might suppose from the play made on women's stockings they were essential to victory. Yesterday a woman bought fifteen thousand dollars worth of War Bonds to get three pairs of nylon stockings.   From the bare-legged women you might think stockings were useless.

John Howard's mother passed along a day or so ago. Just another one of my old patients deserting the s ip and boys are they really pulling out! One after the other like sheep following a bell-wether. One of the sights reserved for old age.

Mrs. Requardt died sometime ago and very greatly enrished the Museum by leaving it a pair of wonderful Robert Adam tables. Genuine and original, designed by Robert Adam and and decorated by Flaxman with beautiful old Wedgewood pieces. Jack called me up to come and see him and told me his wife wanted me to present them, which I think was very sweet and considerate.

The weather has changed again today and we have a young hurrican playing around outside and the thermometer dropping by the minute. A good thing because another week of summertime and our fruit trees would have been blooming - as it is the leaves on the bushes around home were making real progress.

More late.   Love from Ma and

Your

Lt. Col. James Bordley, III.,M.C.0-396822

General Hospital 118

A.P.O. 927, c/o Postmaster,

San Francisco, California, U.S.A.

Series III., No. 35

Dr. James Bordley, Jr.

330 N. Charles St.,

Baltimore -1, Md.,U.S.A.

February 29, 1944

Dear Boys,   The country and trees were beautiful this morning, covered with a wet snow.
It was a surprise because for a week it has been like summertime.   The weather in Washington
has been at times frigid and at others boiling over.   The President vetoed the tax bill and
for the first time in eleven years attacked the Democratic members of the Senate and house
in an insulting blast.   Senator Barkley, the Democratic leader, who for eleven long years
has led every fight for Roosevelt, made a speech resigning the Democratic leadership which
had the fire of Hell in it.   Roosevelt has never been as seriously attacked personally
and politically and he resorted to a telegram of apology and excuses to cover his grave
mistake but it fell on deaf ears.   The Bill was passed over his veto by a three to one vote
in both Houses.   Senator Byrd in a public statement said Roosevelt's real reason for vetoing
the Bill was because it carried a clause forcing the C.I.O. to keep books and pay taxes and
that the President8s domestic policies are all based on C.I.O. orders.   I thought the two
billions in the Bill was too little -- in fact only one fifth asked by the Treasury Department -- but the Congressional report showed pretty conclusively that to increase its size
would require a sales tax and this Mr. Roosevelt objects to and wanted the difference made
up by Income Tax on people in the lower brackets.   The fact is those in the higher brackets
now get taxed as high as ninety-five percent.   You can't get blood out of a turnip.   To
have this occur at this time is terrible   We should all be pulling together against Hitler
but damned politicians never think further than they can see and they all suffer from
extreme nearsightedness.   The people are getting fed up but can't find a leader to direct
them.   When they do, if ever, they will turn things upside down.
          I just heard that Jim is now Commanding Officer of 118. If so, congratulations.
It is nice to know that your work is recognized even though it adds to your worries and responsibilities.   Let us know the facts and tell us whether eagles came along with it. It
will be too bad for me to have to take orders after being a veteran for twenty-five years,
but I gladly salutate my superior.
          Must hurry along now and will write more later.
          With love from Ma and
                    Your

Major John E. Bordley, M.C. O-403012   Dr. James Bordley, Jr.

General Hospital 118
                                        330 N. Charles St.,
A.P.O. 927, c/o Postmaster
                                        Baltimore -b, Md., U.S.A.
San Francisco, California, U.S.A.

                                        March 11, 1944
              Series III., No. 36

Dear Boys,   The maestro has been so busy getting ready for histalk on old Maryland made
furniture and practicing medicine that he could not take the time to write.   It is over now
and I am extricated from another trouble my good nature roped me into.   Well I had a packed
house, with no standing room left and, if I do say it myself, I put on a first rate show.
I told the history of Maryland from 1785 to 1920 as a background and then gave a brief
history of the cabinet makers involved and showed some sixty slides of the motifs used by
them as points inidentification and then illustrated and analyzed two pieces which have been
wrongly classified as English,illustrating the differences.   I have been asked to publish
thestory in two journals but the Baltimore Museum wants me to write a monograph and include
all the illustrations as original material for its library.   The latter appeals to me most
as the article will not have to be re-edited as it would be without the illustrations.
Everybody in Baltimore with a piece of furniture is ca ling by phone to get me to say
whether it is Maryland. Last night I spent on the telephone.   I think the crowds
attending these talks on old things come because they are practically conscious.   If you
know what I mean. They want to hear of the old times, see old things connected with our
history. It is sort of an internal revival.   I saw men at the talks who care no more for
furniture than I do for diamonds, but their sons and neighbors are in the armed forces and
they have a feeling of glorification and want to know what their ancestors did.   It is a
psychological attack.   They tell me that books dealing with our past glories are selling
like hot cakes. People want to know more about their ancestors and their country. It is
the best thing that has come out of the war so far.   Had a talk with Donald ross
this morning. He says his mother is home and looking well and eating better than for a long
time.   He feels she isout of the woods and I hope so because she has had a pretty hard
fight. He says Jim's kidslook fine.   We are having a Red Cross drive. The stated
quote is two and a half millions.   Where in the devil the money comes from I don't know, but
it comes for every war cause.   They asked us all to give 65% more than the last drive and
they are getting it.   The question of cash is a hard one with taxes up so a man in my position pays twenty-five percent. more National, State and City.   Food prices vary in rise
from 10% to 400%, every article you wear, or, need for household use isup from 25% to 100%.
I bought a pair of scissors which usually cost $2.50, they now cost $13.00, a pair of forceps
usual cost $3.00, now cost $12.00. If this is true for me, it must be for everyone else so
Icannot figure out how people find the cash to subscribe more than last year and have money
enough left to pay rent and buy food. Then there is no kicking, everybody goes down deep
with real cheerfulness. The casualty lists, which grow larger daily, have a stimulating
effect I feel sure. So far but few of our acquaintances have been accounted for,   I hope
it holds good.

              With love from Ma and

                        Your

Major John E. Bordley,M.C. O-403012   Dr. James Bordley, Jr.

General Hospital 118

A.P.O. 927, c/o Postmaster   330 N. Charles St

San Francisco, California, U.S.A.   Baltimore -1,Md.

                                          February 7, 1944.

                Series III., No. 32

Dear Boys,

        The newspapers are filled with the South Pacific furloush business but no official
I have tackled knows anything about it.   One Colonel, who probably knows no more than I,
suggested it is an easy way to withdraw troops for some other operation. I know they are
piling in from various places but on what are called limited furloughs.   The public is all
for your Commanding Officer and would raise hell if any of hisforces were withdrawn.
Smith is going to make some inquiries at headquarters,

        Everything is getting shaped up for the coming invasion, and I suppose before
long the thing will roll along.   I am holding my breath because I have a pretty clear
picture of what is going to happen and I have many friends whose sons will be there.
You just can't win a war without casualities and after two years and ten million men involved we have done extraordinarily well. I hope it keeps up.

        Russia is going to save is many losses and without what she has done God knows
how this war could have been won.   I pray for her every night and thank God we have such an
ally. Communism is pretty bad sort of Government for thouhtful people but seems to work
when you need someone to think for you.   It has at least taken the boasts out of their
enemies mouths.   When you think what Germany bit off and how she chewed it, it is really
remarkable.   With the whole world against her she will of course crack, but, what a
stubborn people.

        I am still hard at work but very well except a bit jittery at times.   I have
unnecessarily added to my burden by taking on a couple of lectures, which make me work a
little too late and get up a little too early.

        Everybody is well.   Ma and I send love.

                                Your

Lt.Col. James Bordley,III.,M.C&O-396822 Dr. James Bordley,Jr.,

General Hospital 118

A.P.O. 927, c/o Postmaster,

San Francisco, California,U.S.A.

330 N. Charles St.,

Baltimore -1, Md., U.S.A.

February 12, 1944

Series III., No. 33

Dear Boys, For the first time in two years I have declined to drive my automobile. We had a big snow and then a rain, and now twenty degrees and a strong wind. The pavements are all ice. You see there is no one left to clear the streets and pavements and the stuff accumulates (even the trash and garbage) and it really makes a mess. I would not mind except for the fact that many street cars are being run by the wildest lot of dames who ever turned a crank. Life grows more complex and Hitler knows it and expects us to crack but he evidently never studied the history of our pioneer forebears. We will kick and raise hell among ourselves but hit the first foreigner in the eye who tries to interfere and he is a foreigner. We are all thrilled at the progress in the Pacific. It looks from here that the team play there is better than that across the Atlantic but far be it from me to criticise because I know nothing about fighting wars. It is true we have largely rid the Atlantic of submarines and have greatly reduced the air strength of Germany but our European battle efforts seem puny when compared with Russia. We travel yards where they travel miles, we engage a few divisions while they take on vast armies. Maybe the Germans want to get back to Germany but a lot of them are staying permanently in Russia. At home, we are still playing politics, the President fighting Congress and Congress the President, the Republicans the Democrats and visa versa. It is too sickening but I suppose the price of Democracy. The soldier vote and subsidies are kicking up a hullabaloo. Yesterday Congress voted down all subsidies and tomorrow the President will veto the bill and the day after Congress will try to pass it over his veto (but I think will fail). So with the soldier vote on national issues for the soldiers carried out through a national law. Congress is determined to have a state controlled vote, and declares the President's plan will nullify the election because the procedure would be unconstitional. But with the President in control of the Supreme Court I doubt that. It is a hell of a mess. The boys have put a monkey wrench in the gasoline and food rationing but forged coupons. The rascals are when caught given a few months in jail. If rationing is so essential as we are told, they should be hung.

It has been announced that Eddie Broyles and Edmund keeney have discovered a drug which effectively kills the fungus of athletes foot and are experimenting with fungus in lungs. Eddie is way below his speciality. The announcement came from Keeney. You may know about it.

Maryland is five pe cent. over its bond quota of $200,000,000. This is pretty good in face of rising taxes and food prices.

I must stop and see some more of the multitude.

Love from Ma and

Your

222

Major John E. Bordley, M.C.   J12   Dr. James Bordley, Jr.

General Hospital 118   330 N. Charles St.,

A.P.O. 927, c/o Postmaster,   Baltimore -1, Md.,U.S.A.

San Francisco, California, U.S.A.   February 23, 1944

Series III., No. 34

Dear Boys,   Well I have passed the biblical three score and ten bu I still believe that you are as young as your faith, as old as your doubts; as young as your self-confidence, as old as your fear; as young as your hope and as old as your despair. This is to be my philosophy from now to the end as it has been for a good many years. I hope when you look down from the pinnacle I have reached in age you will see the same green valley, with its flower lined walks of desires realized. Never a great man I have tried to shoulder my burden and deliver it at its destination. I never was troubled with an ambition requiring self adulation. I have only wanted an opportunity to do a first class job well and I hope I have measured up to my opportunities.   The children, with the exception of Jim's, came to my birthday party which added much gayety to the scene. I was sorry Dudy and her flock could not come but the illness of Mrs. Ross has tied her down all winter.   I have no social news to write, have been much too busy and also disinclined to enter into any outside festivities and besides that is the field of the women.

     I think I wrote you that I was to take part in a symposium on the Ancient Arts and Architecture of Maryland. I have gathered together the most beautiful group of furniture illustrations and I hope I can do credit to them. It has been a terrible labor because I have been so busy but I think it has paid. The meetings so far have been crowded and I am looking forward to an appreciative audience.

     Congress and the President have locked horns on many bills and as fast as Congress passes them he vetoes. Senator Byrd said yesterday that the President is merely carrying out a program arranged for him by the C.I.O. as a preliminary to the election and of serious detriment to the country's interests. Even his standbys in Congress and the Senate have deserted his ship. It is a rotten mess and full of portent.

     A sign of hard work is illustrated by the short stay doctors make in the hospitals. You formerly could get a line of gab at either the U.M.H. r the Womans but now they only drop into the doctors' room to get their hats and coats. It really lookslike a deserted village. The gents who used to go to Florida for a winter rest are all on the job which means less bait for the fish and fewer fees for the caddies. The stores open now at nine and some at ten o'clock so as to keep transportation open to the war workers and gosh they are legion! Glenn Martin now has fifty thousand and is building a large addition; the Fairfield shop yard has forty thousand and Bethlehem steel between forty and fifty. Ships are being turnedout so fast they have had to go back to Roosevelt's ancestors for name.

     Mrs. Roosevelt is planning a good will tour to "cheer up the troops on outlying islands", besides she has declared herself in favor of youth military training -- at seventeen for one year -- of all boys and girls. Frank now supports the motion and being unanimous it may be defeated because Congress wants no part of "Hitler's scheme".

                    More later.   Love from Ma and

                              Your

Lt.Col.James Bordley,III.,M.C. 0-396822 Dr. James Bordley, Jr.,

General Hospital 118   330 N. Charles St.,

A.P.O. 927, c/o Postmaster

                                                  Baltimore -1, Md., U.S.A.
San Francisco, California, U.S.A.

                                                  March 13, 1944

                       Series III., No. 37

Dear Boys,   Politically things grow more tangled.   The really serious part of the story is
that in every by-election that has been held this year for Congressmen the Republicans have won
and today the great Democratic majority has been reduced to just one.   In the Senate the Democrats have about sixteen majority with thirty-two seats to be filled at the November elections.
This does not mean that the President has sixteen majority because nine of the Southern Senators are opposed to him, so a change of five seats at most will leave him without Senate support.   Now this will mean after November a Republican Congress beyond doubt and a possible
Democratic President.   Of course, this will seriously interfere with both our war and peace
aims because by the nature of politics they will never pull together.   The only way to stop
the Republican trend is for the Democratic party to nominate a man like Byrd (and there is no
chance) in whom the people have faith.   The personal strength of Roosevelt may re-elect him but
he cannot carry Congress along with him.   His strong stand will be on war issues, his weakness
on domestic policies and it is the latter which will bring in a Republican Congress.   One after
another his domestic policies are being exposed as totally fallacious or inadequate and his
coupling up with the C.I.O. has a mess of Democrats worried.   It is a fact that this branch of
labor today dictates the domestic policies of the Administration and carries them from bad to
worse.   I am branching out as a photographer with John's camera.   I regret to say that
his two rolls of films were dated for Oct.1,1942 which necessitated my buying others.   My old
tripod camera really takes beautiful pictures but is unhandy to carry around.   I am taking
pictures of furniture details and propose writing a complete story of the Maryland product.
The trouble is I have to practice medicine and it interferes a great deal, in fact, leaves me
little time, but, by systematically plugging I will finish in due time.   Ellen Webb is going
to help me as my pictures are in colors which requires a bit more skill than I have.

        Our cook has a cold (so she says) and has been home and visiting friends for a week,
so I am back at dish-washing and bed making.   The damned niggers are the most shiftless, unreliable bunch that God ever made.   Wages and living conditions play no part in their philosophy of life.   The great trouble now is that there is a concerted drive from a great many
directions to help them and the would be helpers do not take sufficient account of their nature.
They are by and large dirty and shiftless and no matter what habitations are built for them
they will never adequately care for them.   Demand is being made to have Southern Colleges receive them as students, that business open its offices to them as secretaries and stenographers
and that industrial plants take them on equal terms with whites.   They are too utterly unreliable to be trusted with business responsibilities.   I mean the rank and file for whom
the Roosevelts are demanding social equality.

                More later.   Love from Ma and

                                    Your

Lt.Col.James Bordley,III.,M.C. O-396822   Dr. James Bordley, Jr.,

General Hospital 118   330 N. Charles St.,

A.P.O. 927, c/o Postmaster

San Francisco, California, U.S.A.   Baltimore -1, Md., U.S.A.

                                                 March 13, 1944

Series III., No. 37

Dear Boys,   Politically things grow more tangled.   The really serious part of the story is
that in every by-election that has been held this year for Congressmen the Republicans have won
and today the great Democratic majority has been reduced to just one.   In the Senate the Democrats have about sixteen majority with thirty-two seats to be filled at the Novembr elections.
This does not mean that the President has sixteen majority because nine of the Southern Senators are opposed to him, so a change of five seats at most will leave him without Senate support.   Now this will mean after November a Republican Congress beyond doubt and a possible
Democratic President.   Of course, this will seriously interfere with both our war and peace
aims because by the nature of politics they will never pull together.   The only way to stop
the Republican trend is for the Democratic party to nominate a man like Byrd (and there is no
chance) in whom the people have faith.   The personal strength of Roosevelt may re-elect him but
he cannot carry Congress along with him.   His strong stand will be on war issues, his weakness
on domestic policies and it is the latter which will bring in a Republican Congress.   One after
another his domestic policies are being exposed as totally fallacious or inadequate and his
coupling up with the C.I.O. has a mess of Democrats worried.   It is a fact that this branch of
labor today dictates the domestic policies of the Administration and carries them from bad to
worse.   I am branching out as a photographer with John's camera.   I regret to say that
his two rolls of films were dated for Oct.1,1942 which necessitated my buying others.   My old
tripod camera really takes beautiful pictures but is unhandy to carry around.   I am taking
pictures of furniture details and propose writing a complete story of the Maryland product.
The trouble is I have to practice medicine and it interferes a great deal, in fact, leaves me
little time, but, by systematically plugging I will finish in due time.   Ellen Webb is going
to help me as my pictures are in colors which requires a bit more skill than I have.
        Our cook has a cold (so she says) and has been home and visiting friends for a week,
so I am back at dish-washing and bed making.   The damned niggers are the most shiftless, unreliable bunch that God ever made.   Wages and living conditions play no part in their philosophy of life.   The great trouble now is that there is a concerted drive from a great many
directions to help them and the would be helpers do not take sufficient account of their nature.
They are by and large dirty and shiftless and no matter what habitations are built for them
they will never adequately care for them.   Demand is being made to have Southern Colleges receive them as students, that business open itsoffices to them as secretaries and stenographers
and that industrial plants take them on equal terms with whites.   They are too utterly unreliable to be trusted with business responsibilities.   I mean the rank and file for whom
the Roosevelts are demanding social equality.
        More later.   Love from Ma and
                        Your

Major John E. Bordley, M.C. O-403012   Dr. James Bordley, Jr.

General Hospital 118   330 N. Charles St.,

A.P.O. 927, c/o Postmaster

San Francisco, California, U.S.A.   Baltimore -1, Md., U.S.A.

                                                   March 16, 1944

                    Series III., No. 38

Dear Boys,

The Hopkins has set up a Unit -- General Hospital -- in England.   As I understand, it is not an official Hopkins Unit but rather a get together of Hopkins doctors. Ben Rutledge is head of medicine and S. W. Moore (of a New York Hospital) head of Surgery; Don Woodruff head of Urology; Gerald Evans, Robert Mason, Paul Lemkin, Marcus Ravitch, Averill Stowell, Douglas Lockard, Arthur Grennan, David Crob and a long list of Hopkins nurses. They had to pretty near build their ownhospital as only the main building was provided and that without prepared spaces.

The Government is having a heck of a time with gasoline rationing. It is said that 45% of the "C" books are counterfeits and it has become necessary to insure coupons with serial numbers marked with the license number of the car. If you could see the number of coupons taken in by the large dealers in one day you could appreciate it will be an endless job of bookkeeping to keep records of sales. I think they should take about a dozen of the black market gentlemen and shoot or hang them. In fact there are black marketsin everything and you can visualize who is running most of them. (The gents whose consciences are not disturbed by profits). Of course the boot-legger of liquor is coming back fast and hisposition is made secure by a nine dollar a gallon tax on whiskey. In my judgment this tax will lose the Government more taxes on liquor than they take in.

The soldier vote law was passed yesterday. It is believed the President will veto it on the groundthat the States cannot carry out its provisions. It is confusing I can form no opinion.

Dudy is coming down Monday of next week for a check of her eyes and teeth. Says the kids are fine. Don was here the other day and says his mother is eating and looking better than for years.

It seems strange to us at home that Russia can smash a couple of million Nazis and the combined Armies of England and France and the U. S. cannot budge a hundred thousand Germans in Italy.   Mud is the excuse but the Russians are not even slowed down by mud deep enough to bog down German transports. Maybe the Italian campaign is a holding affair to keep a lot of Germans busy and maybe the stalemate is entirely doe to the Germans fighting ability. The campaign looks bad when you see the American Navy and Army grabbing everything in sight in the Pacific. Maybe it is too much politics and not enough planning. It is easy to criticize.

                    More later. Love from Ma and
                                  Your

Lt.Col.James Bordley,III.,M.C. O-396822

General Hospital 118

A.P.O. 927, c/o Postmaster

San Francisco, California, U.S.A.

Series III., No. 39

Dr. James Bordley, Jr.

330 N. Charles St

Baltimore -1, Md., U.S.A.

March 20, 1944.

Dear Boys, This is a hell of a day. It snowed all last night, then rained and with a temperature around 20 this morning, the streets were worse than any time this year. I came in on the street car with a mob large enough to fill the Lyric. St. Patrick's day we had snow, hail, rain, a heavy wind and a thunder storm. It lived up to its Irish reputation -- Turbulent. I would not have come to town except that Dudy is coming and I was too late trying to head her off.

I had an afternoon yesterday. People from the Maryland Historical and National Museum spent about five hours going over our antiques and having me explain the diagnostics of Maryland furniture. They were all intelligent, informed persons so it was a very delightful time for me because I know more about it than they did.

We are without a cook and Mother and I are on the loose again, running from one chop suey joint to another getting food. When you come home I will be able to tell you about all eating places, probably including the night clibs. It is disgusting and discouraging especially when you see a gay lot of birds of Paradise sitting around in large groups on the front steps of the negro districts and know that you are being taxed to support them. The negroes had a big parade and demonstration demanding that they be included among private secretaries, stenographers, bookkeepers and clerks. They are the most unstable, unreliable people in the world and when the war is over they will be discharged by the millions. Every man with whom I have talked has employed them on war work and not a single favorable comment to make. About 90% of them are worthless and cannot be trusted on a job. One man said he had one supervisor for every hundred whites and four for the same number of blacks and that the production of the whites was 20% above the blacks. You know what he will do when he can hire white help.

I heard yesterday that Ben Rutledge has always been afraid to go near an airplane and since going to England they have had him flying all over the place. He still does not enjoy the exercise. That reminds me of Homer Saint-Gaudens. He never flew until he got in the Army and since then he has flown back and forth to England twice, to Panama four times and to the West Coast a dozen times. I asked him what he did on the flights and his reply was, "I am so busy raising goose pimples I have no time to even look out".

You know the Government has put the breaks on the wholesale college education for enlisted men. It has left most of the Colleges suspended in thin air. At the Hopkins University practically their whole enrollment has vanished. Being of service age they have bee inducted in fighting units and sent away. I don't know what may happen to the boys who have been studying modern Greek, Italian, French, Spanich and Japanese. They were to be inducted in organization devoted to governmental functions in conquered countries. I guess they will first have to assist in the conquering.

More later. Love from Ma and

Your

Major John E. Bordley, M.C. 0-403012   Dr. James Bordley, Jr.

General Hospital 118

A.P.O. 927, c/o Postmaster   330 N. Charles St.,

San Francisco, California, U.S.A.   Baltimore -1, Md., U.S.A.

                                              March 28, 1944
                                              Series III., No. 40

Dear Boys,   There is nothing on an even keel here except taxes.   The Baltimore Sun says
that until the people realize their own responsibilities they cannot expect adequate response
from Government. Politics we must always have and power politics is only an exaggeration of
the common variety applied on a more intensive scale.   It is up to us to guide its direction
because if it takes a proper course it can be a power for good.   The great trouble is that
we are too small minded to grasp all of its implications, even see in fact only a small part
at a time.

        There is a hot controversy going on here.   A negro organization wants to hold a big
function at the Lyric and the management has declared the hall not available.   The Mayor, a
Republican, is supporting the negroes.   One of the features is a negro woman singer (Bess of
Porgy and Bess) and she has demanded that the Lyric not discriminate in seating whites and
blacks. Mrs. Roosevelt is to be the principal speaker -- and I suspect is behind most of the
trouble. It is now up for a legal opinion because the negroes claim as a subsidized institution every taxpayer has a right to its use. Of course it is a bad precedent, but, I don't
know! The trouble is that once given command the negroes will try and exploit their position.
They always have.   The Roosevelts have provided us with an acute stage in the negro problem and have added fuel to a smouldering Jewish question.   Both a distinct disservice to
both peoples.

        The fighting over in Italy has bogged down badly. Just why seems a mystery without the
Germans were far stronger than was supposed and we had too small an army.   It is politically
bad even though it has taken Italy out of the war and given us airfields from which to attack
German industry.   It shows us what to expect from a Western invasion.

        Bill Fisher is home for probably a year's work in teaching at some naval station. He
saw a lot of the fighting in the Pacific, enough to make him revise downward his idea of the
length of the war. He thinks from a naval standpoint we are tops.

        The casualty lists are beginning to flow in, not so large yet but persistent. For a
long time few of our boys were involved but now it is different. I hope the effect will be
a boost to home morale and a greater incentive to effort which is badly needed.   Employment
does not keep pace with labor drop off. It is a serious problem and should long ago have
been met with a labor draft.   This new man power move to take away twenty-six year old labor
from industry and place it in the Army has brought about a rapid shift of such men from industry to agriculture which is protected by a special law.   It gives you a headache to try
and keep up with the question of man power. The President has been a jellyfish and Congress
is playing politics.

        Secretary Hull and Governor Dewey have been in acrimonious debate over news releases.
Dewey says Hull asked the British Government to censor our news, Hull says it is a lie. Take
your choice. I think our news reports have been pretty fair and accurate.   Of course, not
all that newspapers want, but, still good.
                More later. Love from Ma and
                                Your

Lt.Col.James Bordley,III.,M.C. O-396822

General Hospital 118

A.P.O. 927, c/o Postmaster

SanFrancisco, California, U.S.A.

Dr. James Bordley, Jr.,

330 N. Charles St.,

Baltimore, -1, Md., U.S.A.

April 1, 1944

Series III., No. 41

Dear Boys,   You will be able to vote. Yesterday the President let the bill pass without his signature and the State of Maryland at an extra session of the Legislature approved the plan for a national ballott. Twelve of the States have declined to accept it which brings a serious question of a constitutional election. The bill does not interfere with State laws as to qualifications, it only provides the means of getting the ballots out and in.

The War Department has announced the Germans have definitely stopped our Italian advance and in fact have re-occupied territory formerly occupied by the Allies.   There is,of course some bitter criticism but by and large the people are confident of the Army's ability and await further action.   We could not by pass Cassino because the surrounding land has been a gigantic mud hole all winter which would have forced us to cross two small rivers which would have exposed our troops to a merciless cross fire.   The boys on the beach head are just stuck because they do not number enough to lick a large superior German Army.   No explanation is given why they are there without sufficient strength.   Maybe our Allied staff was just plain fooled.   The comparison of Russian deeds makes one wonder what they have and what we lack.   They are marvelous fo far and travel about as fast as an express train and they always seem to have what they need.   Some people here believe the Germans areretreating because they want to get nearer their bases of supplies, made necessary by a serious lack of railroad facilities and trucks. The only thing against that is theystarted too late and not until Russia demonstrated her superiority. Will she have to recover after the war! And why not, she has shown more guts as a nation than any of us, they thrive on sacrifices and shortages.

Ellen had a nice letter yesterday from   . He is down on Mississippi. We were all interested in reading it. He expects to report in several weeks, and supposes he may get another assignment but does not suggest where.   Elsie is back cooking for us which is a great joy for your mother who really looks less tired already.   She has had a siege but never a word about it has she spoken.   I hope Elsie will stay this time, in fact I amthinking about legally adopting her. We are to have a dinner tomorrow, the first in about two years. Mother is as excited over it as a kid at Xmas.

I have been requested to give a talk at the Museum next month but I got enough in the preparation of the last, but in the end I will probably fall for it. It takes my mind off my troubles, that is one kind of trouble.

At last Congress has decided to draft all 3-Fs and build labor battalions. Sending them where they are needed.   There is talk also of drafting 4-Fs but that would be very unwise because they are mentally or physically crippled and could be of no particular use.   All are to be inducted into the Army and put to work on furloughs.

More later.   Love from Ma and

Your

Major John E. Bordley, M.C. O-403012   Dr. James Bordley, Jr.,

General Hospital 118

A.P.O. 927, c/o Postmaster   330 N. Charles St.,

San Francisco, California, U.S.A.   Baltimore -1, Md., U.S.A.

April 3rd, 1944

Series III., No. 42

Dear Boys,

The third of April and as cold as the middle of January. It looks bad for the fruit. It always looks bad for the farmer but each year we grow a little more. This is a vast country, or, was before the airplane came along, and what does not grow here grows in superabundance somewhere else.

Well Ma had her party and it was a gala occasion which b ought out the old silver and glass and china. It was a real thrill after a lay off of some two years. You felt like opening the windows and shouting to the world that you intended to be normal for one day. Hannah Lowndes, Mrs. Hawkins, Peter Blanchard and his wife, etc. Everybody seemed to enjoy it from the Manhattans to the coffee. It made me feel sort of guilty but as it is more fun tosin than go to chu ch I soon forget my conscience. Mrs. Hawkins showed me a letter telling about John's operation on her grandchild and seemed very happy that he had done it but could not understand how it could have been fixed up.

I hear they have a wonderful chap over at Walter Reed fixing up plastics in conjunction with the pastic surgeons. He has worked out a very pliable material which men tell me is a most remarkable substitute for skins. Even under close examination a new nose or cheek bones cannot be told. He was the make up expert at Hollywood. Everybody in medicine is going over to see him work. I suppose his experience in making girls pretty comes in handy.

We are still bogged down in Italy while Russia goes chasing along. It is a bit discouraging after years of preparation but in the end we will prevail Maybe we could borrow a few generals from Russia. They certainly have a unique technique in destr ying enemies. Maybe they are not trying too hard to conserve their own soldiers. The Sun is publishing a series of articles by their former reporter in France who has been interned in Germany two years. They give his personal impressions of the reactions from defeats and bombi both the German people and Army and outline the procedures the Nazis are taking to preve depression. The articles are very interesting but give little hope for civilian collapse. He thinks the destruction has worked in reverse and boosted German morale. This hardly sounds like a normal German reaction.

I saw Tommy Water wife on Saturday. She looked particularly pretty. I had no chance to ask her about Tommy and I do not know where he is. I usually see him around the Club but I get there so seldom I suppose I have missed him.

We have a le up in rationing now. Things have piled up so fast there isno cold storage space for the coming crops. This sounds to me like they underestimated supplies and that in the face of the fact that hundreds of thousands of people are eating more than ever before. In fact I think our nation is living as never before. I have no patience with the growlers and there are plenty of them.

More later. Love from Ma and

Your

Series III., No. 43   April 10, 1944

Dear Boys, Wendell Wilkie took an awful licking in Wiscons͟   ͟s tragic but American. he
withdrew his name from further consideration. I am not surprised because I am convinced this
country is slowly but surely being lead back to isolationism. It is a profitable venture for
those who make money out of a high tariff and a telling argument with farmers who want to ex-
port but not import food stuffs. The swing to the Republican party is only a sign and it is
very definite that the swing is toward the ultra conservative element in that party. I am convinced that Wilkie has definitely given birth to a new trend of thought and that his services
have been of great value. It takes a generation for new ideas to percolate through the body
politic. It is timid and clings to what it has no matter how insufficient rather than experiment with new ideas. Four things worked against Wilkie: he was in favor of more taxes to hold
down the national debt, wanted them now because of the enormous national income; he told the
people what he thought, irrespective of its effect uponthem; it was currently believed he
favored many of the plans and ideas of Roosevelt; he plead for a foreign policy giving the
nations international responsibilities. In other words he believed in the acceptance of national and international responsibilities and this country is not now prepared to accept the thesis,
no more prepared thanin the time of Woodrow Wilson. This may come as a shock to our Army which
believes it is fighting for what Wilkie stands for whether for or against the man. Or,does it!
Maybe the individuals inthe armed forces are still activated by political considerations of a
ward variety while fighting for sound principles. I don't know. While not surprised I am
shocked. I want Roosevelt defeated but if the Republican party does not give us a strong candidate on a strong progressive platform I shall vote for Roosevelt. It isonly half a loaf but
it is better than none. His domestic policies are bad and his foreign policy poor but I will
accept them rather than return to the days of Coolidge and Hoover. (Two days later). Secret͟
Hull spoke in extenso yesterday on our foreign policy. It was straight from the shoulder
very clear and quite rational. I think the nation will back it 100%. The only criticism that
is adverse is in the non-recognition of the French Committee of Liberation. His position is
that the French people must elect their own officers and establish their own Government and that
no Committee outside of Continental France has a right to represent France except in so far as
the Allies require guidance. It is the purpose of the Government to consult with the Committee
but not attempt to make it supreme in France. Both England and Russia are willing to accept
the deGaulists 100% and same t ink with an invasion impending the voice should be unanimous.
I am sure Mr.Hull's statement has made the President's position far more secure and gathered in
some hundreds of thousands voters. I do not mean to imply the speech was for that purpose. I
believe Mr. Hull a high minded public official who would not stoop to questionable tricks. The
people were demanding information so he gave it to them.   Yesterday was a beautiful Easter day. Ma and I went out to the Weebs to hunt rabbit eggs with the kids. It was lots
of fun but a bit hard on the legs and back. There was the usual parade of finery up Charles
St.,hardly suggestive of the great air battle being fought over Eastern Germany at the time,
but I suppose it was not a bad idea. People are less troubled and troublesome when they are
occupied.   More later.   Love fromMa and
                              Your

231

Major John E. Bordley, M.C.O-403012

General Hospital 118

A.P.O. 927, c/o Postmaster

San Francisco, California, U.S.A.
Series III, No. 44

Dr. James Bordley, Jr.

330 N. Charles St.,

1
Baltimore, Md., U.S.A.

April 14, 1944.

Dear Boys,   Just had word that Worthington has a Purple Heart.   I wonder whether he is
with your outfit. I suppose not as he was a long way from you. He wrote a very scratchy
letter, short with no details and said as soon as he was able to write he would tell more
about himself.   Evidently the European invasion is not far away, or, maybe it is only a
gesture to draw Germans away from the Eastern front.   The bombing pattern is distinctly
changed so it looks like business.   I really believe the people here are more alert as the
time grows shorter.   So many families and friends are involved that it makes the war seem
nearer to a large proportion of our population.   Ther is a lot of parlor criticism of the
general strategy.   It reminds me of the old women who butt in on our patients and tell th m
how badly they are being treated.   It takes a very wise man to understand his own limitations
and he is a wiser one who never advised about things he knows nothing of.   I never say one
critical word about the Armed Forces because I am sure they have an over all pattern of which I
am entirely ignorant.   You should see the boys scampering for cover now that all eligibles
not in key positions in critical industries are being called -- married and single.   They have
had two years to get into a helpful position but preferred to hold their status and make money.
It is over now and how they scamper trying to find cover.   I am losing no sleep over them.
I can't tell you how many of such of their families have tried to get me to help them dodge.
My specialty has been to try and help those get in who have been turned down but really want
to help and I have had some success.   I never help dodgers in any way.   I must say the Army
has taken in some whose eye sight and hearing is pretty terrible.   I know one boy who has
only one eye and not over twenty percent vision in that, who holds a very important job on
the front.   It is beyond my imagination how he gets away with it.
            This is another cold April day, in fact we have had freezes for the past two nights
and I am afraid the advance gardeners will have to replant.
            I sold our home last night. Charles Garland, now in with Alexander Brown, came over
to the house last night at nine o'clock, stayed until eleven, and left with a contract.   He
had never seen the house before and of course was pleased with it.   Said he, "This is the
first house I have ever seen with everything just as I like it."   He was Vines doubles partner and won a lot of cups on his own and I am sure the squash court played a major role in the
sale.   I got five thousand dollars more for it than all the real estate men said I would get.
In fact the best price paid in twelve years for a Guilford house.   While it was nothing like
the cost, or, value it was satisfactory.   Now what in the devil we are going to do with all
our stuff is beyond me but I guess we will be able to store or sell what we will not need.
I am going to take an apartment if I can ever find one and if I cannot, we will go over to
McElderry St. as the lease on that house is out in September and we will not have to get out
until October 1st.   I sold it to save your mother. The servant problem is so bad that it
kept her nose right down on the grindstone, which worried me all the time. I am going to
try and get in some apartment house where meals are served so if we have no cook we can still
eat without mother's cooking.
            More later.   Love from Ma and
                            Your

232

Lt.Col. James Bordley,III., M.C. 0-396822   Dr.James Bordley, Jr.

       General Hospital 118   330 N. Charles St

          A.P.O. 927, c/o Postmaster   Baltimore -1, Md., U. S. A.

       San Francisco, California, U.S.A.   April 20, 1944.
                              Series III., 45

Dear Boys,   Your little orphan parents have no home.   Every apartment house is filled
and no prospects.   I have appealed to some of my friends who own establishments but without
results.   I still own the little house over by the Hopkins and am holding back its rental
until we are sure of our location.   I am distributing my library, giving the medical books
to the Library of the Maryland University, except those belonging to you and some rare edi-
tions which I am keeping for you. I am sending to the little Centreville Library all the
standard works and such current novels as I have; to the Museum the works of art.   I am keep-
all the biography, history and antiques.   There are quite a number of your books which are
set aside for you.   We are not going to disperse the liquor until you come home so you can
each get your share.   Many other things will find their way into your wives' hands so you can
enjoy them when you get back, that will include furniture, etc.   We are keeping enough to
furnish an apartment and only enough.

          This is a terrific break but neither your mother nor I are worrying about it. It
had to come and we both knew it. We have had a wonderful life and no cause for regrets. And
it is a voluntary choice and nothing forced upon us so it is easier to be philosophical. The
whole truth is we are too old to assume the burden and worry of a big establishment, to be in-
adequately run by inferior servants (when we can get them).   It will not be long now before I
close the office and spend the balance of my time in pursuits of interest without responsibility. I have many things I want to do and less time each day in which to do them.   So don't
worry about us or have any illusions about out attitude. We will be happier when we are
settled.   We are going to get Dudy to bring the children down in a couple of weeks. I want
Bay to remember the home.

          We are preparing to have a big fight for the next Senator. Tydings is up against
strong opposition in his own party and even stronger from the Republicans.   Charlie Webb
thinks he is going to get a good licking to which I do not subscribe. I think he will get the
support of all the independent vote and that is always the determining factor in this State.
I must say I am a bad prognosticator so maybe Charlie is right. Tydings and Willis Jones
his Democratic opponent had a debate last night and while the fur flew I think Tydings much
more than held his own. Charlie thinks he has a swelled head since marrying a rich wife and
that he is posing too much for the average voter. The most damaging thing of which he is
accused is that he has used his office to promote his law firm.   I think he pretty well
spiked that last night.   And what do you think: The President wrote him a letter thanking
him for his cooperation.   Politics is lousy!

          Mrs. Lambden has sold her home and left Sam and gone to New York to live. This
will permit Sam to spend more time at home.   Maybe she has her eye on some new Adonis.

          More later.

                         Love from Ma and
                              Your

                                                                              233

Major John E. Bordley, M.C. O-403012

General Hospital 118

A.P.O. 927, c/o Postmaster

San Francisco, California, U.S.A.

Dr. James Bordley, Jr.,

330 N. Charles St

Baltimore -1, Md., U.S.A.

April 24, 1944

Series II., No. 46

We were thrilled last night by Gen. MacArthur's radio message of the move against
Dear Boys,
the Japs.   It was remarkable that he could surprise them socompletely and wondeful that he
could do it with so little loss.   My, what a gigantic thing this war has developed into.   The
countless lives it has cost and countless treasure expended and expending. This country alone
has amassed a debt of three hundred billions, so great a sum staggers the imagination but what
does it amount to when you think of the human loss.   And all to satisfy the ambitions of a
sign painter!   What a world, what a civilization, what a travesty on intelligence.

Ma and I are trying to find a place to live, so far no luck, but by and by will discover something. We hope. It is remarkable that every apartment house is full and each has
a waiting list of from fifty to a hundred. Servants, or, lack of same; no gas or not sufficient to taxi back and forth to the country; pressure of business requiring a closer residence
and high taxes constitute the reasons for the prosperity of apartments. The prosperity is not
very real however as service costs have exactlydoubled in two years and the services are so
inferior that more supervision is demanded and rents are frozen on a 1941 basis. You can
never imagine the attitude of a large portion of labor, the war to them is just a Roman
holiday, more money, more clothes and more fun. Nothing out of Pandora's box can equal them.
The Secretary of War in speaking before a Congressional Committee epitomized the situation; T
The nation sends its young manhood out to fight and then declines to take its own portion
of the war seriously, the first requsites of which are stability of labor, full cooperation,
and a desire to help keep the nation on an even keel.

I am very uneasy that the Isolationists are making inroads on our post war intentions.
They are working day and night to control the Republican party and to writeits platform. So
far Congress has not fallen for its bait, if you can judge by its acceptance of the gold
standard -- not yet voted on to be sure; the world stabilization fund of seven billion dollars;
and the appointment of a joint committee of Senators to work with the State Department on post
war plans so as to obviate the difficulties of bi-partisam discussions and differences.
Old man McCormick of the Chicago Tribune is the chief devil among the isolationists and is
going so far as to defend a bunch of Seditionists now on trial for helping the Hitler cause.
He should be hung along with the balance.

The United States Chamber of Commerce has selected as its President a man by the name
of Johnson from the Pacific Coast.   He is developing into a national leader and great force
and power.   A remarkable fellow indeed and the dark horse in the Republican Presidential
derby. He is more outspoken as to our shortcomings and our dangers than any one other than
Wilkie, has done more to influence labor and Congress than any other person. He is a tower
of strength for the good and I would love to vote for him. He is a comparatively young man
and full of vim and fight but with a real flare for diplomacy. Even the President has had to
call him in from time to time to help straighten things out but eventhat does not influence
him not to speak his mind.   I had a talk with a man yesterday who write a syndicate column
for some thousand newspapers and he is convinced that Johnson would sweep the country in a
general election, receiving the full support of both labor and business.

More later.   Love from Ma and

Your

234

Major John E. Bordley,M.C. O-40?012   Dr. James Bordley,Jr.,

General Hospital 118   330 N. Charles St

A.P.O. 927, c/o Postmaster

San Francisco, California, U.S.A.   Baltimore -1, Md., U.S.A.

April 24, 1944

Series II., No. 46

We were thrilled last night by Gen. MacArthur's radio message of the move against
Dear Boys,
the Japs. It was remarkable that he could surprise them socompletely and wondeful that he
could do it with so little loss. My, what a gigantic thing this war has developed into. The
countless lives it has cost and countless treasure expended and expending. This country alone
has amassed a debt of three hundred billions, so great a sum staggers the imagination but what
does it amount to when you think of the human loss. And all to satisfy the ambitions of a
sign painter! What a world, what a civilization, what a travesty on intelligence.

Ma and I are trying to find a place to live, so far no luck, but by and by we will discover something. We hope. It is remarkable that every apartment house is full and each has
a waiting list of from fifty to a hundred. Servants, or, lack of same; no gas or not sufficient to taxi back and forth to the country; pressure of business requiring a closer residence
and high taxes constitute the reasons for the prosperity of apartments. The prosperity is not
very real however as service costs have exactlydoubled in two years and the services are so
inferior that more supervision is demanded and rents are frozen on a 1941 basis. You can
never imagine the attitude of a large portion of labor, the war to them is just a Roman
holiday, more money, more clothes and more fun. Nothing out of Pandora's box can equal them.
The Secretary of War in speaking before a Congressional Committee epitomized the situation: T
The nation sends its young manhood out to fight and then declines to take its own portion
of the war seriously, the first requsites of which are stability of labor, full cooperation,
and a desire to help keep the nation on an even keel.

I am very uneasy that the Isolationists are making inroads on our post war intentions.
They are working day and night to control the Republican party and to writeits platform. So
far Congress has not fallen for its bait, if you can judge by its acceptance of the gold
standard -- not yet voted on to be sure; the world stabilization fund of seven billion dollars;
and the appointment of a joint committee of Senators to work with the State Department on post
war plans so as to obviate the difficulties of bi-partisam discussions and differences.
Old man McCormick of the Chicago Tribune is the chief devil among the isolationists and is
going so far as to defend a bunch of Seditionists now on trial for helping the Hitler cause.
He should be hung along with the balance.

The United States Chamber of Commerce has selected as its President a man by the name
of Johnson from the Pacific Coast. He is developing into a national leader and great force
and power. A remarkable fellow indeed and the dark horse in the Republican Presidential
derby. He is more outspoken as to our shortcomings and our dangers than any one other than
Wilkie, has done more to influence labor and Congress than any other person. He is a tower
of strength for the good and I would love to vote for him. He is a comparatively young man
and full of vim and fight but with a real flare for diplomacy. Even the President has had to
call him in from time to time to help straighten things out but eventhat does not influence
him not to speak his mind. I had a talk with a man yesterday who write a syndicate column
for some thousand newspapers and he is convinced that Johnson would sweep the country in a
general election, receiving the full support of both labor and business.

More later. Love from Ma and

Your

Lt.Col. James Bordley,III.,M.C. O-396822

Dr. James Bordley,Jr.

General Hospital 118

330 N. Charles St.,

A.P.O. 927, c/oPostmaster

Baltimore, 1, Md.,U.S.A.

San Francisco, California, U.S.A.

April 27, 1944

Series III., No.46

Dear Boys,

The medical pot is boiling. The U. S. Health (Oublic Health) is trying to force through a bill to control th practice of medicine, hospitals, medical education and fees. It is having strong opposition but may pass. The Governor -- O'Connor --has appointed a State Commission, the rep rt of which is just announced, placing the indigent under the medical supervision of the State Department of Health which will keep U.S. Public Health out of Maryland Medicine.   Arthur Shipley is head of anoth r Committee to report for the Medical Faculty its plan for the care of the indigent.   This report comes today. The State plan is very comprehensive and offers adequate medical, hispital and nursing care. It further more does not attempt too much monkey business with the profession.   It is to be under control of the State Health Officer, with county decentralization of control by the County Health Officer.   Over all is a commission embodying public health, medical care, nursing, mental hygiene, tuberculosis, social diseases and hospitals.   It makes agreements with the profession for fees for various services and does not attempt any control of hospital or medical schools.   It will furnish on requisitions approved by its board such money as hospitals and medical fees for the indigent may require. It looks to me like a sensible plan and is not a vote buyer like the U.S. Public Health plan. In other words, one must be entitled to free service before he gets it.

(The next day)

The Medical Faculty has accepped in toto the State plan for medicine and has agreed to work out the essential details such as hospitilization, medical insurance, distribution of physicians in under-staffed localities, etc.   I am delighted that the profession has worked out with the State its own plan and divorced itself from the Nationalset-up. This means freedom of thought, action and education,the three cardinal essentials for a high grade peofession.   Editorially the Baltimore Sun and News are for the plan a hundred percent. and it has the full concurrence of the State Planning Commission (which is doing a fine job for Maryland.   This is interesting as a demonstration of what can be done politically when fine citizens agree to do a political job. Left to their own devices the politicians would have made a mess of the whole thing.   This plan is only for the counties.   A special Commission is preparing a plan for Baltimore. It is essentially the same Commission dealing with a more complex problem which requires special study.   Then another Commission is studying the care of chronic diseases. All these Commissions are under the same wise guidance.

We have been unable to find an apartment but we are not worried because I am holding the little house over by the Hopkins until I know that we can do better.   It is very comfortable but will hold a very small part of our old furnishing.   We will not definitely know about the apartment until July. It is a tedious business making an inventory of our belongings. God only knows where we got so much stuff and why.

More later. Love from Ma and
                    Your

236

Major John E. Bordley, M.C. O-403012   Dr. James Bordley, Jr.

General Hospital 118

A.P.O. 927, c/oPostmaster   330 N. Charles St.,

San Francisco, California, U.S.A.   Baltimore -1, Md., U.S.A.

                                              May 4, 1944

                        Series III., No. 47

Dear Boys,

      Summer is here and the trees and flowers are taking on their greatest charm. The weather has been rainy, too much so for the farmers who are about three weeks back. The Mississippi and Missouri rivers are on their annual rampage and destroying the handiwork of man but all these put together have not raised the rumpus that Attorney General Biddle raised by marching the Army into Montgomery, Ward to demand a contract for the C.I.O. Nothing the Administration has ever done has brought about as much bitterness and Congress has never had as much mail since the President tried to pack the Supreme Court. The Attorneys for the Government pleading before the Supreme Court yesterday said the President had the authority to put even a corner grocer out of business even though there was not a complaint against him. He could confiscate his stock and even his place of business if he saw fit. This will lose Mr. Roosevelt millions of votes and is the most dastardly thing ever done by a President. Done he says for the purpose of suppressing opposition to the Government it has done more to bring disunity than anything that has happened. This show of personal power reminds one unpleasantly of Hutler.

      It appears that Worthington's wound was not serious and he is on deck again. One of the boys just back said Worthington is Commanding Officer of one of the Admiralty Islands. I take this with a hand full of salt.

      Had a letter from Madison saying he had just received his first mail in five months. He touched where Worthington is stationed and looked him up only to find he was away for the day. He did not say where he was so I have no idea where he expected to find Worthington.

      Ma and I are up to our eyes getting things together for moving.

      I don't know whether you have heard of the "forward step" of the Hopkins. They have advanced the nurses training to a post graduate course and will take only women who hold college degrees. This is a long way from the old wet nurse. Some of the administrative nurses at the Hopkins are wondering what will happen and where the graduate are to come from and what they will do when they finish with the new degree. John Gibbs gave a very enthusiastic statement to the papers and seems quite confident as to the outcome. I have always thought there should be a special course given for administrative nurses as the one way to find new methods and inculcate new ideas but I feel such women should be handpicked. My experience with the average woman college graduate is she does not rate any higher than the man graduate and few of them are mentally equipped for executive positions. It is interesting and I am sure no institution other than the Hopkins could put it over.

      More later.

              Love from Ma and

                    Your

Lt.Col.James Bordley,III.,M.C. O-396822

General Hospital 118

A.P.O. 927, c/o Postmaster

San Francisco, California,U.S.A.

Dr. James Bordley,Jr.

330 N. Charles St.,

Baltimore -1, Md.,U.S.A.

May 8th, 1944.

Series III., No. 48

Dear Boys,   For the first time for a long while I have only a handful of patients and what a relief as I had two operations this morning and it takes a lot out of me.   Every day there are from two to four new patients.   Where and why they all come from God knows.   I am losing my desire for work and if you were home I would quit.   This is the psycological time for me to stop.   I have had nearly fifty years of unusual success and happiness in medicine, I still have a fine practice and to stop now will leave a good taste in my mouth.   If I hang on until I get kicked out, it will spoil the whole show.   Going into smaller quarters and getting rid of a lot of financial burden and worry really give me an opportunity to stop.   I am only working for the Government as it takes a major portion of my income to pay taxes   Since January 1 have paid between three and four thousand dollars and the year is not half over and taxes only one quarter.   I know the country needs the money and I am perfectly willing to do my part, in fact that is my only reason for working.   I am ashamed tostop while so many men are making so many more tragic sacrifices.

The President is home after a month's rest down in South Carolina.   He is truly a remarkable chap and can stand a lot of punishment. I often wonder how he gets away with it. He has some serious domestic problems on his hands, the least of which is not the Montgomery Ward business.   All of this could have been saved if the Government had appealled to the Courts for help instead of the Army.   The crux of the whole dirty mess is whether the President had the power to sieze a non war plant.   The Courts could have told the Attorney General and as long as he has now appealled to a New Deal Judge it is a foregone conclusion that he will get the authority.   The facts are this country is now run on executive orders and not constitutional law.   I ca not argue against the Government during the war but I do wish it would do somepracticing as well as preaching constitutional Government.

We still have no place to live but if we can get priority to put in an oil heater we will go to the house on Guilford Ave. occupied by Worthington.This will beonly until we can get an apartment inone of the nicer apartment houses where there is a dining-room.   You know houses are at a tremendous premium, that is two story city houses.   Since you left literally thousands of new houses have been built, whole new towns within the City limits and still the demand shows no let down -- this in spite of the fact that hundreds of war workers have gone home.   The Sun says the colored people are all staying but the whites are leaving.   Well maybe they are but you cannot notice it.

We hear again Jim is Commanding Officer and Wink in charge of Medicine.   We have heard it so often we just disregard it.

More later.   Love from Ma

and

Your

Major John E. Bordley, M.C. O-403012   Dr. James Bordley, Jr.

General Hospital 118

    330 N. Charles St.,

A.P.O. 927, c/o Postmaster

    Baltimore -1, Md. U.S.A.

San Francisco, California, U.S.A.

    May 12, 194

Series III., No. 49

Dear Boys,   The President is back and the Ward concern has been returned to the Company, and the CIO has been voted the Union representative. So all the rashness resulted in exactly nothing except to stir up the country. It is a good riddance. Thousands of workmen are out on strikes in essential plants. The strikes they call unauthorized and against organized labor policy. The court took action against two labor leaders, indicted them, found them guilty and ordered them to jail. They appealed and probably that ends the law as the Supreme Court disregards all precedent and does not much favor the laws. Justice Roberts says with the present attitude of the Supreme Court no man knows where he stands and what are his rights. So much for a Court of the present competency.

I understand Dr. Wise's house is for sale and if he sells it will bring new people to the entire neighborhood. The Johnsons have not occupied their house for nearly two years. Samm Crowe's friends sold to a restauranteur from Highlandtown and Miss Whiteley sold to the Sages. You see our old neighborhood has got to start all over again. Up until this Spring you could not sell a large house and now they are in demand but by an entirely new group of persons. I thought it was because the small house market was exhausted but the real estate men tell me it is new people with rolls of cash and a social desire. I have not seen a "For Sale" sign in Guilford in the past two months and before that I think it conservative to say that one-third of the houses were for sale. I believe when the war is over a lot of these houses will be for sale again. The enormous profits will vanish in the period of readjustment and after that large houses will be a drug on the market. One hundred and seventy-two thousand men from Maryland are in the Army and hundreds per day are now being inducted. This is a good share for our little State of some two million souls. This does not include the Navy and Marine nor the women. It will bring us up to about fifteen percent. making allowances for children and old people, the sick and helpless you can visualize what stock is left to keep up production (and the quality of that production). A similar state of affairs during the Civil War accounts for the backwardness of the South. Even three generations have been unable to greatly elevate the calibre of their stock.

Tomorrow is Preakness Day. Every room in every boarding house and hotel is jammed and the crowd will go out to Pimlico and bet some two millions. Pensive is the favorite since winning the Kentucky Derby but a horse owned by Widener, the experts say, may win. I don't know enough about it to bet my money so I will go out to the Club and play golf for drinks or less.

I went over to the Hopkins last Sunday and in Clifton Park there were thousands of people watching a lacrosse game. I noticed particularly the younger element from say sixteen to twenty-two or three. Where they came from in such huge numbers I can't divine without they were the strangers within our gates who are doing war jobs. Possibly some military although I noticed no uniforms.

Dick Shackelford is home. Had to stop off in San Francisco for a final check up and will not be permitted to return to the South Pacific. Thinks he will have a little time off but how long does not know (on the authority of his father-in-law). Priscilla spent three months down in Florida trying to shake off a sinus infection but being unsuccessful "had a major operation" a few days ago by Sam Crowe. I don't know exactly what.

More later. Love from Ma and

Your

General Hospital 118

A.P.O. 927, c/o Postmaster

San Francisco, California, U.S.A?

330 N. Charles St

Baltimore -1, Md., U.S.A.

June 1, 1944

Series III., No. 52

Dear Boys,   We have had a great time with the children at home and I think they too, have enjoyed themselves. We had the whole Hollyday family around yesterday(Sunday). Jim became quite struck on Dick Hollyday. The children were in a great show-off spirit which is remarkable when you want it. Every time Jim sees me he says "more beer". You might think we are profound topers instead of just steady drinkers. Pat won't touch the stuff, says it "is not nice for little girls but nice for little boys". Well they have brought the home and the old folks to life and we will be sorry to see them go. I know Ma will miss them because Jim makes love to her all the time. It is funny to watch him with her. He looks so much like his daddy that I think it brings back memories of his childhood to Ma. Pat was given a birthday party and had five or six children in to eateggs and toast, cake and ice-cream. She was very cute at the head of the table and entered into the spirit of the occasion.

We heard through aMajor from Down Under this morning that the Army is planning to move your Unit. He said that such things take place slowly and it might be months before you go. He did not intimate where. We hear so many rumors that we disregard them until something official comes along. We know that most of the war around Australia is about finished but there must still be a lot of troop activity and as long as there is I feel you will stay. The war in Italy is getting along well and we are all on our toes waiting to see the Russians start to move and then the Western invasion. May the God of justice stick by us and stab the Hitler gang.

Two days have elapsed since I wrote the last sentence. I have been so busy with so many things I am disgusted. Yesterday, I had a complete inventory made of our furniture with values. It was an eye-opener to me who came through the price rising period of 1927 - 29. They were a mere song as compared with what things bring now. If I were sensible I would sell everything and retire with plenty -- but I am not sensible. The man who made the inventory advised me to sell any junk I owned especially glass, pewter and silver. He thinks there will never be such a market again. He estimates that as compared with the twenties there are now at least twenty times as many purchasers. A large proportion of the fine sales are made to Jewish Refugees who are investing their money in commodities which thru thick and thin maintain a high value. Many of them were European dealers and they are searching the land to find salable things when and if they become established in their old homes.

We were heart-broken to have Dudy and the children leave this morning. They have been more than a ray of sunshine and came at a good time. They were going to stay longer but Dudy found it impracticable to help with the children and pack her belongings. She is coming back the first of the week and store her belongings. We could have a man do it, but she thinks it better to come herself and I guess she is right. Jimmy and I are firm friends. He spend much of the time making faces at me and playing peek-a-boo. Honestly he is a card and the best natured thing I know. I hope you will soon be home to see him.

With love from Ma and

Your

Major John E. Bordley, M.C. O-403012

General Hospital 118

A.P.O. 927, c/o Postmaster

San Francisco, California, U.S2A.

Dr. James Bordley, Jr.

330 N. Charles St.,

Baltimore -1, Md., U.S.A.

May 24, 1944

Series III., No. 51

Dear Boys,

Well, Jim's kids are here and what kids! Jimmy weighs four pounds less than Pat .
thirty-one pounds, is a gay creature in spite of his size. Knew us all by name within the
hour. He is a magician, can slip Pat's toys right from under her nose but takes the trouble
to beat it lest she attack. His hair, which is not in paternal scarcity, just missed being
red. Pat remembered the house and even the ex-servants' names. She knew just where to go
for what she wanted and just what she and I used to play. I think that is pretty smart after
a year away from us. Dudy looks very well but not as fat as she used to be. Says she never
enjoyed better health. I should think carrying Jimmy around would keep her lean. She has
an excellent nurse whom the children seem to like very much. It is a treat to have them
with us. If they could stay, I would never have sold the home.

Ma has been busy making Brucie and Anne little play-suits. They are quaint, pretty
costumes and they both seem crazy about them. I can't describe them except to say they
remind me of the costumes of the Dutch children. Brucie was delighted with hers, I think,
particularly because the waist looks like those of the older children. She isgetting qui+
grown up.

(Another day)

You have got to keep en eye on your son Jimmy. I was having a quiet bottle of beer
out in the butler's pantry when he hove in sight looking for me. I asked him to join meand
to my surprise he, after his first sip, came right back with "more Pop". He hung around
like a fellow hoping for a treat until Dudy carted him off. Pat came in to see what was
going on and when I asked her to join me, she said "it wan't good for a little girl, but it
was all right for a little boy", and you thought you had a modern girl!

Mrs. Roosevelt was over to talk to the negroes in one of their churches a night or
two ago. Her usual inflammatory stuff. Yesterday, they went on a rampage as they always do
after her visits. Today our cook and maid did not show up, it has not yet failed. Yesterday
one of the large plants here discharged a hundred and twenty of them for refusing to take
orders. There is surely coming a day of reckoning and they will have the Roosevelts to thank
for their troubles. The Baltimore Sun has assumed a curious attitude toward the negroes,
calls them, Mr. &. Mrs. & Miss, defends them for their actions. I am sure it is not helpful
in bringing them to a realization of their shortcomings. They are ignorant and arrogant, need
helpful advice and constructive criticism.

Must stop. Love fromMa and

Your

General Hospital 118

330 N. Charles St

A.P.O. 927, c/o Postmaster

Baltimore -1, Md., U.S.A.

San Francisco, California, U.S.A?

June 1, 1944

Series III., No. 52

Dear Boys,   We have had a great time with the children at home and I think they too, have
enjoyed themselves. We had the whole Hollyday family around yesterday(Sunday).   Jim became
quite struck on Dick Hollyday. The children were in a great show-off spirit which is remarkable when you want it.   Every time Jim sees me he says "more beer".   You might think we are
profound topers instead of just steady drinkers. Pat won't touch the stuff, says it "is not
nice for little girls but nice for little boys". Well they have brought the home and the old
folks to life and we will b sorry to see them go. I know Ma will miss them because Jim makes
love to her all the time. It is funny to watch him with her. He looks so much like his daddy
that I think it brings back memories of his childhood to Ma.   Pat was given a birthday party
and had five or six children in to eat eggs and toast, cake and ice-cream.   She was very cute
at the head of the table and entered into the spirit of the occasion.

     We heard through a Major from Down Under this morning that the Army is planning to move
your Unit.   He said that such things take place slowly and it might be months before you go.
He did not intimate where.   We hear so many rumors that we disregard them until something
official comes along.   We know that most of the war around Australia is about finished
but there must still be a lot of troop activity and as long as there is I feel you will stay.
The war in Italy is getting along well and we are all on our toes waiting to see the Russians
start to move and then the Western invasion. May the God of Justice stick by us and stab
the Hitler gang.

     Two days have elapsed since I wrote the last sentence. I have been so busy with so many
things I am disgusted.   Yesterday, I had a complete inventory made of our furniture with
values. It was an eye-opener to me who came through the price rising period of 1927 - 29.
They were a mere song as compared with what things bring now. If I were sensible I would sell
everything and retire with plenty -- but I am not sensible. The man who made the inventory
advised me to sell any junk I owned especially glass, pewter and silver. He thinks there will
never be such a market again.   He estimates that as compared with the twenties there are now
at least twenty times as many purchasers.   A large proportion of the fine sales are made to
Jewish Refugees who are investing their money in commodities which thru thick and thin maintain a high value. Many of them were European dealers and they are searching the land to
find salable things when and if they become established in their old homes.

     We were heart-broken to have Dudy and the children leave this morning. They have been
more than a ray of sunshine and came at a good time. They were going to stay longer but
Dudy found it impracticable to help with the children and pack her belongings. She is coming
back the first of the week and store her belongings.   We could have a man do it, but she
thinks it better to come herself and I guess she is right.   Jimmy and I are firm friends.
He spend much of the time making faces at me and playing peek-a-boo. Honestly he is a card
and the best natured thing I know. I hope you will soon be home to see him.

     With love from Ma and

          Your

Major John E. Bordley, M.C. 0-403012

Dr. James Bordley, Jr.

General Hospital 118

330 N. Charles St.,

A.P.O. 927, c/o Postmaster

Baltimore -1, Md., U.S.A.

San Francisco, California, U.S.A.

June 7, 1944

Series III., No. 53

Dear Boys,   I have the women in the family down on me because they are afraid I am going
to Guilford Ave. as a permanent residence.   We have been unable to get an apartment and we
have to find some place to live and while I am going to fix the houseup, it is to make us comfortable while we are waiting and the house is so in need of repairs that without a change I
could never rent it. (Just one of the signs of family appreciation for services rendered).
I sold the home to keep your mother from working so hard and just a change from house to
house will not effect any objective, so to an apartment we go when and if we get one, which I
feel sure will be nigh on to a year and maybe more.

Dudy is down packing up to store her belongings, I wish our problem was as simple.
She goes to York Harbor in a few days with the children and her mother.   Don has taken a
cottage for them for the summer which will free Dudy of a lot of responsibility, as Mrs.Ross'
nurse is to be with them.

Since I started this the long expected invasion has started.   We are sitting around
holding our breath. It is a gigantic undertaking and may it please God to make us worthy of
the men who are making this sacrifice for us.   Yesterday all the bars in the City were
closed and all the churches open and at eight-thirty the President prayed a fifteen minute
prayer of hisown composition.   He told the Lord a lot I took for granted He knew.   It was
not so much a supplication as a review of our achievements.   An "independent Congregational"
minister gave vent to one of the most beautiful prayers to which I have ever listened. Its
humbleness and supplication was a classic. This, too, was over the radio. All the commer-
cials were laid aside and some quite splendid patriotic programs were substituted, inter-
mingled of course with reports and summations of the day's happenings. Altogether it was the
most impressive day of the war for those at home.

The impression grows that Germany's great effort will be to stop the Russians of whom
they have a holy fear of reprisals and God knows I hope they get their anticipations. Their
brutality to the Russians is one of the world's most damnable stories. The thought prevails
that if they must surrender it will be to the AngloAmerican contingent of the Allies.
Personally, I don't believe this will help them -- that is the leaders -- very much.
Churchill says this has ceased to be an ideological war -- that does not hold good for the
American public.   It wants victory with a stable peace and the elimination of Fascism and a
re-establishment of Christian civilization.

It is unfortunate that this should be an election year. The country is filled with
politics and rumors, a most unholy alliance when we should be thinking only of winning
the war.

More later.   Love from Ma and

Your

P.S.--Sergeant Schnapper was here this morning and Ellen and I know more about the Unit than
ever before.

Lt.Col.James Bordley,lII.,M.C. O-396822   Dr. James Bordley, Jr.

General Hospital 118

A.P.O. 927, c/o Postmaster   330 N. Charles St.,

    San Francisco, California,U.S.A.   Baltimore -1, Md., U.S.A.
Series III., No. 54

Dear Boys,   The invasion on the second day looks good but it is a long hard road to Berlin. I have every confidence in our ability to lick the Germans but it is a pretty good feeling to know that the Russians are over in the East and the Allies in Italy. The Germans are a stubborn people and this time I hope they really fix them up for at least a hundred years. They are a menace to our civilization and have be n since they settled in Europe, but, right now, there are people pleading their cause. This I can never understand because after all who are their leaders but the offspring of the same stock and who have always been their leaders and what guarantee have we they will not breed the same kind of skunks again. I hope we kill them off by the millions and then send in the Poles and Jews to marry their women and change their stock. They are able scientists but perverted inventors and remind me of a genius we had in Bay View, when I was there, who was continually inventing contrivances to destroy the attendants and buildings.   Baltimore has a first class ball club this year. I have not seen them in action but listen to the games at night ove the radio. They are an aggregation of sluggers. Yesterday three of them were classified One A and it looks as if the team will be broken up. About half of last year's team was taken for the Army. It is O.K. and you never hear a word against it even by the fans and sports writers.   The people outside of organized labor are all for winning the war and they do any and all things requested. Labor right now has ten or twelve strikes even though the fight in Europe has started and every bit of war material is sorely needed. It is dishusting and the people are really fed up. Thomas, head of the Automobile C.I.O. Union gave organized labor hell and told them if they expected to keep labor unions in existence when the soldiers come home they had better get down to their jobs and quit striking for any cause whatever and he urged workers not to regard picket lines but go through to work. It was the first real blast against existing coalitions I have heard from any Union leader. Most of them defend the unions and point out only five or so percent. are on strike, they fail to say that only a hundred and sixty crane operators at the Fairfield ship-yard struck but twenty thousand workers were made idle and they fail to say that we have had twice as many strikes in the first half of 1944 as in the corresponding period of 1943. The real truth is that labor has been so spoiled that it resents orders even from its own leaders and knows no obedience either to duty or country. It would be interesting to know the proportion between old labor union workers and the new crowd who belong to unions only because they want to work to help them win the war, in the promotion of strikes. Another thing for which labor isresponsible in a sense is the increased mortality from automobiles. These workers get all the gasoline they want to take them not only to and from their work but for nightly joy rides. It is again the National law (and now this State) to drive over thirty-five as a means of conserving gasoline. Last Saturday night a hundred and twenty were arrested and everyone proved to be a plant worker. The fines were from ten to two hundred dollars and only six had to be jailed for non-payment. One crew went thru a congregation of people at 90 miles an hour and killed five and injured ten or twelve others. Charlie told me the order had gone out sometime ago to excuse speeding by war workers so as not to keep them away from work. He said then it would be discovered and abused by the workers. Now something has to be done.

          Love from Ma and
            Your

Major John E. Bordley, M.C. 0-403012   Dr. James Bordley, Jr.

General Hospital 118   3.0 N. Charles St.,

A.P.O. 927, c/o Postmaster
                                              Baltimore -1, Md., U.S.A.
San Francisco, California, U.S.A.

                                              Series III., No. 55

Dear Boys, We are much excited over the way our troops managed to get inside the German Coastal defenses.   We realize a hard fight will be coming but we have faith in our youngsters and
in our general officers.   The plans were slow maturing but they seem adequate, I hope so.
Already the talk has turned to Japan and what we will do.   Personally, I do not like too much
cockiness because it may have a far reaching effect upon our production at home.   All this
talk about plans for post war development and the nearness of defeat of our enemies is driving
a lot of war workers to peace time jobs. It has grown so serious as to require the ManPower
Board to hold everybody on the job and even to shift jobs after July 1st. Why wait until July?
Nobody will be able to get a job except through U. S. Employment Bureau, a labor organization,
or a business group -- such as the Manufacturers Association. The last two represent politics
and not sound economics and should never have been included.

        You know I have so little family gossip that I feel my letters are not very satis-
factory.   I will have to tell you how the brother-in-law of James Hollyday frequently ended
his letters: "Perhaps you want to know something of the family, well I am depending upon the
women to keep you, as they keep me, informed.   In fact they tell me many things but I almost
invariably forget them".

        Jim Farley has resigned as the Chairman of the Democratic Party in New York.   I was
told today he is down in Texas organizing the State against Roosevelt.   His companions on the
job are a partner of Mr. Clayton and an associate of Jesse Jones.   Their object is to nominate an uninstructed delegation to cast the states vote in the Electral College.   This has
never been done before but is smart politics of the election is close because the Texas vote
can be cast either way. In the Democratic Convention in Texas the Roosevelt delegation bolted
when they were outnumbered three to one.   They will carry a protest to the National Convention and ask to be seated.   If they are, I am told, Texas will cast an overwhelming vote
against the President.   There is bitt r opposition to a fourth term in South Carolina (which
too has elected an uninstructed delegation to the National Convention) in Mississippi (also
an uninstructed delegation), and in Tennessee where the election will be very close. Roosevelt expects the negroes to elect him in the doubtful states of Illinois, Indiana, Pennsylvania and New York. Mrs. Roosevelt is working day and night among them.   This ribs the
South.

        The vested interests are trying to upset price control. They are a lot of asses
for without it we will certainly have a serious commodity inflation. It is bad enough as it i
is but will be infinitely worse. Congress is not inclined at the moment to interfere and
yesterday gave them a spanking.   I hope it does not change its mind.
                        With love from Ma and
                            Your

Lt.Col.James Bordley,III.,M.C. O-396822   Dr. James Bordley, Jr.

General Hospital 118
                                         330 N. Charles St.,
A.P.O. 927, c/o Postmaster

San Francisco, California, U.S.A.   Baltimore -1, Md., U.S.A.
                                              June 19, 1944
                     Series III., No. 56

Dear Boys,   Have just had a hard argument with Ellen Fisher on greatness and its constit-
uent elements.   It is queer to me how few people agree with my definition: A great man is
one who understands the needs of his fellow men and makes substantial contributions to their
welfare and happiness;   This requires erudition on a borad scale, because, how can a man
know his fellow men without he is familiar with their tendencies and history.   No general is
a great man just because he wins battles, if he has not a profound understanding of the basic
cause of his action he is simply a good general, fine tactition, or an exceptional mechanic.
I believe Gen. Eisenhower has the making of greatness.   I am much impressed by his understanding.   I hope I am correct. Jefferson was a great man, Dr. Welch was too.   I have
never met but two great men -- Dr. Welch and Mr. House. The nearer you get to so-called great
men the smaller they become.   With really great men their greatness becomes more manifest
with contact.   One o He t Senators from Texas has been acclaimed as great.   I heard him make
a speech the other day indus ch he attacked labor unions and called this "a white man's
country". He showed n howed standing of the alteration of labor's status since changing from
the farm to industry; its is jus d protection from exploitation and its essential right to a
living. He showed even le s is erstanding of Democracy when he called this a white man's
country.   He is just an op more st and an exceptionally successful politician.

          This is another ttingyesterday was hot -- 97° and humid (about 110). Of course
I had to leave my more or less ughte rtable home and go out to a dinner given to Elizabeth
Hollyday who is getting married is v ly.   The man (whose name I do not recall) is much her
senior and has a daughter gettin ince ied a we k before.   He is a fine fellow so the in-laws
say and I can add he is very agre rmise.   Milton Hollyday is here on a ten day leave, has been
working on a bomber since he left unkn bout a year or more ago. Has been made a lieutenant
from the ranks so I surmise he is p   helpful. He knew all the fellow who went to Japan.
He is leaving for parts unknown in a rp w days. Said he might see you before long. He is a
bright fellow.

          Just h d a sharp storm and the air is cooler. Gosh! we need it, because today too
is a hot one.

          Work keeps up and I do also but I am longing for a good rest.   I have had so many
serious complaints to look after that I am fed up with the responsibility.   Then too getting
ready to leave our home for parts unknown is a very taxing job. I don't kno where we got all
the things we possess. We could start most any kind of a store from silks to metal.   All
these have to be culled over and distributed and in the end we will have to send much to the
auction room, things the family cannot utilize.   If we sold all we do not want to move I
think we could start a bank on the proceeds.   Mother is loading the girls down with all kinds
of Madeira textiles, glass and china with some pieces of early furniture, etc. They take it
away by the automobile load and still we do not miss it.   The man who bought the house wants
to buy the things in the old kitchen, but Ellen Fisher and Ellen Webb each wanted one of the
corner cup-boards.   I do not wish, nor have to, sell anything the family wants.   I confess
I am weaned from the home which was my dream for forty years but I have a dread of moving
into a small interior house.   I will be happy when we get into an apar ment with a dining-room.
                    More later.   Love from Ma
                              and Your

Major John E. Bordley, M.C. 0-403012   Dr. James Bordley, Jr.,

General Hospital 118   30 N. Charles St.,

A.P.O. 927,c/o Postmaster   Baltimore -1, Md., U.S.A.

San Francisco, California, U.S.A.   June 21, 1944

Series II., No. 57

Dear Boys, Good old Maryland weather.   Yesterday boiling, today quite cool.
Estelle Hollyday died yesterday. Had a cancer and been ill for about three months.   Her
hisband has not shown up yet but probably will be on to claim his part of her estate.   He is
a rotter.

The newRobot plane of the Germans is being widely discussed.   I did not know until today
that we made a similar one four years ago and after extensive trials it was abandoned as of
no major value.   Experiments are still going on but the question of control over wind drift
and gravity have not been conquered for long fights.   Our plane could be sent up and down at
a given point but for short distances only. It is expensive and a veritable waste of material
so I guess it has a short life in Germany where the pinch of raw materials must be very great.
Anyhow it is not half so important as a strong foot Army fully equipped and protected big
fighter planes and this the Allies have as can be seen on the Channel Beachhead.

The sensational fight of the week was the air battle in the Pacific with the Jap's loss
of three hundred planes. That is really thrilling and shows how the Japs feel about the Islands
near their home shores. Bit by bit we are biting off the enemies' territory in every sphere
of action, soon something will reach their bloody hearts and the sooner the better.

I go by a blood donors center every morning and since the invasion started there are
lines of donors crowding the entrance and adjoining streets. Last week we exceeded our quota
by over a thousand pints. This week will be even larger I am sure. There is a manifest
change in the civilian attitude since the invasion.   It is really quite marked. People are
more serious about our efforts. Well in the main we have been a long way from the war but
the thousands involved and the large casualty lists are beginning to trickle through even the
average mind.   I don't mean that black markets and crooks and selfish politicians have been
eliminated. They are just skum which must rise to be destroyed.

The medical profession isputting up a real fight on the Senate bill for socialized medicine. Its supporters are flooding the country with misinformation but it is being promptly
met with the truth.   Senator Tydings who is working with theprofession does not believe the
bill will pass but the vote will be close.   Its advocates -- the New Deal -- will not force
a vote until afterthe election because they are afraid of the reaction.   I think they are
going to get the reaction in spite of that because the profession is aroused.   As most commentators see the political situation now Roosevelt will be nominated and try and force the
the acceptance of Wallace as Vice-President. The story going the rounds is that as soon as
the war is over Roosevelt will resign and Wallace will appoint him Minister Extraordinary
to the Peace Conference.   I doubt a Roosevelt resigning any power and I also doubt the Convention's acceptance of Wallace. It will be a big fight as most of the Democratic leaders
have no faith in the ability of Wallace and fear his social New Deal tendencies and pronounce-
ments.   The flash has just come in of a probably major naval engagement off the Phillipines.
We are praying for a substabtial victory. The dirty rats had to come out of their hole and I
hope they never get back We have perfect confidence in our representatives.

More later. Love from Ma and

Your

Lt. Col. James Bordley,III.,M.C. O-396822   Dr. James Bordley, Jr.

General Hospital 118   330 N. Charles St

A.P.O. 927, c/o Postmaster   Baltimore -1, Md., U.S.A.

    San Francisco, California,U.S.A.   June 24, 1944

                         Series III., No. 58

Dear Boys,   Yesterday George Finney had a party at the Ruxton Club.   At the party were most of the men of the Hopkins who served in the last war and a group of George's contemporaries. It was strictly a Finney Party as John's children served the juleps and sandwiches, made the drinks and entertained the guests.   It was a very nice affair, followed by a terrific thunderstorm which lasted for two hours and a half.   The Lord certainly showed his fireworks but treated us better than our neighbors in Garrett County, Cambridge, West Virginia and Pennsylvania where he treated them to a series of cyclones which killed and injured some hundreds of people.   It was a day of intense humidity, but not very warm, there was a blue haze, such as I have never seen before, all the afternoon.   Everybody at the party wanted to know what your Unit was doing and whether any of you were coming home.   Did I tell you that a young Sergeant working with Fox spent a morning with us at the office. We gained the first comprehensive idea of the workings of your Unit. He told us in extenso of the work in the various departments and was enthusiastic over his opportunity to serve in the outfit.   The Republicans are boosting Senator Byrd for Vice-President on their ticket.   The Senator was entered in a Democratic primary contest in Florida, without his sanction and without his aid, on a ticket in opposition to a fourth term.   Roosevelt beat him only by the skin of his teeth after a moststrenuous campaign. Add to Byrd's vote the Republican vote and he would have swamped the President. I don't believe he would accept a place on a Republican ticket although he has made some caustic speeches about a fourth term.   I wish he could be nominated on the Democratic ticket for first place.   I think he could sweep the country and save what is worth saving out of the present administration -- such as Cordell Hull and our Secretary of War, Jesse Jones, Mr. Clayton and Mr. Nelson of the O.P.A.   What stupid asses are politicians. The Republican Convention is meeting in Chicago with the nation wide open for a fine candidate andplatform. What do they do? Turn down the most important thinker in the country, Wendell Wilkie and, write a platform that makes for future war. We are to negotiate with England, Russia and China but as an individual and not as a member of the United Nations.   In substance I see no difference between the Treaty of 1918-19 and the Republican platform as now proposed. Then Grundy is out there working for a high tariff plank. I knew it would come because both industry and labor are fearful of competition. Governor Landis has at least temporarily put a stop to Grundy but the latter represents the sinews of war in the coming election and money talks. What a travesty, what a cinch for Franklin Roosevelt. He will win in a walk.   What a choice for the voters: Roosevelt with a wreck the country domestic policy and a strong foreign policy and Gov. Dewey with a bowl of jellyfish. The Republicans are confident they have the election in the bag, I think they are in for a great surprise. They don't know, or do not appreciate that Wilkie resurrected a buried corpse and gave it new life and vigor. As soon as the party was able to crawl they kicked him out. What the leaders see now is really a ghost. I don't give a tinker's dam for myself but I will not vote for anyone who puts profits before the lives of my grandchildren. My river is nearing the ocean but theirs is still a little trickle.   We have had some excitement at home. Yesterday, a New Yorkedealer dropped in and offered us -- and we accepted -- thirty-five hundred dollars for one of the pie crust tables. Boy, what a price.   Don't tell anyone but I paid twenty-five dollars for it. He made us unbelievable offers for all of the fine pieces but he only got the table and some o thepieces we did not need and the girls do not want. We are seeling only about $8,000 worth of trifles,mostly pine,glass and old iron.   Love fromMa and your

Major John E. Bordley, M.C. 0-403012

General Hospital 118

A.P.O. 927, c/o Postmaster

San Francisco, California, U.S.A.

Dr. James Bordley, Jr.
330 N. Charles St.,

Baltimore -1, Md., U.S.A.

June 30, 1944

Series III., No. 59

Dear Boys, Well Dewey is the standard bearer of the Republicans. Accepted last night in a speech that impressed me with three points: He will keep General Marshall and Admiral King and give them his every support; he will name a non-political commission for the peace and strongly favors full cooperation with our allies in its settlement short only of yielding our objectives, and he favors a strong force for the maintenance of peace; last but not least he will form a cabinet of young men and take on none of those grown old and tired in politics. he has a reputation for carrying out his promises. The plank I was worried about as reported did not materialize in the platform and was subtle propaganda by the opposition. Of course, I have little faith in platforms, my trust is put only in men, men who can see and who can learn, men who are not afraid to do what is right because it gibes with politics. Governor Bricker of Ohio accepted the Vice-Presidential nomination. He is a level headed fellow with both feet on the ground and a successful administrator. I was told by a Democratic politician from Tenn. that he made a fine impression in his State and he thought, in the South, he was stronger than his party. I hate politics and politicians. I hate anyone who does not play the game straight. Politics means compromise and compromise means yielding principles. This is one glorious opportunity to clean up and start a less crooked game. I mean a successful young man who has been drafted for every office he has held comes on the stage without a promise and beholding to no man. If he will surround humself with clean young men, untainted by the present rotten politics maybe we can start a new era. I wanted Wendell Wilkie, also a young man and new to politics, of vision and sound judgment but he was defeated by the powers of reaction. They accepted Dewey only because they dared not name one of their own ilk and they hated Wilkie for his candor. The ones who controlled the Convention are not those who will elect Dewey, they are merely trying to stay on the band wagon while the forces of progress and order drive. If the war was over and only the New Deal was before the people Dewey would win in a walk. They have had enough of regimentation, dictation, Franklin Roosevelts, Frankfurters and Blacks.

The second front is growing into a real success. Pity we had to have forty thousand casualties, pity we only destroyed the help of seventy thousand Germans but we have made an auspicious start.

The Baltimore Museum inherited a large sum of money and other valuables from Mr.Cone, brother of Dr.Clarabel. It came at a good time. Mrs. Daingrfield left the Museum about a hundred thousand dollars in pictures and we have recently had several other substantial legacies and gifts, including the Chinese collection of the former President of the Hopkins-- a very valuable addition.

I just heard Charlie Austrian was carried to the Hopkins following a cerious heart attack. I know none of the particulars and it is of recent origin.

Donald Symington, the Franklin Roosevelt of Baltimore banking, is dead of an inter-cranial hemorrhage. It is quite remarkable how quickly he came back after being busted, if he had lived longer he would have been busted again.

Beale is in the 29th Division which carried the bulk of the effort of the beach landings. Their casualties were ery heavy. So far no bad news.

More later. Love from Ma and

Your

Lt.Col.James Bordley,III.,M.C. O-396822   Dr. James Bordley, Jr.

General Hospital 118   330 N. Charles St.,

A.P.O. 927, c/o Postmaster   Baltimore - 1, Md., U.S.A.

San Francisco, California, U.S.A.   July 5, 1944

                                    Series III., No. 60

Dear Boys,

        Well another 4th has come and gone and the arguments of Thomas Jefferson are being
defended as vigorously and in a much wider space than in 1776. Liberty and Union! I wonder
whether we can stop wars without both?   And if we get the latter how much of our sovereignty
will be have to give up, and how much will it change our liberty and prosperity?   I heard a
debate on the subject by a group of students (voting age) which was one of the most enlightening debates I have listened to. Most of the adult debates have a basis in party politics
and are not free from suspicion, but, not so the kids.

        The Oriole grandstands and bleachers burned down in the early morning of the 4th.
It is distressing because it afforded good healthy sport for some thousands of our war
workers. The team is in first place with the best club it has had since Jack Dunn's days.
Even mother knows the names of all the players and is an ardent rooter, that is, around
the radio.
        Yesterday was a duplicate of John's wedding day, in fact the weather has been
strikingly good for June and July with the exception of a few very hot days. We have a new
weather man and the new system of weather reporting will start before long.   It is said to
be far more accurate and enlightening.

        Have you used any Tyrothricin? Tell me something your experience if used in acut
antra or acute superficial eye diseases. A lot os being published but I have seen no one
who has used it.

        Charlie Austrian has been in the Hopkins for a month. He sees no visitors and has
not been out of bed but he is expected home in two weeks. His condition is considered
satisfactory, so his Secretary tells me.

        The war rolls on and we are getting nearer and nearer the original sources of the
troubles   It has been officially reported that heavy shipments of gold have gone from
Germany to Spain. This money is marked for the Hitler club, so we are told. If the report
is correct and I guess it is, the rats are trying to get off a sinking ship. If England
and this country permit the escape of these rascals through neutral intervention we should
hang our rulers. If we are ever to stop international or any other kind of war we have got
to punish the responsible parties. The fear of hanging will be more effective than prayers.
So far the casualty lists have carried none of our intimates although many are on the
fighting fronts.   I hope the good record holds.
                        More later.   Love from Ma and
                                        Your

Major John E. Bordley, M.C. O-403012

General Hospital 118

A.P.O. 927, c/o Postmaster

San Francisco, California, U.S.A.

Dr. James Bordley, Jr.,
330 N. Charles St.,
Baltimore -1, Md., U.S.A.

July 10, 1944

Series III., 61

Dear Boys,

We are in the midst of a typical July hot spell with middle ninety temperatures. It must be hard on the old folk because it even bothers me.

De Gaulle is here to see the President who does not like him very much. He is not after immediate recognition of the French Committee as the Government of France but to enlighten the President on the activities of the underground. There is a definite division here on recognition and much denunciation of the President for his attitude. It seems to me that we are under obligations to support the President in all matters of foreign policy -- provided they eminate from Secretary Hull. They certainly have more accurate information than we, the outsiders, possess. Of course, the attitude toward Vichy, Spain and Fascist Italy are not helpful to the President especially when all the propaganda has been directed to stifle such opposition to Democracy. Oh, well if the prosecution of war is not interfered with the harm will not be very great! The about face which I looked for in coming peace is slowly taking place and the isolationists are in my judgment slowly gaining ground. I wish I could order them, one and all, on the firing line for first hand information as to the value of cooperative effort.

George Finney will not return to the Pacific. He is ordered south to create some sort of organization and will be sent to the European theatre in due course. I have only the facts and none of the particulars. The question here is what will happen to his old outfit. We hear Brune is to return (if not already in Oregon). Only gossip. Joe has gone to the Coast but she told me it was to keep house for her brother. I think the rumor probably originated there. I saw by the paper that a private in Saipan tuned in on San Francisco when he wanted to know how the troops were getting along on the island.

Beale has been in the thick of it in France. His mother has had several letters but no particulars as to his activities. We heard he was driving a jeep for a General officer but this seems queer as all of his training has been on big guns. He wrote that he now knows the meaning of war. His father and mother are staying with us while they wait to get in a new house they recently bought. It is a cute little affair for large enough for these days. It is out near our Brown cousins. We are fixing up the house they lived in but will not move so Ma says until Sept. 15th or after. We have to be out of our home by Oct. 1st. This is a great experiment but I guess it will be comfortable until we get an apartment where there is a dining room and no niggers to worry about.

Mrs. Roosevelt is loud in her demands for negro equality but never mentions negro responsibility, honesty or interest in their jobs. It just does not dovetail to make the white race responsible for the moral shortcomings of the negroes.

More later. Love from Ma and

Your

Lt.Col.James Bordley,III.,M.C. O-396822   Dr. James Bordley,Jr.

General Hospital 118   330 N. Charles St

A.P.O. 927, c/o Postmaster   Baltimore -1, Md., U.S.A.

San Francisco, California, U.S.A.   July 15, 1944

Series III., No. 62

Dear Boys,

        Well the Donkey has brayed and the American public has been overwhelmed with
surprise at the drafting of Roosevelt. The real truth is the puppet jumped up and down when
Roosevelt pulled the strings.   The papers are trying to play up the fight over the Vice-
presidency but when the Boss speaks it will probably be Wallace, without the Boss is convinced he will be a liability. The facts are Texas, South Carolina, Mississippi and Tennessee
threaten to leave the party if Wallace is named, why they select Wallace instead of Roosevelt
I don't know.   Roosevelt is "accepting bowsas any other soldier to the will of his Comman-
ing Officer, the American public."   So he is now running, asthe Baltimore Sun put it, as a
self confessed one-A.   It is plainwhat he plans to do to make the voters overlook domestic
issues.   I cannot size up the election. There are powerful forces opposing Roosevelt.   In
this State, and it may be a real sample, such men as Mayor Jackson have publicly announced t
their intention of opposing Roosevelt and I hear that in the underground the fight against
him will be heavy. Still there is a war going on and being darn well conducted -- of course
by the Military -- but under the Administration of the President. I have heard many people
who have never voted for Roosevelt say they will this time because they want no disturbance
in our war effort.

        Yesterday was one of those days! Hot as hell, an office full in the morning,
operated all the afternoon and was called to U.M.H. to stop a nose-bleed in the middle of the
night.   Boy, was I tired, but only healthfully tired as any youngster would have been. This
morning up early so as to get to the hospital by eight and not a nigger in sight and to date
none have shown up. Tomorrow they will come with a story of illness and draw their money just
as if they had worked all of today.   I long for an apartment and a self-conducted dining-
room.   Our grass has been cut but once this year, the front lawn twice.   You talk about
your jungles, you should see ours. It is gently raining for the first time in weeks.   For
last two weeks the temperature has gone to about 95° with a parching dry wind with dust. The
wheat crop came through O.K. and will be enormous but the corn and vegetables are having a
hard time to survive. We may not have inflation but the prices are from one to four hundred
percent. above normal for staple food products.   Soft crabs, for instance, at six dollars
a dozen against fifty and seventy-five cents. The oyster men and professional fishermen to
avoid service are working in war plants at less money. The Kansas wheat is in the field
because of no labor and still the administration refuses to act on a man power bill. It is
a damn mess.

        Bruno's mother died of intestinal obstruction. She has been in Gundry's for some
months and her death is a relief.

                More later.   Love from Ma and

                                Your

Major John E. Bordley, M.C. 0-403012   Dr. James Bordley, Jr.

General Hospital 118   330 N. Charles St.,

A.P.O. 927, c/o Postmaster   Baltimore -1, Md., U.S.A.

San Francisco, California, U.S.A.   July 24, 1944.

                                Series III., No. 63

Dear Boys,

        I wish you were home because I could supply you with some nice jobs. Believe me
I am rapidly lesing my mind. This thing of clearing out a house and disposing of the odds
and ends is an interminable job.   Today we have a morning visit from an antique buyer,
this afternoon a visit from a New York dealer. This takes hours and patience. Of course,
they always want to buy what you do not intend to sell and haggle over the things the can
buy. We not only have antiques but as we distribute antiques among the family, moderns are
returned and they must be sold. If I ever buy another piece of furniture, it will be for a
padded cell in Spring Grove, or more probably from a padded cell.

        John has the worst trained golf clubs I ever used. They never hit the ball in the
right place. Having sent my clubs to Rye, and I had to get some kind of a plausible substitute, and oh boy, what a travesty after playing with real ones.

        The first of the casualties among those we know well came in yesterday. They were
wounds and apparently not serious.

        The Government is getting tough about vacation travel and may ban it entirely, so I
am told, on account of troups and casualties. Then everything is coming East for shipment   a-
to Europe and the railroads are badly taxed. I am selfish enough to want them to let me go
but I will cheerfully abode by the rulings as I know the importance. The travel difficulty
is the sudden influx of money onto pockets before empty. These people are on the go constantly and week ends the stations are so jammed that it is worth your life to try and buy
even a newspaper. Four thousand automobiles are being retired every hour so I hear and
second hand ones are so in demand that you can sell them for double and treble their origir
cost.   The Government has now put a ceiling on them but the bootlegger keeps on buying and
selling I suppose. Our car situation is really serious. If yours breks down it is hell even
to get it repaired because the Government has taken over practica ly all the younger mechanics
and a large proportion of the older men. Now they have reduced the octane of gasoline by
stopping the use of chemicals and t is new gas is terrific on the motors. You can't drive
up such an incline as our alley without the metor knocking its head off.

        I started this days ago. My time has been so filled that my mind is going around
like a top.   We leave tomorrow for Rye Beach and glad I am to get away from patients, carpenters, painters and constructors, and I might add the U.S. Government departments with their
rules and regulations.

        Charlie Webb, Jr. was tickled with his letter from Jim. He shows it to everybody
and refers to it on all occasions.

        I will write you next from New Hampshire.

                        Love from Ma and

                                Your

Vol. #IV

Notes on Letters to Jim and John 1942-1945

Nov. 28, 1944 Hull resigned for health reasons.

Dec. 14, 19, and 28 all numbered #16.

Oct.12, 1944 Note the tone of his letters after they moved. He is more upbeat and enthusiastic.

May 2, 1945 Official signing of German Surrender

June 5, 1945 Dr Firor was on Hopkins staff, as was Dr George Eaton, an Orthopedic Surgeon. Walter Buck, not a physician, was a longtime friend of J.B. jr who had been on Board of St. John's College with him. Bruno is Dr. Hills.

Aug. 6, 1945 Hiroshima Bomb

Aug. 9, 1945 Nagasaki Bomb

Sept. 2, 1945 Official Japanese surrender

Last letter from Baltimore was typed on July 2, 1945.

They went to Rye Beach on July 9 for 2 months and the war was over before they returned.

An interesting note is on June 2, 1945, Dr. Longcope had requested the Army send J.B.III back to Hopkins. The country was being told the Japanese would be able to continue a defensive fight for some time, and the request was denied.

Lt.Col.James Bordley,III.,M.C. o-396822

General Hospital no. 118

A.P.O. 927, c/o Postmaster

San Francisco, California,U.S.A.

Dr.James Bordley,Jr.,

330 N. Charles St.,

Baltimore -1, Md.U.S.A.

September 14, 1944

Series IV., No. 1

Dear Boys, Well we are back home and hard at work packing up to move temporarily down to
2630 Guilford Ave. It is a very great task because there are so many angles.   We are sending
to the auction room all modern stuff - furniture, iron, etc.; selling privately a lot of old
glass, the Liverpool pitchers and some old furniture which we cannot use and which none of you
will want the responsibility of keeping.   If all the sales go through we will have money
enough to much more than pay for the alterations on our new home which will make it easy to
rent when we get out of it. The girls go away with a car full of stuff on every visit and Ma
is setting aside things for Dudy to balance the account.   I saw Dudy and the kids at York
Harbor.   Jimmy has adopted as his name "Bordley". Tells everybody that is his name. Sort
of snobbish but with the greatest smile I ever saw.   He is a peach and everybody is crazy
about him.

Ellen and her crew are well and had a vacation at Atlantic City. Ellen Webb and
her crew are now at Rehoboth which worries me because a tropical storm of great intensity
is due to strike the coast at noon today.   I hope she will have the wisdom to move inland.
In most places the Government is requiring the transfer.

I had a wonderful vacation. Never was as well in my life the whole time I was
away.   Enjoyed much golf and quite a few parties.   Of course, we were limited with no
automobile.

Walter Hughson was found dead in a pit near his Hospital and the official report
was "died of meningitis". He left the Hospital to go home and was not found for several days.
Where he was in the interim no one knows. I guess his old trouble was responsible.

The war is making rapid progress and nothing delights me more than the fine work
of Gen. Patton. He started with a handicap of his own making but with the full confidence
of his Commander and he has redeemed both. I always felt he was overworked and just did a
very silly thing but with a full apology to his Army I felt the incident should be closed.
Well, he is made of fine stuff and I get a great kick out of his victories.   You probably
know his daughter lives here and her husband, one of Alzy Waters' sons, is a prisoner of
Germany.

It looks like Gen. MacArthur is on his way to the Philippines and we are wondering
whether it will change our status.   It was announced that an over-all Commander is to be
appointed for the Pacific Theatre.   The rumor is that he will be an Admiral, we all hoped
it would be MacArthur.   Dewey made a plea for his greater su pose by the Administration
which probably means he will not get the job.

More later. Love from Ma and

Your

O-403012

General Hospital

A.P.O. 927, c/o Postmaster

San Francisco, California,U.S.A.

Dr. Jam.   Md..U.S.A.

Charles St.,
Sept.

Series IV., No. 2   .A.

Dear Boys,

The moving goes apace.   I feel lonely without a package under my arm, I have
carried so many that my muscles are as hard as iron.

I suppose you have heard the sad story of Guinney Williams.   He isout with T.B.
Had a hemorrhage as his first notice of trouble. Murray Fisher is keepinghim here in bed
to get a line on the best thing to do for him.   The poor fellow has worked himself to death.
You really have no idea of the pressure under which the family doctor is working.   It is
terrific punishment, one by one they ave to haul intheir signs.

Mother is waiting for your Christmas requests.   The boxes have to be mailed before
October fifteenth.   She has collected some things but is waiting to move before mailing
hoping to hear from you.

Charlie and Carroll have the whooping cough. Charlie pretty bad.   The complication is the doctor situation out at Pikesville. They were at ehoboth when the hurricane
struck there but the wind was their only threat as they were on high ground and not
threatened by the forty and fifty-foot seas.   A tree blew down on th ir house but no one
was injured.   Ellen said it was terrifying.

The war goes well for us and the time is getting shorter.   How the devil the
Germans find the men and material to put up such a fight is a mystery to me but they
are licked.

Dewey is making progress in his fight and i hope sufficient votes will be found
to elect him.   If this country is not strong and governed by men interested more in national
interests than politics we will not establish a s able world peace.   The present administration has divided our people as never before, management agains labor and labor against
management; white against black and visa versa; agriculture against industry. If this is
carried over into peace we will never be a potent factor and i we ar not there will be no
real peace.   We must be pulled together, our differences composed, our economy made stable.
This is essential to political solidarity and that is essential for a stable world peace.
Roosevelt has built up a powerful organization but it built on the shifting sands of
personal ambition and not founded on our national welfare.

More later.   Love from Ma and
Your

Dr. James Bordley, Jr.

Lt.Col.James Bordley,III., M.C. O-396822   330 N. Charles St.,

General Hospital No. 118

A.P.O. 927, c/o Postmaster   Baltimore -1, Md.,U.S.A.

San Francisco, California, U.S.A.   October 4, 1944
Series IV., No. 3

Dear Boys,

    Things have been moving fast for Ma and me. We have moved, fixed up a new home, sent a lot of things to storage, divided up a lot of other property, shopped, practiced medicine, met our neighbors and done everything except have fun.

    Frannie Cromwell called up a day or so ago. She came on to have their home fixed up and put it up for rent again. Said the family was fine and Charlie now a Major and located somewhere in Wisconsin. I don't know where or why.

    Dudy was down for the dentist yesterday who found a dead tooth and took a lot of Xrays. Has not yet determined what to do so she will come down again around Election Day to vote and be fixed up. Dudy looks remarkably well and says the children are fine.

    Our Baltimore base-ball team is cleanin up. It is astonishing the interest and excitement it has created. They draw crowds of twenty and thirty thousand every game on the play off for the junior world champions ip. Such batters you have never seen, home runs two and three in a game. Various organizations are showering the players with war bonds, last night alone thirty odd were distributed among them, besides they get sixty percent. of eighty percent of the attendance proceeds. They are reallycleaning up. It is not a great team but a colorful and winning organization.

    We hear authoratatively that Base 18 has gone to India. Ben Baker I hear is in Washington. I don't know whether that is correct. I hear a lot of their nurses had to retur and they could not stand the tropical climate. That is a fact.

    Beale sent home a decoration of some sort to put away for him. He is with the advance forces in or around Germany. Says he has had so little time to enjoy France and Paris, he may stay over for a while after the war.

    The reports from the correspondents in France and the low countries are very different from what could be expected. The people are not so bad off as to food, habitations or clothes; the bombing damage is much less than supposed and the people are not half as resentful as one would expect. They are hanging a fe of their traitors but not molesting the Germans.

    I was stopped a thousand times and I must give up and go.

          With love from Ma and
              Your

Major JohnE. Bordley, M.C. 0-403012

General Hospital 118 (Unit No. 1)

A.P.O. 927, c/o Postmaster

San Francisco, California, U.S.A.

Dr. James Bordley, Jr.

330 N. Charles St.,

Baltimore -1, Md., U.S.A.

October 12, 1944

Series IV., No. 4

Dear Boys, This town is base-ball crazy. Night before last in the play off for the minor league championship fifty-two thousand paid to see the Orioles lose by a five to four score. Last night they came back and won ten to nothing putting them one game from the championship and with twenty-thousand watching. You never such an aggregation of sluggers in your life.

We hear that General Hospital 18 has gone to India.

Our new little home is very comfortable and I must add quite attractive. Everyone who has come to see us has been delighted. I have the cutest book room and for once the coziest sitting room I ever possessed. I have gathered together a l my papers and as soon as I finish my index files they will be available for immediate reference. I will use the room as my dressing room as I have a large cupboard for my suits and a high boy for other things. Mother has a nice room with bay window and western exposure with two large closets. Our only handicap is one bath-room and no place for a second. Still we can get along except when we have guests. Quite a contrast to the old home with five bath-rooms.

Since writing the above Baltimore has won the minor league championship before some twenty-thousand people. You never heard such a din even in battle.

Mother has sent each of you three Xmas boxes. She has never heard whether the last boxes sent have ever arrived. Better write her. It issome job tofind and collect all the stuff she sends and she works very hard to get what you ask. You know special foods in packages are almost non-existent so some she gets from Boston, New York and Baltimore.

Hugh Young just called me to say that Jim's secretary (or once was) Garey (?) has n not been heard from for about two years and his family is a mile up inthe air. You might suggest a little consideration.

The campaign for the Presidency goes along but not too impressive. Roosevelt wise cracks and Dewey criticises. I see no signs of any enthusiasm. The national registration is setting an all time low -- in proportion to the eligibles. This makes for Roosevelt's advantage. The real problem is the soldier vote and the migratory war workers. How many will vote is hard to guess. In some States the national ballot -- out of the country votes -- is illegal, so another complication. The negroes and Jews are about unanimous for Roosevelt. They are a misguided crowd because what Roosevelt has done will bring a serious reaction to both, in fact the re-action is well along. He has succeeded in giving us a negro and a Jew problem and in the midst of an overwhelming white, Christian people who eventually require obedience to its own code of ethics.

More later. Love from Mother and

P.S.--Wendell Wilkie died of coronary thrombosis, a great national loss.

Lt.Col. James Bordley,III.,M.C. 0-396822   Dr. James Bordley, Jr.

General Hospital 118, Union No. 1   330 N. Charles St.,

A.P.O. 927, c/o Postmaster   Baltimore -1,Md.,U.S A

San Francisco, California, U.S.A.   October 13, 1944

Series IV.,No. 5

Dear Boys,   Another rainy day. We have had lots of them this Fall but needed them too as the wells are dry and our city water supply very low.

The City has just had a survey made for a way through the City on the north and south route. It is proposed at a cost of forty off millions to have a sunken way so that cross town traffic will not be interfered with. I think it will be a go. Then we are to bridge the harbor so as to make a quick trip to the Curtis Bay district. The cost not yet determined. It means City borrowing of about thirty millions and a substantial increase in taxes. These are post war preparations to give jobs during the trasition period from war to civil industry. All corporations are holding back improvements, railroads, street cars and even the clubs (Elkridge is in for twenty-two thousand). The State has two hundred millions available for roads, buildings, etc. and the City a substantial sum. The State this year had a surplus of many millions.

This is all good sense and may keep us out of a post war jam. The soldiers are to be given preference in all jobs. The National Government will match dollar for dollar in all public improvements and the State will help Baltimore. I hope the other States have as keen organization committees as we have. I am proud of Maryland which has been first in nearly all the war undertakings: Bonds, Red Cross, the blood donations, etc. Now this is business not politics and it just shows what can be accomplished when the best brains are brought into jobs.

Mr. Clayton has resigned because he could never have his recommendations carried out. According to all the daily papers his resignations is a serious loss to the Government. I knew that he was very unhappy and when they appointed him on a three man commission to apportion help to the States -- post war -- he promptly got out. He argued for a one man board and no division of responsibility and when he was overruled he quit. We have lost some wonderful men from the Government service and have taken on some of the finest rif-raff.

Al Smith passed on a few days ago. He was a remarkable chap. A New York lawyer told me that Smith had a better grasp of New York Corporation law than any lawyer at their bar although he was not a lawyer. I glory in seeing the old American system from poor boy to worth while citizenship work, and Smith was an excellent example.

No recent word from either Worthington or Beale. I suppose they are all right. A secret: Ann Bordley is going to be married to a young fellow by the name of Riggs Jones. He is a teller in the National Bank of Baltimore. He seems pretty young but a fine fellow. She has had several serious beaux in the past year but preferred Riggs I suppose. One was a wealthy chap, a Captain in the Army.

More later. Love from Ma and
Your

259

Lt.Col. James Bordley,III.,M.C. 0-396822   Dr. James Bordley, Jr.

General Hospital 118, Union No. 1   330 N. Charles St.,

A.P.O. 927, c/o Postmaster   Baltimore -1,Md.,U.S A

San Francisco, California, U.S.A.   October 13, 1944
Series IV.,No. 5

Dear Boys,   Another rainy day. We have had lots of them this Fall but needed them too as the wells are dry and our city water supply very low.

The City has just had a survey made for a way through the City on the north and south route. It is proposed at a cost of forty off millions to have a sunken way so that cross town traffic will not be interfered with. I think it will be a go. Then we are to bridge the harbor so as to make a quick trip to the Curtis Bay district. The cost not yet determined. It means City borrowing of about thirty millions and a substantial increase in taxes. These are post war preparations to give jobs during the trasition period from war to civil industry. All corporations are holding back improvements, railroads, street cars and even the clubs (Elkridge is in for twenty-two thousand). The State has two hundred millions available for roads, buildings, etc. and the City a substantial sum. The State this year had a surplus of many millions.

This is all good sense and may keep usout of a post war jam. The soldiers are to be given preference in all jobs. The National Government will match dollar for dollar in all public improvements and the State will help Baltimore. I hope the other States have as keen organization committees as we have. I am proud of Maryland which has been first in nearly all the war undertakings: Bonds, Red Cross, the blood donations, etc. Now this is business not politics and it just shows what can be accomplished when the best brains are brought into jobs.

Mr. Clayton has resigned because he could never have his recommendations carried out. According to all the daily papers his resignations is a serious loss to the Government. I knew that he was very unhappy and when they appointed him on a three man commission to apportion help to the States -- post war -- he promptly got out. He argued for a one man board and no divisionof responsibility and when he was overruled he quit. We have lost some wonderful men from the Government service and have taken on some of the finest rif-raff.

Al Smith passed on a few days ago. He was a remarkable chap. A New York lawyer told me that Smith had a better grasp of New York Corporation law than any lawyer at their bar although he was not a lawyer. I glory in seeing the old American system from poor boy to worth while citizenship work, and Smith was an excellent example.

No recent word from either Worthington or Beale. I suppose they are all right. A secret: Ann Bordley is going to be married to a young fellow by the name of Riggs Jones. He is a teller in the National Bank of Baltimore. He seems pretty young but a fine fellow. She has had several serious beaux in the past year but preferred Riggs I suppose. One was a wealthy chap, a Captain in the Army.

More later. Love from Ma and
Your

Major John E. Bordley, M.C. 0-403012   Dr. James Bordley, Jr.,

General Hospital 118, Unit No. 1   330 N. Charles St.,

A.P.O. 927, c/o Postmaster

San Francisco, California, U.S.A.   Baltimore -1, Md., U.S.A.

                                             October 23, 1944
                        Series LV., No. 7

Dear John,

        I was invited to lunch by Polvogt on Saturday -- 21s .   I had no idea why the
invitation but he soon enlightened me.   It was a long story which I will write briefly
because I think you should be informed.   Crowe's health has been very precarious and two
years ago he made up his mind to resign.   Polvogt dissuaded him for the time being.   Now
the Hopkins is preparing extensive plans forphysical changes as soon as the war is over and
included is a design for a new and much enlarged surgical building on the ground of the
present structure.   Crowe has l st all interest in the department and will not make the
slightest effort to see that his unit is properly placed.   He wants to quit but again
Polvogt has had him defer action until he can turn over a better equipped establishment to
his successor.   He has declined to take any part in getting the necessary funds for
equipment which will be between fifty and a hundred thousand dollars.   He will, however
permit the use of his name.

        Both Crowe and Polvogt are working to have you made head of the reorganized
department.   Polvogt says he will not take it if it is offered to him, because, he feels
it is work for a younger man, but, Crowe has placed the entire responsibility of reorganiza-
tion, including raising the funds upon his shoulders.   He wanted to talk the plans over
with me and get my advice and help, so the invitation.

        While I think it wise for you to keep your own council and offer no suggestions
you can write me freely and I can use th information.   Do it now as the plans will soon
be out for bids -- on the building in which must be housed all clinical, operating and
laboratory space.   You might make a little drawing of the arrangement you would prefer
and what of modern fixtures, etc. you would prefer.   Don't delay.

        I know nothing of Crowe's financial arrangements or his income.   I understand
he has outside wealth.   Whether you feel that you can afford to take it, or even whether
you would take it is of course none of my business but some information from you would
greatly influence my personal efforts.   I am not young and I am very much overworked but if
you want the job I will work hard to see that at least the physical plant is worth while
so let me know without delay.

        I must run.   Love and best wishes,

                                             Affectionately,

P.S.--Suggest in full and as much in detail what youwould like to have.   Disregard any
consideration except your judgment of what is best.

Lt.Col.James Bordley,III.,M.C. O-396822

Dr. James Bordley,Jr.,

General Hospital 118, Unit No. 1

330 N. Charles St.,

A.P.O. 927, c/o Postmaster

Baltimore -1, Md.,U.S.A.

San Francisco, California, U.S.A.

October 26, 1944

Series IV.,No.8

Dear Boys,

The election grows hotter and hotter. The New York Times has come out for Roosevelt on his foreign policy. As both Dewey and Roosevelt have agreed on a foreign policy and Mr. Hull and a Republican Congressional Committee have agreed on every point and have organized a working agreement, it seems far fetched to assign such a reason. Of course it has stirred up a hornet's nest among the Jew baiters because the Times is wholly owned and controlled by Jews and from this clan Roosevelt is having very active support. It does look fishy after the Times' campaign against him and his foreign policy only four years ago, pointing out among other things, the dangers from a third term.

Mr. Jamison from up in Greensburg, Pa.and the largest independent mine owner in the country says Dewey he thinks will carry Pa. by about 800,000. That Lewis has served notice on all the mine workers it is Dewey or C.I.O. and they are falling over themselves getting on the Dewey band wagon. Mr. Roosevelt has certainly lined himself up with the worst elements in the country and as I believe the honest far-sighted patriotic people outnumber the crooks and rascals I think Dewey stands a good chance, certainly there is a big swing toward his candidacy. Of course the resident has great political foresight but to tell you the truth I think he is worn out and not the old master he once was. Certainly his speeches while they lack nothing of the old assurance and cunning lack much in fire. He looks dreadfully sick, or, tired and his speeches reflect it. He had painful difficulty in completing his last speech, it was pitiful really to listen to. Dewey on the other hand has grown bolder and bolder and his efforts have drawn great approbation from all ranks.

By the time this reaches you the question will be settled and we will know whether we have a Dictator or a President.

We are all thrilled at MacArthur's move into the Philippines and trust everything will go well for him. It is interesting that some of the most acute politicians think his move will gain Dewey thousands of votes by drawing attention to MacArthur who the home folk feel has been badly treated by the Administration and who has demonstrated what can be done without the cooperation of the Commander in Chief.

In Europe everything seems to be shaping up well though there is some disappointment that the war there has not made more rapid progress. I do not feel that way myself because the obstacles to overcome were many.

More later.

Love from Ma and

Your

Major John E. Bordley, M.C. 0-403012   Dr. James Bordley, Jr.,

        General Hospital 118, Unit No. 1   330 N. Charles St.,

    c/o Postmaster, A.P.O. 927,   Baltimore -1, Md.,U.S.A.

        San Francisco, California, U.S.A.
                                                        November 1, 1944.
                        Se ies IV., No. 9

Dear Boys,
        The closer the voting the hotter the election and the greater the change in the
betting odds. Starting at six to one on the President it is now twenty-seven to twenty-one
and the betting commissioner in St. Louis, the largest of the crew, says that a single large
bet would change the odds to Dewey.
        To save my life I cannot understand those who are voting for Roosevelt as an
insurance for a stable peace. He has provoked nothing but controversy in all his dealings,
he has disrupted his party, driven out of authority every able man, connected with him, but
Secretary Hull whose Southern support and influence the President dared not offend --
although he did egg on Welles in the hope Hull would quit. He can no more harmonize the
people in this country whom he has constantly and intentionally offended than he can convert
the heathen to Christianity, (a poor simile seeing he is the heathen). Now he has further
offended his party and the intelligent people of the land by turning his campaign over to
Sidney Hillman and Browder both offensive, communist Jews and has ordered all efforts cleared
through them. Such an outstanding Democrat as Byrd of Virginia declined to speak for him
and thousands of lesser light Democrats have left the ship.
        There has been a sudden tremendous registration and a growing silent vote. What
it means no man knows but that it will have a tremendous effect upon the election is clear.
The war will hold many people to Roosevelt there is little doubt, thousands of these people
would otherwise vote against him and at the last minute they may change their minds and vote
for Dewey. In a week from today we will know the answer.
        It is clear to an old timer that the thinking of this nation is undergoing a vast
change. I think that it is an augury for good because it had gotten in the rut of self
satisfaction. A revolution in thought is as portentious as a physical revolution and is as
necessary to cure vicious drifts. Of course the pendulum always swings too far in mass
movements as a result of its own momentum, but, before long it comes back in balance and I
hope the balance this time will be a strengthening of our constitutional democracy. We
have taken too much for granted and we needed a strong poke.
        Yale has a strong team, so far so good. She has three half-backs who apparently
have the stuff and so far have run wild. I hope they keep it up.
        It was a glorious victory for the American Navy and apparently a great stroke for
Gen. MacArthur. I knew we would slash them at the first opportunity.

                I must run.   Love from Ma and
                                Your

Lt.Col. James Bordley,III. M.C. O-396822

General Hospital 118, Unit No. 1

A. .O. 927, c/o Postmaster

San Francisco, California, U.S.A.

Dr. James Bordley, Jr.

330 N. Charles St.,

Baltimore -1, Md./ U.S.A.

November 2, 1944

Series IV., No.10

Dear Boys,

 An Australian who saw you three weeks ago called up Ellen and told her of your farewell party and your immediate destination and your future prospects. We have heard intimations and rumors but this was our first direct information. I am afraid you are swapping off a fine stand for a doubtful one, but, at least it is a step nearer home and shows progress.

 We have heard much about the good will you all distributed in Australia. It must be a very satisfying feeling to know that you have completed a very successful undertaking in spite of troubles and worries. It must be equally pleasant to know that your services are appreciated by a large number of informed persons.

 Base 18 is on the Lido Road so Ellen tells me, from direct information. They are occupying a deserted Pennsylvania Unit, native, mud hut hospital. They are not enthusiastic but just take this like the rest of their bad deal.

 The Gallup and the three other leading polls have declined to make a choice in the election. It is so close they say that popular vote is now secondary to State considerations and no man knoweth. The odds went up on the President but last night the prop was knocked from under,a betting commissioner said there should be even money.

 Dewey was here yesterday and his point was the Communist attempt to seize the Democratic party. This is a real favor among many prominent Democrats. Two Democratic Congressmen have already declared for Dewey and sent out a blast against Hillman.

 The Medical profession has centered the fight because the President and Sidney Hillman are working overtime to pass the Wagner-Murray bill to socialize and hamstring the profession. It is serious because most of the questions involved are local and State and not national and the proposed national tax for the support of the measure cuts directly across the fine work in progress by most of the States -- which have passed recent and excellent rules covering all phases of medicine. It is just another step in the regimentation of the people.

  More later. Love from Ma and
    Your

Major John T. Bordley, M.C. O-403012

General Hospital 118, Unit No. 1

A.P.O. 927, c/o Postmaster

San Francisco, California, U.S.A.

Dr. James Bordley, Jr.

330 N. Charles St.,

Baltimore - , Md.,U.S.A.

Series IV., No. 11   November 17, 1944

Dear Boys,

We read a letter from one of your nurses about your change. It is I imagine not like the old atmosphere, physical or otherwise. I guess you are on your way to other and more active fields. Has your post-office address changed? Mother is worrying about your Christmas boxes which were sent a long time ago. I hope you get them.

The election is over and the "people have triumphed" according to Mr. Roosevelt, (but by only two millions out of forty-six). It was a close race and carried by the Communists who worked night and day and piled up a substantial vote in New York, Michigan Illinois and California. Too bad but too true. The balance of power has narrowed itself down to the worst elements in our country. The only disadvantage to our two party system.

Tydings ran away with the Senatorship far exceeding Roosevelt's majority in the State. I thought the friends of Roosevelt and the disgruntled Democrats would lick him. Apparently both voted for him. I still believe a strong independent Democrat could have beaten him but against Randall, a weak Republican he had a cinch. The war was the principal factor, add to that five million Government employees and their families, and the solid south, and you have a hard combination to beat.

Well we are all good Democrats so the election settled the question of who should govern us. There was in fact a unanimous consent in both war and peace both parties agreeing on the general principles and promising support to the vistor. It is really a step toward square politics when the country is put ahead of political victory. Dewey made this his theme and he carries out of the election a much bigger man than he was when he went in.

The Japs must have more ships than we thought. The story of our sinkings runs on endlessly, anywhere from five to seventy-five a day. Where did they keep such an outfit? It was a glorious battle -- the Philippine Sea. Our boys can certainly tuck them away when they show up. I thought their Navy would outstrip their army but just the reverse has happened.

My old friend Patton seems to be holding his own with Germany's best. He is truly old Blood and Guts. Now he takes Metz which in five centuries has fallen but once before. He had a narrow escape the other day but his luck held out, thank Heavens

The home front is having its troubles with strikes and deserters from war plants. Most of the industrials to whom I have talked are opposed to labors conscription but how the situation is to be handled otherwise I don't see. The fear it would result in industrial chaos. The Government has allowed too many plants to partially convert to peace time work and many workers, looking to the future, are flocking for jobs. The Government threatens to close them down, but only threatens.

    More later.

       Love from Ma and

         Your

Major John E. Bordley, M.C. O-405012

General Hospital 118, Unit No. 1

A.P.O. 927, c/o Postmaster

San Francisco, California, U.S.A.

Dr. James Bordley, Jr.,

330 N. Charles St.,

Baltimore - 1, Md., U.S.A.

November 28, 1944

Series IV., No. 12

Dear John,

I received your letter of the second of November a day or so ago. There has been some hitch in the new building. I don't know the circumstances but Bill Rienhoff told me it was held up in telling me a story of the "new plans". The Otological plans were to be shown me but so far they have not materialized. Of course I will never discuss the circumstances under which you will serve. That should come only from you direct. I was just not sure where you could afford to take the place. I do believe that a substantial salary would not be bad insurance for the next few years. Maybe I am a bit pessimistic but I fear the doctor is in for a radical change in his income for the next several years, if not permanently.

We have lost the services of Cordell Hull as Secretary of State. This is the most severe blow the country has sustained. Not indispensable of course, but, he stood for things which are essential to the well being of mankind and he was a powerful advocate, one in whom all had confidence. He was replaced by a able young fellow (which I believe in, as this younger generation should take over). Not so experience as Mr. Hull he has nevertheless been welltrained in the art of diplomacy by that gentleman and knows Mr. Hull's objectives. He is acceptable to the country inspite of his association with the U. S. Steel Corporation.

I am convinced that Roosevelt has lost his right arm and just as convinced Mr. Roosevelt would not have been elected if the resignation had been in before the election. Thousands and thousands really voted for Cordell Hull.

I went down to my farm for my annual visit last week. The new farmer is really doing a good job and bringing in more profit than his predecessor. Even at that I am glad I don't have to live there in the wintertime. He has five fine children who never have colds in spite of the heating ofonly one room. It may be healthy but it reminds me too much of my own early days and makes me cold to think about it. From what I have heard you might enjoy a little of such wintertime.

The war ismaking progress, but to those as far away as I it seems very slow, especially in Germany. Of course we have but scant knowledge of the necessities and the reasons, but I believe we all have fullconfidence in our leadership in both the Army and Navy. The home front is not up to the Army in the performance of its duty. Our war plants are crying for help, the various black markets flourish and the consumers of gasoline go merrily on their way. There is more grouching about the cigarette shortage than of the lack of small arms and ammunition, and morecomplaints against ration points than against the lack of seaman. I suppose this is not extraordinary when you realize how far the war is away, but it does give the really patriotic sleepless nights. Too much stress is being placed on our wonderful industrial showing and too little stress on how much better it could have been with everybody's heart in the job.

More later.

Love from Ma and

Your

Lt. Col. James Bordley, M.C. C-396822

A.P.O. 72, c/o Postmaster

San Francisco, California, U.S.A.

Dr. James Bordley, Jr.

Home: 2630 Guilford Ave
Office: 330 N. Charles St

Baltimore -1, Md., U.S.A.

December 2, 1944

Series IV., No. 13

Dear Boys,

Ma had a long talk last night with Mr. Robertson of Richmond. He said that he hadonly recently left New Guinea and had seen you both and that you were well and looked fine, that he thought your ultimate destination had been settled and was further north, that your stay on New Guinea would be brief. As we have heard nothing tothe contrary we are using the same address. If there is a change let us know.

Ma is worried for fear you may lose your Xmas boxes. Be sure to write as soon as you receive them to set her mind at rest.

We are fully established in our modest little home and it is on the inside, quite attractive. I have set up a little shop from which emanates much useful stuff. We have had more visitors in a month that we had all of last year. I am not sure curiosity has not drawn more of them th n Ma and me. Anyhow it is very nice to have them.

Today is Army-Navy Day in Baltimore. The game should be a thriller with two such great teams. Maybe it will be a fizzle. I have seen great teams play rotten football. It is clear and cold -- very cold. There was heavy snow all around us but none here. I would hate to have my head bumped on the frozen ground.

Yale went thru the entire season with no losses. Virginia tied her last Saturday. The virginia team is rated one of the finest in the country and has been licking them all big and little.

Princeton has had nothing worth mentioning having been beaten by small colleges. Harvard had only a midiocre team and has played but two or three games. This should have been Yale's year.

Since writing the above this a.m. Jim's letter telling of his arrival has come in. So Mr. Robertson was correct in his prediction.

Now you will see war at first hand and have the privilege of looking immediately after the wounded, which I think is a great honor in spite of the drive and extra toil and responsibility. May you have the greatest of luck in all your undertakings. I am sure you both have the ability to do the job and we are all proud of what you have and may accomplish.

More later. Love from Ma and

Your

267

Lt.Col.James Bordley,III., M.C. O-396822

General Hospital 118, Unit No. 1

A.P.O. 72, c/o Postmaster

San Francisco, California, U.S.A.

Dr. James Bordley, Jr.

330 N. Charles St.,

Baltimore -1, Md.,U.S.A.

December 9, 1944

Series IV., No. 15

Dear Boys,   A real let us in work for the past two days and what a relief.   Pop is beginning to feel his oats and a little respite is very helpful.   If the world would only settle down i would feel strong and young again but just as soon as I get the old craft on an even keel something else happens.   I have learned for the first time in my life to take things as they come and worry only about the present and not the future.

The home folk are much riled by the conduct of England in Greece.   We all believe in self determination with no outside interference.   Of course we do not know all the facts but what we do know we don't like.   Churchill has a lot of rebel in his make up and he should appreciate the efforts of the Greeks to determine their own interior problems.   Our Secretary of State senses the danger and has sort of begrudgingly expressed an opinion adverse to the British stand.   I don't think he was strong enough but maybe he feels a word to the wise sufficient and Churchill up to now has been very wise.

We were thrilled by the news from Leyte in yesterday's communications.   It was a bold move to get back of the Japs but it paid rich dividends.   We are wondering whether Worthington was in the party as the report said the action was carried out by the dismounted cavalry. we know he is with them.   Our progress in Germany is slow except for General Patton.   Old Blood and Guts seems to know his way around.   I am always tickled when he goes places and I believe that feeling is shared by the country.

I wrote you on Jim's birthday to congratulate him and had so many interruptions while writing that I closed my letter without saying a word about it.   It still holds good however and I congratulate you and wish you the pleasure of being home on the next anniversary.   As I cannot send you a present, I am buying a hundred dollar War Bond for each of your kids and I have done the same for John's on his birthday which at the time I confess I forgot.   I am not so hot in remembering birthdays and other celebrations.   I depend upon Ma for information.

President Roosevelt has nominated Mr. Will Clayton for Assistatn Secretary of State. The Senate sent his name back to the Committee for further investigation because he is a multi-millionaire.   In other words they shy away from successful men as they may spoil their stock stories to their contingents.   He is to represent us and have charge of all economic questions involving the State Department, and if I am not mistaken he will be a busy man as the whole peace settlement will have an economic base and that is where we will miss Secretary Hull who had a firm fundamental knowledge of worl economy.

The Army is asking for three thousand more doctors.   Where they are to come from is hard to say as most communities are already on the minus end.   We had a State meeting a few days ago and there was but one doctor found available and four counties are working with four doctors and one with two.   Chesney says next year the teaching will be at an all time low as the result of an inadequate number of instructors.   Some how,somewhere the three thousand will be found.

Long lines of people can be seen at nearly all the tobacco emporia every morning, hoping and trying to get a package of cigarettes.   They say in New York those at the head of the lines can sell their positions for real money.   Matches, too, are on the demand list and very hard to get.   I think this unwise and the Government should end it.   Matches may be a luxury with smokers but they are a necessity in many other places, a real necessity which cannot be done without.

Love from Ma and

Your

Lt.Col. James Bordley,III.,M.C. O-396822

General Hospital 118, Unit No. 1

A.P.O. 72, c/o Postmaster

San Francisco, California, U.S.A.

Dr. James Bordley, Jr.,

330 N. Charles St.,

Baltimore -1, Md., U.S.A.

December 19, 1944

Series IV., No. 16

Dear Boys,

We have enjoyed your letters which come much quicker than from Australia,very much. We often speculate on how you and the heat and the mosquitoes are getting along together but I guess youfind more tempestuous enemies than were the little fellows with nasal swords.

Gee, MacArthur is really doing a big job and so is the Navy. Killing Japs and sinking their boats must be making a real impression on the Sons of Heaven (God forbid the name). Keep it up is our constant prayer.

Have you received any of the boxes sent you from home? The editor of the Nurses Journal told me yesterday th t Base 18 has been ordered home. All are to come who originally went out. The youngermen of later arrival are tostay in Assam. She said the report was that something had happened but just what she had no idea. She asked the sensor for confirmation and the right to release the story and was given permission to say the Unit would be home sometime in February -- only that and that it is now stationed in Assam. She could not find out whether the nurses are included in the shift. This was a great surprise to me as I thought they would be badly needed. A father of one of the members told me they were treating no casualties We feel these fellows have had an unnecessarily hard time.

Things are O.K. for Christma , that is all except my present for Ma. She is a Sphinx.

More later.

Love from Ma and

Your

269

Major John E. Bordley, M.C. O-403012   Dr. James Bordley, Jr.

General Hospital 118, Unit No. 1   330 N. Charles St.,

A.P.O. 72, c/o Postmaster   Baltimore -1, Md., U.S.A.

San Francisco, California, U.S.A.
                                         December 28, 1944
                    Series IV., No. 16

Dear Boys,

           Christmas has come and gone and old Santa was very kind to me, not only in the
presents but in the kids who kicked me around for some few hours. Those birds don't think
I have grown up and I often wonder myself. We had a small tree placed on a table but it
quite lovely even if I did help to dress it. Under the table mother placed a village with
church, cottages, trees, dogs and cards. You have no idea how much prettier it looked on a
table than on the floor. We had a mob all day in spite of constant rain. I think people
have some curiosity to see how we can live in a two by four after living in the large house
in Guilford. Well, to tell you the truth I think our present home is quite lovely and
everybody seems to agree and be surprised. I really have never regretted the change as I
feel under far less strain and am under far less expense. Tinsel does not look so pretty
when you get old, especially when it comes with a strain.

           Anne is enthusiastic over the change in their Christmas tree. Mother divided her
Christmas tree ornaments with our kids. You know you cannot buy any of the really pretty
things. Anne says their tree never looked more than half dressed before. Of course the
kids all had fun but I missed the noise because there were no horns or drums. Can't buy such
useful things any more.

           Another sleet storm last night. Boy, what a mess of ice we have so far had this
year. It is one of the great comforts of living in the City that you can go around the
corner and take any one of half a dozen street cars.

           We were all flabbergasted at the German drive. Of course, it unleashed a thousand
fantastic rumors, probably all lies. We were making slow progress and I guess this will slow
us down still more. I am not worried about the outcome because I know we can lick any
German Army ever put together. We must expect a few thorns among our roses as we are not
exactly omnipotent. My old friend "Blood & Guts" Patton is showing the Germans a few tricks.
He can do it.

           Well, Leyte is free from a Jap menace and that makes us at home breathe easier.
At least we hope it is.

                    More later.   Love from Ma and
                                        Your

If you ever get a Christmas box write
your mother about it.

Major John E. Bordley, M.C. O-403012   Dr. James Bordley, Jr.

General Hospital 118, Unit No. 1

A.P.O. 72, c/o Postmaster   330 N. Charles St.,

San Francisco, California, U.S.A.   Baltimore - 1, Md., U.S.A

                                             January 10, 1945.

                    Series IV., No. 18

Dear Boys,   We are much excited over the report that landing on Luzon has started.   Of course
this comes from Japan but we hope it is no exaggeration.
        I saw Guinea Williams yesterday. He is slowly getting back into harness. Says
he started with a hemorrhage which lasted intermittently for several days,, with bloddy ex-
pextorations for another two weeks. The T.B. bug has never been found nor do the Xrays reveal
anything.   They just conclude it must have been a very small focus immediately surrounding
a blood vessel. He looks very well and his rest was much needed because his gang have certainly been hittin the high spots of prodigious work.
        Murray Fisher's baby -- 18 months old -- had a close call. "An attack of croup
complicated by a penumococcus laryngitis". (I would put the horse before the cart).   A quick
operation and massive doses of Penicillin did the trick and he is all right now.
        Another sleet and snow storm lasting all last night.   Boy, we really are having
some winter.   I am conveniently located for the U.M.H.   I had to go there this morning to
see an old man whose cataract I removed a day or two ago. My, when I see such old fellows
their decrepitude touches my heart and makes me thank God that I can still do a day's work
and then play a round of golf. This old bird is six months younger than I but has all the
ear marks of veneration -- looks, acts and thoughts.
        The President has asked for a national draft law -- universal -- but with
particular emphasis on twenty thousand nurses, all 4-Fs in the regular draft and all farm
workers under twenty-six.   This is a bomb shell for labor but it had it coming. Turnover,
absence, shifting of residences and worhtlessness on the job called for action months ago
but the Germans did us the favor of clinching the argument.   Now, don't think I am condemning
all labor because the vast majority have beenfaithful and produced a wonderful job.   It is
the rotten apples in the barrel which have frustrated too many of our plans.   There will be
no lowering of wages, working conditions or seriority but everybody will be given a job and
will be asked no questions whether it be to New York or NewMexico he will go when told.
There are hundred of thousands of young men in political jobs who sould be in the military
services or doing essential war work but I am betting my last cigarette they will never be
touched.
        The President made the speech of his life last night, even I applauded, but
with the mental reservation that only actions help the war and peace efforts.
        Beale is in a Hospital in England. The reason no one knows. He said there was
no use writing because the censor would delete. He added he was rounding into form and
would soon be with his old outfit.   He is in the 9th Army or is it the 7th?
        Ellen Fisher and the kids will be here for dinner. Everything os well with the
family.   Dudy and her kids postponed their visit because her nurse had a vacation.   They
will be here soon.
            More later.   Love from Ma and
                    Your

Lt. Col.James Bordley,III.,M.C. 0-396822   Dr. James Bordley,Jr.

General Hospital 118, Unit No. 1

A.P.O. 922, c/o Postmaster   330 N. Charles St

San Francisco, California,U.S.A.   Baltimore -1, Md.,U.S.A.

                                            January 11, 1945

                    Series IY - No.19

Dear Boys,
            If you could get even a part of the enthusiasm resulting from the invasion of

luzon you could realize the intense home interest in the Pacific war.   Everybody was hanging
on the radio after the first word until late in the night and when it was flashed that a large
body of troops and supplies had been landed there was general rejoicing.   The Sun this morning printed a map of the Jap landing and said it was as faithful now as then of troop movements.   I cannot understand why the small preparationthe Japs reception committee made, they
must have expected MacArthur. Maybe they are playing fox. We have no doubt of the ultimate
result but expect much hard fighting.   It looks like you all may be very busy in a short
time, maybe taking a trip yourselves.
            The President has asked for eighty-four billions, making in all a half trillion--
so far.   Not a single kick, we are ready to mortgage the old place if it will help win the
war and save lives.   Our fine home record has been blurred by a fraction of our people.
Well, I suppose it is hard to weed out selfishness in the world and until we can substitute
for it the philosophy of Christ we will never have peace at home or abroad.   When I think
of the joy riders, the black market,the strikes and those who try in other ways to take advantage of the world's misfortune, it makes my blood boil.
            Well, my little carpenter's shop is getting along fine and I am having a grand
time with it.   Even Ma trusts me tomend things for her -- furniture, glass, etc.   That is
really progress. Ma made Anne and Brucie each a fancy dress, just in case they go to a fancy
dress party.   Charlie and Carroll were made an "ermine" trimmed robe each -- King and
Queen.   The only trouble is nobody is giving any fancy dress parties but I guess they can
get together and have fun.   They love to play with each other and generally leave the old
home a shambles but we don't mind as long as they have fun.
            Everybody is tickled with our little home.   The trouble is we live in a com-
munity where every house, on the outside, is a duplicate of every other.   Even I have tried
to make illegal entries.
            More ice and snow. For the first time in my career, I staid home one day
because of the dangerous walking.   I am too old to be bouncing up and down on the street.
My old bones are too brittle for that kind of amusement.
            I don't see many of our old crowd of youngsters often.   They are so busy trying
to keep their flocks they have little time for social gaieties. It isinteresting though
thatwe have had more people of the ancient variety for meals than for a long time. The new
Ford coupons will I fear bring it to an end. We are allowed fifty tickets each per month
and with butter requiring twenty-four and beef twenty one per pound and canned goods as much
as sixteen per can, you can see we have not the where-with-all for a banquet.   Mother is as
fine a banker with her coupons as Morgan & Co. with their bonds. It would drive me crazy
to have to fool with the coupons and figure a month ahead what I could eat.
                    Love from Ma and
                        Your

Major John M. Bordley M.C. O-403012   Dr. James Bordley, Jr.

General Hospital 118, Unit No. 1   330 N. Charles St.,

A.P.O. 72, c/o Postmaster,   Baltimore -1, Md.,U.S.A.

San Francisco, California, U.S.A.
                                            January 12, 1945
                    Series IV., No. 20

Dear Boys,
        The new continues to filter in of the Philippines campaign. We get very little
real news, only the beachhead landings and a push inward or four or five miles but no real
information. Of course, we understand and appreciate the reason but that does not dull our
desire to know more. The Pacific isbeing given the right hand front page of the papers
and the editorials on war are now dealing with the same. It is interesting how much the
changed conditions abroad have stimulated things here. Thousands applying for jobs, practically no strikes, the Government getting busy to strengthen its foreign policy -- which
has grown woefully weak. The President is getting ready to sign off Hillman just as he did
John L. Lewis. The signs are perfectly clear. The election over, the money spent and all
the dreams of the C.I.O. are needless, so why not? Friendships are only of transitory use
to the President, thenthey go. The President says he is "down the road and just a little
to the left". I think he is getting nearer the middle and especially when one of his
closest henchmen says the Wagner Act is just a C.I.O. club and should be repealed.
        Have not heard a word about Worthington, have you seen him? He was on Leyte.
The family had a letter from Madison. He is still sailing the Pacific. Just where of
course he did not say. Maybe near you?
        This has been a tough winter and if it keeps up it will establish a bad record.
The Legislature isin session, with Charlie Carroll as usual on the wrong side of most
questions. He is a Roosevelt dyed in the wool, with no imagination nor stability.
        We are having a bit of coal shortage. Have had to cut down on plant consumption,
on train service and no illuminated signs are permitted, with a demand for sixty-eight
degree temperatures. Most people who could converted their oil to coal furnaces and how sore
they are now that we have plenty of oil and only a little coal. The O.P.A. has restricted
reconversion. It costs from ninety to a hundred and fifty dollars to convert but at the
Government's request thousands converted to coal. The boys are using strong language.
        There is no one on the Government who can see more than one day ahead, if so
lots of conflicts, headaches and grouches could have been avoided. Pop did not get
caught this trip, because I have no faith in the patriotism of John L. Lewis and his unions.
        Everybody keeps well and your children continue to be fine youngsters. What
their Pop would do without them he does not know.
                    More later.
                            Love from Ma and
                                    Your

Lt.Col. James Bordley,III.,M.C. O-396822

General Hospital 118, Unit No. 1,

A.P.O. 72, c/o Postmaster

San Francisco, California, U.S.A.

Dr. James Bordley, Jr.,

330 N. Charles St.,

Baltimore -1, Md., U.S.A.

Series IV., No. 21

January 16th, 1945

Dear Boys,   Another God awful day -- snow, sleet, rain and ice.   The old home front is
vying in winter with the Western Front except we lack the tragedies -- we have some as a result
but not so many.   Ellen read me John's three latest. They were very interesting and some of
the stories about mud inside and outside reminded me of the first six months of my own experience, except of course we were not expecting Jap bombers at the time.   It is very difficult to practice medicine and do surgery under such conditions but it is just as hard to
change conditions.   I suggested a few letters previous that you get one of the radio
commentators to tell us something about the men and I mentioned Folster whom your letter said
you were having over for cocktails.   There are so many Baltimoreans in your Unit it would delight hundreds of persons here to hear something about what you are doing.   I would get
Paul Patterson to make a note of the broadcast in the Sun if I could know when it was coming
and I would call up a lot of people and have a notice posted in the Hopkins bulletin board.
As he talks on a commercial it would not hurt their business. Westinghouse puts on a similar
thing three times a week and everybody listens to it hoping to hear something of their boys.
(I just heard Folster from Luzon, so I suppose he has left you for good).
        Admiral Halsey's sweep over the China Sea shows above everything else the intrinsic
weakness of Japan. If she has not exhausted her resources she is playing a curious game.   I
mean not so much her men and material as her leadership and ingenuity.   She played a strong
hand once but behind it was a moral instability the ultimate effects of which is shown in defeat after defeat. Of course we have put up a great fight and won but on the other hand with
every opportunity to prepare adequate defense she has lacked ingenuity and brains.   She does
not hold a candle to Germany which is fighting the combined armies of the world's three most
powerful nations and making it everlastingly hot for them, making them use not only three best
but pretty nearly their all.   Work keeps up at a killing pace. New patients,
difficult operations and hosts of old patients.   Pop gets very tired but keeps on going as it
is all I can do to help and after all my work is small as compared with the drugery of the
older general practitioners. Their lives are really tough.   The Government has played a
dirty trick on those who have been trying to help it conserve food. It rescinded hundreds of
coupons for food after promising to honor them at any time. Of course those whose only interest
is self cashed all their coupons at once and those like your mother who working to help have
lost their coupons and been left out on a limb with insufficient coupons for food requirements.
It is similar to a Bank which takes your money and then declines to honor your checks. It is
inexcusable for the Government to set such a precedent.   The Army has been financing a
"Cadet Nurse Corps". Sending girls into Hospitals for training, laying all expenses and giving
each girl a liberal monthly allowance. I just heard that out of seventy graduating only twelve
of them went into military service. It is pretty bad and shows rotten management not to know
what the girls could be depended upon to do after graduation.   I have had a nice
carpenter's bench built for my shop but I am so darned tired when I get home I can do precious
little. I have some good schemes and I hope I can get up the pep to make them.
                   More later.
                        Love from Ma and
                             Your

Major John T. Bordley M.C. 0-403012

Dr. James Bordley, Jr.

General Hospital 118, Unit No. 1

330 N. Charles St.,

A.P.O. 72, c/o Postmaster

Baltimore -1, Md.,U.S.A.

San Francisco, California, U.S.A.

January 17, 1945

Series IV., No. 22

Dear Boys,

Weather report: Rain followed by sleet and snow all last night. For those who have artistic sight the scene is surpassingly beautiful, but for one whose life is filled with chores it has far from a cheering appearance. The trouble is I have no one to put chains on my auto and that I will not do. The wheels of my car will not take the separate links and the full chain is a hard job.

I hope your nurses have arrived. I hear they have been packed up for a month and long to get to you. Their stay in New Guinea made them more wedded to 118. It seems funny that with all the demands being made for nurses that they are not courteously treated in our foreign hospitals. Major George Bordoin of the marines who is just back from the Pacific Islands says they need nurses and all he saw were enthusiastic in the work. He suggested if they were looking for husbands it was a fine opportunity.

Ellen is my right bower. Neither rain nor snow nor ice keeps her away. She is remarkable in her attentiveness and interest and has been a Godsend in these days of slack man and woman power. I am getting her well trained so that when John comes home he can give her a permanent, hardworking job. She can stand it!

Young MacMillan, the one who married a Roosevelt is just home from the European theatre, was wounded three times and has won a bunch of medals and ribbons. His wife has taken the place of some man down in the West Indies so as to relieve him for combat duty. (Strange Roosevelt she got no publicity).

The full medical plan has been laid before the Legislature. I am sending you under separate cover the newspaper report. It will give you an idea of the scope of the intended operations. Take it all in all, I think it an excellent step forward. If politicians can be kept out it will succeed, if they get in it will fail. It is a rich plum for vote getting and will have to be eternally safe guarded. This I hope will keep the iniquitous Wagner bill from operating in this State.

I am ashamed of the lack of current home news in my letters but really there is hardly a thing doing, even gossip is at such a low ebb it is either scandalous or abscent. I never was a good hand at collecting news outside my own sphere. Maybe I take too little interest in other people's business but after all it does not concern me, so why should I hasten to gossip.

Betty Atkinson Reynolds was just in here and asked me to send her love as an old friend and wish you a speedy return. Her husband is playing Secretary to Senator Saltonstall of Mass. Says the latter was elected by the largest majority even given a public official in Mass. and everything he stood for was defeated. Shows the thinking power of the average voter.

We have a new cook, Elsie like most of the niggers got beyond the pole. One day she rang the door bell, coming in at 10.30 a.m. Mother had to pile down the steps to let her in. When asked if she had forgotten her key, she replied: "No, I just like to have someone open the door for me now and then." Well, that afternoon she got her walking papers. That is only one minor sign of what everybody has been putting up with from domestics. They are entirely out of hand, with no regard or consideration for those who pay their wages. The new cook is a bit unpolished but a fine cook with a nice cooperative disposition. I can stand her hair if she keeps up her good work. More later. Love from Ma and

Your

DR. JAMES BORDLEY, JR.

Lt.Col. James Bordley, III., M.C. 0-396822
PROFESSIONAL BUILDING
330 NORTH CHARLES STREET
BALTIMORE, MD.

General Hospital 118, Unit No. 1

A.P.O. 72, c/o Postmaster,

San Francisco, California, U.S.A.

Dr. James Bordley, Jr.,

330 N. Charles St.,

Baltimore -1, Md., U.S.A.

January 18, 1945

Series IV., No. 23

Dear Boys, The thing of greatest moment at home is that we had a beef steak last night. Two weeks ago mother put it in the freezing compartment of the ice box and boy was it good. It is the first one since the birth of Adam and Eve's second baby. Now chickens are out except where you can find a farmer with charity in his heart. One by one our food items shrink up and the coupons become more valuable. Now we are to be given cigarette books. This is an invention of the cigarette companies and is not sponsored by the Government. Each person is to have one and each package punched. You will be able to buy only one at a time and only so often. I don't think it will work any better than prohibition. Even with the Government there is a black market in spite of heavy penalties. The companies can only decline to sue the dealer who violates company orders. No good!

I will give you a tip if you keep it quiet: when you have to walk on ice put some strips of adhesive plaster on your rubbers. There will soon be a shortage of such plaster here because everybody is doing it and it is really great. By the way I would gladly trade you some winter for some summer, I am sick of the former.

To give you an idea of scarcity we had to send to the Virginia quarries to have a laundry tub made and it took just three months to get it. It is made of slate and used to cost twenty dollars, now the cost is ninety. They are making them of concrete but they are so brittle they are not worth buying. No more copper ones are allowed.

I started to get my car our yesterday and had to shovel the now and ice in order to move the doors, then I got ou in the alley and got stuck and had to shovel a path so I could turn. I went up to see Mrs. Tinsley, Jr. and got stuck in front of her apartment and had to shovel my way out; then I went to see a patient on John Street and again had to shovel my way out. I foolishly stopped at the U.M.H. and there I really got in trouble and but for a good landlady bringing me some ashes I would have been there still. The lady told me to look on her front porch as she always keeps a bucket of ashes because so many doctors get stuck. The filling stations are so short handed they will not put chains on and I just can't put them on myself. I tell you winter medicine is no fun for an old bird.

Mr. Cutler has resigned from the Safe Deposit & Trust. "For personal reasons" which none of us understand. I saw him quite often last winter but not once this. He was having much difficulty getting to town on account of the gas shortage. A group hired or bought a bus and chipped in the gas, but, he told me the bus was not heated and was having so many break-downs it kept everybody with bad colds and he thought he would have to give it up. If he had trouble last winter he must have had much more this winter. Maybe he was discouraged.

Railroads are slashing passenger trains. Shortage of coal and man power and the necessity for faster freight movement are given as reasons. Every train has been packed to capacity with war workers who are jumping from place to place and trying to spend their money. Not the unions are demanding higher wages as a means of curing the scarcity of labor. Money is the principal reason for the scarcity. Two days' work a week nets enough to live comfortably, so why work.

More later. Love from Ma and

Your

Col. James Bordley,III., M.C. 0-396822

Heneral Hospital 118, Unit No. 1

A.P.O. 72, c/o Postmaster,

San Francisco, California, U.S.A.

Series IV., No. 24

Dr. James Bordley,Jr.,

330 N. Charles St.,

Baltimore -1, Md., U.S.A.

January 19, 1945

Dear Boys,   Congratulations Jim on your promotion.   Now you outrank me, so I am in the

position of salute.   The highest rank ever held by a Bordley in the Army of the U.S., not so

bad after three years' service. I began to think you had been lost in the shuffle but am glad

I was wrong.   I suppose before long you all will be on Luzon with the main body of the forces

The Japs are taking a good beating and I hope the good work will keep up.   It is interesting

to hear the speculations as to the numbers of MacArthur's forces. It varies from one to five

hundred thousand. Nobody knows any more than I and I know nothing.

The Russians are going to town. Traveling a mile an hour. It sounds to me as if

the Germans are withdrawing to the Odor River, where they will make a final stand and I hope

it will be their final and the Russians will be in Berlin before the Spring thaws.

There is great unanimity in the Senate as to the peace aims.   For the first time

in my recollection politics is out.   Of course such men as Senator Wheeler have things to

say but they are rare birds and very effectual.   We still have our isolationists but they

too are less talkative and offensive, maybe when the tariff is considered their ranks may grow.

Everybody is very well.

Love from Ma and

Your

Major John E. Bordley, M.C. O-403012   Dr. James Bordley, Jr.

General Hospital 118, Unit No. 1   330 N. Charls St.,

A.P.O. 72, c/o Postmaster   Baltimore -1, Md.,U.S.A.

San Francisco,California,U.S.A.
                                             January 24, 1945
                    Series IV.,No.25

Dear Boys,   More snow flurries this morning and last night but thank God for turning on a
little heat and the snow is gone. We still have three inches of ice in the alley back of
the house and it is still difficult to get the car in and out of the garage. Miss Everist
and Miss Rusk came out for dinner Sunday, they were followed by Uncle Dick and his wife, and
before the night closed down we had had ten guests for the day.

          The President has kicked out Jesse Jones to make room for former Vice President Wallac .
He wrote Jones it was a present to Wallace for his activity in the election. It was the
rawest bit of politics that can be imagined and the man is totally unfitted for the job as it
carries with it the lending agency of the government and forty billions of dollars. The office
is Secretary of Commerce. He may be confirmed but it will require more votes than show at
present   Senator George has asked that the lending agency be divorced from the Commerce Dept
before the confirmation, if it is not Wallace will not be confirmed Iam sure. Wallace represents the C.I.O. and is now the leader of the radical left wing of the Democratic party. The
appointment under the circumstances has shocked the country and is a wedge driven in to disturb the unanimity of the country in its support of the President. It is sad.

          I have a bunch of operations this week and I am tired of doing them. Indeed, wish John
was around so I could turn them over to him. They are well-to-do people so he could make a
nice profit.   You would be surprised in a walk through the hospitals to see who have taken
jobs. At lunchtime at U.M.H. it looks like a photograph of the social register, as old as
seventy and as young as fourteen. Really these women have saved the situation and their
work is really surprisingly good. They do every kind of job which will save the nurses steps.
I am sure that scores of these women never carried a tray from their kitchen to their dining-
room but they push whole carts loaded with food, keep the water pitchers filled in the rooms,
help post the charts, run errands and do a thousand little things which add up to big jobs.
Stout told me that the Woman's Hospital would have to be closed except for them and he has
succeeded in keeping more of his old professional and domestic help than any other superinten-
dent. He gives them parties and dances and keeps them otherwise stimulated. Even gave a
cocktail party last week in the nurses home. The greatest trouble is to get the consent of
the parents to let their daughters accept nursing jobs abroad. I suppose it is a natural thing.
Katherine Bordley is doing missionary work among them,tells the fathers and mothers that their
boys in the armed forces expect and want to see intelligent young women of their own social
circle on duty in their hospitals. She is accomplishing things.

          Hollister Davis has light up his old T.B.   The boy has been the only anaesthetist
on duty at the U.M.H. for two years and has worked himself to a shadow. He has trained
several nurses and has at last been persuaded by his friends to go home and to bed at four
and stay there until late morning. He then comes over and supervises the work and occasionally gives an anaesthetic. He is gaining weight and his doctors think his T.B. quieting down.
He is a fine chap and one we could ill afford to lose.

          Ellen is taking the morning off to see Anne do her stunts in a play. Whether the
lass is the lady on the flying trapeze I don't know but that is her natural style. And boy
is she a husky -- strong as a mule. I know because I tackled her the other day and came
nearing taking the count.
                    More later.   Love from Ma and
                                   Your

Col. James Bordley,III.,M.C. 0-396822

Dr. James Bordley,Jr.

General Hospital 118, Unit No. 1

330 N. Charles St

A.P.O.72, c/o Postmaster,

Baltimore -1, Md.,U.S.A.

San Francisco, California, U.S.A.

January 25, 1945

Series IV., No. 26

Dear Boys,   More snow flurries and temperature 8° above, wind 35 miles an hour, ice in abundance on pavements. What a winter!   Walter Graham wrote their Unit is coming home and bringing no glad tidings with joyful people. They have had a raw deal. It makes me tired the Army is demanding more doctors and asking Congress to draft nurses and then it fails to utilize the services of those already in. It holds as good for the University Units as for 18. There are a number of units which have never left this country and they are really het up. About ten thousand nurses have gone in since the draft has been before Congress and the Surgeon General has raised the anti and asked for twenty thousand additional. The original request was for only twenty thousand. They don't seem to know how many they want. If they wait a little longer the Russians will solve the difficulty by getting to Berlin. What a tribe of men and women they are, nothing stops them. Of course it is due to total mobilization which we should have had and would have had except for organized labor's influence with the President. A congressional Committee yesterday endorsed a bill for total mobilization - whether it will pass is a moot question.   The Jones - Wallace affair waxes hot. Jones testified yesterday that the economic fate of this nation is locked up in the lending agencies of the Government and when asked the direct question whether Wallace was competent to handle the vast sum of money involved said, No. In that the whole business community agrees. It is really a show down whether Congress or the President will control the post war finances of the U.S. By our Constitution it belongs to Congress and it was only by a Hitlerism Executive decree that these vast agencies were put in the hands of one man. Fortunately, it was Jesse Jones who has kept the faith by making the agencies non political business organizations. So far out of forty billions expended the Government has not lost a penny, and to turn the agencies over to a scheming dreamer would be a national tragedy. Of course, the C.I.O. is working for Wallace because his theory of spending fits into their scheme of Government control of industry. If this appointment of the President is a sample of the appointment to be made on the peace commission, God help the peace. How can we advocate international peace when we cannot even establish national harmony. Roosevelt travels too far with the old crowd of power politics in Europe to make me have any faith in the ultimate outcome of the efforts for world peace. He is constitutionally opposed to seeking the advice and help of able men. He keeps Perkins in his Cabinet and discharged Jones. One has accomplished nothing and has not the public's confidence; the other has accomplished the impossible and hold's the public's faith.

        Anne was not the strong woman of the play but a mere "plate on the table". What a job for an athlete.

        Wait until you see my cabinetmaker's shop and its output. You have a real treat in store for you if I can keep Ma living in the house until you get back. She is set on an apartment but thank God none are available.
                        More later.   Love from Ma and
                                Your

Major John E. Bordley, M.C. 0-403012

General Hospital 118, Unit No. 1

A.P.O. 72, c/o Postmaster

San Francisco, California, U.S.A.

Dr. James Bordley, Jr.
330 N. Charles St.,
Baltimore-1, Md.U.S.A.

January 26, 1945
Series IV., No. 26

Dear Boys,

Weather report: ground covered with fresh snow, temperature 10°, wind twenty-five miles an hour.

Things are not going so well here for peace and harmony. Roosevelt is on the rampage. His son, Elliott's dog was given priority on a plane going to California which resulted in kicking off of three service men. There has been much severe criticism and justly so. Last night he named Elliott for a promotion -- Brigadier General. It has brought more severe criticism from both the papers and radio. It was just a slap at those who criticised the dog and came not from usual sources of promotions. What he is thinking of -- if he ever thinks -- I don't know. The times demand harmony and he seems intent upon throwing in a few bomb shells. If his recent appointments are indicative of his peace commission he will never get national support.

The Western front is bringing along its heavy toll in casualities but to my surprise the number killed in the Germany drive was surprisingly small in comparison with the German loss. Nearly four to our one and in total casualities, including prisoners, two to one.

The Russians are certainly creating the impression that Germany is a set up for them but I don't yet believe it without Germany has been able to fool everybody about number of their men and the quantity of their ammunition. Russia has a long line to get down with supplies and but few German prisioners have been reported. The longer th line the greater the peril for Russia. They travel about as fast as if no Germans existed. I hope they are as small as they seem.

The tax bills are all at hand and you fellow certainly require a lot. The funny thing is you never hear war caosts mentioed, it seems to be perfectly satisfactory to everyone. I think those who would like to kick are ashamed to do it. Of course the damned politicians are letting such people as negroes and domestics get away with murder when it comes to paying taxes. I think it would have a salutary effect if they were included among the taxpayers. It would give them a better idea of the costs of war. All they do is spend, spend, spend and save nothing.

It is getting increasingly hard to get certain essentials of food and coupon values keep on rising. I don't know how people on a limited budget make ends meet either in coupons or money.

We all remain well and grow increasingly anxious to see you all at home.

Love from Ma and
Your

Col. James Bordley, III., M.C.

General Hospital 118, Unit No. 1

A.P.O. 72, c/o Postmaster

San Francisco, California, U?S.A.

Dr. James Bordley, Jr.

330 N. Charles St.,

Baltimore -1, Md., U.S.A.

January 29, 1945

Series IV., No. 28

Dear Boys,

Weather report: another ice storm, roads filled, walking atrocious.

Ridge Trimble is home. He called us yesterday and said he was off for thirty days and was coming around to see us and tell us all about it. Thinks things are going O.K. in the Islands. We will be delighted to get some first hand information. Three years is a long time on both ends of the line when you are waiting. Unfortunately Ma and I grow no younger as time passes.

Stalin says Russia is out to clean up Germany and end the war. Some say by April they will be in Berlin. God forbid such a long time. At their present rate of travel they s ould be there in two weeks or less. The Germans are a tricky crowd and maybe they are fooling but I don't believe the Junkers would ever have given up East prussia without a struggle except from sheer necessity. We will soon know.

Charlie, Jr. spent Saturday afternoon and Sunday with me working in the shop. We are a hot team of carpenters. He said when I got stuck, "Were you ever a carpenter before or are you just learning?" I had to confess it was my first outing and I think I lost caste at once. I am laying out a couch, sort of a day bed for my little sitting room. It is a folding affair and holds books on the front and looks like a bookcase. If I ever get it finished I may get a patent on it because I am sure it will be unique. Ma just laughs. I have made some pretty little stools for my workshop and have done most of the fine carpentering around the house. Bill Hubner gave me a set of thirty-two moulding planes -- antiques such as were used before the Revolution. I can make any kind of lovely moulding. The trouble is all lumber has to be acquired on a priority so my only source is what I can find among friends. Bill Hubner had a nice stock of mahogany and maple and gave me quite a nice pile.

I took Charlie over to spend the time with Anne while I went out in the country to see a patient yesterday -- Sunday. They always have such a good time together, only fuss a normal amount and both are tom-boys. I had an argument on my hands when I got back to get Charlie away. Anne seems devoted to me and always shows me a lot of affection. She is growing like Jack's beanstalk.

Dudy has not yet arraived with her kids but expects to come soon. The railroads are so congested and the weather has been so bad that it has been bad for traveling. In fact the railroads have stopped all freight except war frieght because there is not enough coal even to permit ordinary business concerns to operate. All public schools and buildings have been requested to close. The Mayor here says public organizations have enough coal on hand to continue for the present so instead of taking the coal for more important functions I suppose they will go along. Poor business.

More later. Love from Ma and

Your

Col. James Bordley,III.,M.C. 0-396822

General Hospital 118

A.P.O. 72, c/o Postmaster

San Francisco, California, U.S.A.
Series IV., No. 32

Dr. James Bordley, Jr.

330 N. Charles St.,

Baltimore -1, Md.,U.S.A.

Februay 28, 1945

Dear Boys,

We listened over the radio last night to the return of the Philippines Islands to their owners. It was very impressive and full of portent. What must the other countries occupied by Japan be thinking of the comparison? How it must increase their faith in our intentions and desires. It shows up the brutality of Japan as nothing else that has happened. It made me very proud of my country and thankful that my sons played even a part in this historic event.

Things are going well with our armed forces but damned badly at home. While Congress plays around with the Manpower Bill we are having a series of ghastly strikes in important industries and more threatened -- John Lewis and his coal miners. What we need is a few men of guts instead of a bowl of jellyfish in Washington. I heard a slant on the closing of the night clubs which had not occurred to me. It is said to be the fine hand of the prohibitionists. Last night Fulton Lewis analyzed the racket and showed that no fuel would be conserved and no man power conserved and predicted an extension of the liquor ban on hotels and restaurants.

We have been warned against the shortage of gasoline, a few days ago all the filling stations were supplied, for the first time in months, with high test gasoline and an oil man told me it was the result of a tremendous surplus with all available storage space occupied and the necessity for more room. Why does the Government lie to us. We are, with few exceptions, willing to do our part so why not tell us the truth. The change would be helpful I am sure to the health of the nation.

I am still so busy that I have to write you between patients and as there is nothing worth recording of family interest, my letters must be short.

Love from Ma and
Your

Dr. James Bordley, Jr.

Major John F. Bordley, M.C. 0-403012   330 N. Charles St.,

General Hospital 118

A.P.O. 72, c/o Postmaster   Baltimore -1, Md., U.S.A.

San Francisco, California, U.S.A.   March 1, 1945
                                           Series IV., No. 33

Dear Boys,

I understand that the war has brought about a change in human anatomy:
A G.I. with "two nerves" in his right eye endangering his life. They were growing so
close together there was danger of their touching and if they did it meant suddendeath.
Oh, yes the eye was taken out to end the danger! What kind of stuff is the M.C. trying to
pull off, or, was it just a mother's explanation?

The public is raising more hell about the closing of the night clubs than about
the strikes and shortage of war materials. I think I will take a crack at this shocking
attitude in the Sun.

We went to a nice party at the Trimbles. The Colonel was a genial host and the
party was a great success. Nearly all the wives of the 118th were present and Ma and I
were included. It was a very nice thought which we greatly appreciated. Unfortunately,
Mrs. Trimble had a sudden attack of lumbago so we missed the pleasure of seeing her.

All thegirls are excited over the rotation and making many guesses as to who
and when the first contingent would arrive. Of course we all hope that you both may soon
be included as we feel three years is as long as you should be asked to stay away from
your famalies, provided replacements can be found.

I have been suffering from an infernal bursitis and its usual pain. Today I can
move my arm a little more freely. I have worked right along as I have too many sick
people on hand to stop but I must confess I have had my difficulties.

Well the President is back and is right now talking to Congress. I have no radio
here so will miss the explanation of the agreements reached by England, Russia and the U.S.
I suppose we have already been given the gist of the story. I think the settlements were
fair, just and promising. If we could bottle up such politicians as Senator Wheeler, the o
outlook for full cooperation would be better. He, the Isolationist, blames the President
for not making the world a family of nations like the U.S. Some transformation for an
isolationist, but even he senses the desires of the American public in its attitude toward
cooperative peace but has not sense enough to cooperate.

                    More later. Love from Ma and
                                        Your

Col. James Bordley,III.,M.C. 0396822

General Hospital 118,

A.P.O. 72, c/o Postmaster

San Francisco, California, U.S.A.

Dr. James Bordley,Jr

330 N. Charles St

Baltimore -1, Md., U.S.A.

March 6, 1945
Series IV., No. 34

ar Boys,

 I am certainly longing for Penicillin. They have given the hospitals some but
ive never made it available for the drugstores. I have been putting patients in the
ospital in order to use it and I turn them all over to Murray Fisher. The iritis cases
et brilliant results in three or four days even the chronic recurring type. I have just
ad a case of panophthalmolitis following a cataract extraction. The patient became
iolently nauseated in twenty-four hours following the operation and tore open his corneal
ncision and b came infected with pus streaming from the interior chamber. Penicillin
n twelve hours stopped the pus and in forty-eight hours was well.
 (P.S.) Murray just called me to say the patient has just had an extensive
emorrhage from an old peptic ulcer and they are giving him a trandfusion. That is the
kind of worry that will sooner or later drive me out of medicine. An old man can't take
it like a youngster.

 Mr. Migel is going to spend some time with me tomorrow afternoon. You may
remember him as the good angel of the blind in the last war and head of my French
organization.

 I just heard that Randolph is at Velley Forge looking after the blind there. I
don't know what that means unless he is looking after their medical needs. A recreation
centre has been established I understand for the blind in Connecticut but so far as I am
informed no serious effort is being made for their re-education for jobs. Randolph says
he hears t'at all th medics who have served in the U.S. for two years will be sent abroad
to re-place medics who have served abroad for a like time. This must sound pretty good
to you fellows who have been away for three years.

 Unit 18 is coming home with a few exceptions. From what I heard they have already
started. Those who come by plane will be here in a few days, those by ship in about two
months. My understand is they will be re-assigned to hospital in this county after
thirty days at home.

 Have you ever received your Christmas boxes? if not, do you want something
sent you?
  Love from Ma and
   Your

Dr. James Bordley, Jr

Major John E. Bordley, M.C. O-403012   3.0 N. Charles St.,

General Hospital 118   Baltimore -1, Md.,U.S.A.

A.P.O. 72, c/o Postmaster

San Francisco, California, U.S.A.   March 8, 1945

                                              Series IV. 35

Dear Boys,   Well the nurses' draft has passed the House with excellent prospects of
passing the Senate.   Single nurses between twenty-one and forty-five are all included. Some
of the nurses are scared to death. They never came up against any similar proposition.   I
don't know whether it is wise or not. When I hear of the Units which have done absolutely
nothing and think of the nurses tied up in their midst I can't help feeling that the military
forces are not taking advantage of the immediate supply and how far that would go if utilized
I do not know.   I know no practical steps are being taken to help the blinded. There is a
"center" in California, one at Valley Forge and a "recreation" center in Connecticut but
Mr. Migel who is President of the American Association for the Blind tells me that no practical steps for their training has been undertaken. He induced the California and Valley
Forge centers to let him send them a fine teacher for a limited period, it was such a success
that both are clambering for more such help. He spent last evening with us and left for
Washington to see what could be done about it.   Forty-nine "blind shops" have produced
sixteen million dollars worth of articles for the Army and Navy and it has been written into
the law that their products be given precedence (price being equal).   Machines have been
invented controlled by an electric beam to automatically stop if the blind make a false move.
With these machines they have made over five million pillow cases without an accident,
five million brooms, five million mops and thousands of other complicated articles.   Henry
Ford has adopted the machines and put a lot of blind persons at work and so far not one has
lost his job.   This bears out my theory of twenty-five years ago that with a little ingenuity of invention and sound training the blind can be included in available labor.   The
blinded soldiers who number about twice that of the last war should have these tricks made
available to them.   I have done my best to wake up the authorities but to no avail.   If the
Surgeon General expects credits for good work he must expect criticism for lapses.

          Point values on most foods have been raised and this makes housekeeping a very
difficult job for everybody but Ma who takes it in her stride, utters no complaints.
Honestly if I had to do the job of looking after coupon books I would go crazy. Ma's cross
word puzzle training has fully equipped her for the job.

          Madison was in for a visit a night or so ago. He reports back for duty Saturday.
He will not go back to the Pacific but expects an increase in rank and a better assignment as
a result of his record. He looked very well and is a much changed -- improved -- fellow.
Told us some interesting facts.

          The President's plan for unity -- before Congress -- greatly impressed the
country and everything was swinging his way and then he sent the names of two near Communists to the Senate for ratification for important jobs and in doing it he rocked the country.
Such a fool.   He expects and asks unity and then prevents it by his own actions.
I don't get him.

          Most of the Hill Billies have gone home. We see a few now and then but as far
as they are concerned the war is over and the fun through. I must say most of them did
pretty well, their worst trouble was they took a fancy to traveling. They saw the country
while the money was flowing in. A butter man told me the other day that 80% of them had never
eaten butter before they came and they lived on it as long as their coupns lasted and when
they were gone they started buying clothes. I wonder if they will ever be satisfied again.
I doubt it.   Love from Ma and   Your

Col. James Bordley,III.,M.C. 0-396822

General Hospital 118

A.P.O.927, c/o Postmaster

San Francisco,California,U.S.A.

Dr. James Bordley, Jr.,

330 N. Charles St.,

Baltimore -1, Md.,U.S.A.
March 15, 1945
Series IV., No. 56

Dear Boys,   We had a nice long letter from John and were delighted to get it.   We also
read Ellen's latest letter telling about Gen. Kirk's visit, etc.   These are the first

authentic stories we have read.   My understanding, gained by talking to those in authority,
that when you come home your assignments will be in the U.S.   This is due to a spreading re-
sentment that many of you have served overtime abroad and many have served overtime in this
country.   You know that even the Army has to listen to public opinion.   It is a long time -
three years - to keep a married man away from his family when there are available single men
at home.   The war goes on apace and with the blows now being dealt Germany she cannot last much longer.   I heard an informed commentator say last night that the first of
July would see the end of organised opposition in Germany and it would not surprise him if
six weeks would end our opposition.   The mystery to me is that the Germans stand for the
destruction of their own towns and villages by their own Army.   They have done almost as
much damage as our bombers and artillery.   Hitler says he will destroy Germany rather than
let it surrender and he is for once keeping his word.   The blows of our Air Force against
his transportation is a mystery to me.   For months they have hammered it but the Germans
seem able to move troops and supplies at will.   Of course their terminals must be shambles
but they seem to find ways around them.   Think what New York would be like with Grand
Central and the Pennsylvania stations out of commission.   Our crossing the Rhine must have
been a hard blow to the Germans but so far as I can see it is a limited operation and the
location gives us a long haul to important German bases.   Still from the standpoint of
morale it must give our enemies a bad headache.   Caesar and Napoleon are our only rivals
in the exploit.
        I am sorry that one of the commentators working the radio in your neighborhood
does not tell the country about the little individual exploits of the men.   Every report
from Europe tells about the fellows there, just human interest stories.   No matter where
you go people excuse the interruptions to listen, they are afraid their boys will be mentioned and they might miss the story.   It is the only means of finding out whether their
boys are alive.   It is a wonderful thing and much appreciated by the public.   We listen
to the communicique from General MacArthur's headquarters and always feel that something is
lacking.   The public generally is more interested in its children than the battle reports.
Stir up your friend Folster and see whether he can do something about it.   It will greatly
stimulate public interest in the Pacific battle area.   Malone who reports for Westinghouse
 devotes his entire broadcast to stories of the boys.   He was just home for a week and had
invitations from all over the U.S. to speak, etc.   Everybody knows him, and more about
the products of Westinghouse than ever before.
        The Manpower Bill is in the hands of the damned politicians and they are playing
for time hoping the German war will soon be over and they will not have to tell American
labor it is only a part owner of the country.
                        Love from Ma and
                                Your

286

Major John E. Bordley, M.C. 0-403012

General Hospital 118

A.P.O. 72, c/o Postmaster

San Francisco, California, U.S.A.

Dr. James Bordley, Jr.

330 N. Charles St.,

Baltimore -1, Md., U.S.A.
March 20, 1945
Series IV., No. 37

Dear Boys,

Well I have taken a step which has sort of shocked me.   I have given up operating on cataracts. In the past year I have done quite a few and each one takes a little more out of me and I decided to be sensible and quit.   You know cataract operations carry an especial worry and anxiety and for once in my life I want to dodge trouble.   Before long I will stop all operating and live like a gentleman. I have served a long apprenticeship and am entitled to a rest.   Bring home a good eye man and I will give him all my operative work.   I want to see the fellows who have made the real sacrifices get real opportunities and any help I can give them will add to my happiness.

Ma and I are going to take a long vacation this summer, up at Rye, of course. I really am ready for it now but will have to wait a while for the Hotel to open.   Don't think from all this I am down, to tell you the truth I am only tired.

Bruno arrived yesterday. Brought home twenty-six nurses and left all but six I understand at Miami.   Says he has no finger nails, ate them on his way home as the trip was pretty rough and he was not paticularly familiar with the eccentricities of air planes. I have not seen him personally but Guinea told me the story.   His vacation not starting until today he had to report to Camp Meade.   I am very anxious to see him and we will probably have a little party for him.   I don't know who came with him, I understood Walter Buck was to share the sameplane.

I saw one of the B-29s a day or so ago. What a gigantic contraption.   It was flying relatively low so we got a fine look at it.   The Mars is the only plane I have seen to compare in size and itsstubby wings kept it from looking as large as it really is.

We have a curious condition of affairs. The National Government has decreed the curfew for night clubs as twleve o'clock. Mayor LaGuardia of New York has decreed one o'clock. It wasan economy request by the Government so it leaves it out on a limb.   I think the Mayor is rotten and unappreciative of the effect of his disregard of the Government decree. But he is only one in some millions who are more interested in their own well being than in that of the community.   How people can read or even just see the long lists of killed and wounded andthen think of their pleasures as transending these terrible sacrifices is hard to understand.   What we need is a man at the head of things with guts enough to tell the law breakers where they get off and mean it.   The rank and file areunderstanding and responsive and why the others should be permitted to go their own sweet way is exasperating.

Some three hundred of Base 18 are home. I have not yet seen any of them. I suppose they are sticking around at home and I don't blame them after three years away.

Love from Ma and
Your

Col. James Bordley,III.,M.C. 0-396822

General Hospital 118,

A.P.O. 72, c/o Postmaster

San Francisco, California, U.S.A.

Dr. James Bordley, Jr.

330 N. Charles St.,

Baltimore -1, Md., U.S.A.

March 23, 1945
Series IV., No.38

Dear Boys,   The possibility of seeing you in the near future is a great relief and pleasure to all of your family.   Personally, I think your long stay has been pretty exacting and especially when you have growing families.   I must say for your wives they have been most attentive in their loving care of your kids and not without the trials that come in a household.   They are fine women and whether your good judgment or plain luck you are extremely fortunate, much more so than some others.

The evidence of decadence of German arms grows.   It looks the beginning of the end although such well informed men as Watson of the Baltimore Sun warns against undue optimism He says there are thousands of first class fighting men still left in the interior of Germany and a number of first class generals.   Still with Silesia, the Saar Basin and the Ruhr lost there must be a great decrease in supplies.   If it takes all of our plants working night and day to supply our needs the loss of such a vast number of plants to Germany must be a real blow.   Then the attacks on the home Islands of Japan gave us a real thrill and a better sense of our power and Japan's weakness.   Maybe the Lord is getting tired of the war and intends to stop it.

Ann Bordley is getting married the latter part of April.   Of course she is full of enthusiasm and joy.   I hope everything goes well with her as she is a nice girl.   The boy is rather young but a good hardworking, steady fellow.   Ann is just wishing for Worthington. he has certainly been the mainstay of that family and I hope he comes through all right. His would be a serious loss.   The casualty lists grow rapidly and particularly the Maryland group.   It is the one thing that has brought anxiety and sobered the people at home.

I heard a debate on the Forum of the Air on the continuation of professional sports last night.   The opponents I think were a bit bitter.   I could not help remembering what a Commentator told me of an interview he had in a fox-hole with a Marine.   He asked him how he felt about the continuation of such events at home while the Army and Navy boys were away fighting.   His reply was: "What the Hell do you think we are out here fighting for? We want to go back to the same old country unchanged."   Well, that about answers all the questions and he was right.   With people herded together in strange places it is wise to provide some outlet and I think base-ball and foot-ball are about as innocent amusements as can be provided.   The Selective Draft says who can play and who can fight, so after all it is up to the Board to give the answer.   I do not believe favoritism has played any important part in the draft.

Love from Ma and
                    Your

Dr. James Bordley, Jr.

Major John E. Bordley, M.C. O-403012   330 N. Charles St.,

General Hospital 118

A.P.O. 72, c/o Postmaster   Baltimore -1, Md., U.S.A.
                                              March 28, 1945
San Francisco, California, U.S.A.   Series IV., No. 39

Dear Boys,

We were glad to hear from Jim yesterday and gain a better idea of your work and living quarters. I hope before a other rainy season sets in you will be comfortable at home.

Frank Chew did not send you the box. It was from Ma, she used FrankIs name because her quota was filled and the Postmaster said it could be sent in that way. His gave his consent but none of the material. He only gives what he picks up onthe street. If there ever was a miser, his name must have been Frank.

Young Jim Foster is marrying Walter Ruth's daughter on Monday. Dorothy did not include any of our family except Ma and me, but, Mrs. Ruth sent Ellen an invitation and telephoned her. Dorothy is such a sweet woman with a heart full of charity.

Mary Garnett was in to see us about her eyes this a.m. Her husband is abroad in the Army and she has a civilian Army job. She helps formulate the plans for the re-education of the Class F 4's who are to take the places f able bodied men in clerical jobs. I imagine she is quitecapable.

Well another Easter is poking its nose out and with it has come lovely spring weather. Pop is taking off a couple of days and expects to spend most of the time in bed getting a long rest.

Beale has been shifted from the combat forces and given a clerical job in the forces in England. He had quite a nervous reaction two weeks of first line duty including D day in Normandy. A y ung woman wrote Kathering she had been to see Beale and that while he was still pretty jittery he was coming through all right.

Did I tell you Jack legg was given some medals and a fine citation for his exploits in and around Italy.

Anne Bordley's wedding is the excitement among the women folk these days. I get a belly full of it every day It comes off on the twenty-first of April (or is it the twenty-third). She is getting more stunning looking every day.

What a licking we are giving the Germans. It is freely predicted in high circles that thirty to sixty days will end all organized resistence. They are not supermen but boy they are almost, What a fight they have put up against the world. I only hope this fact will not make the world soft hearted but you know how we in this land cheer the defeated.

                    Love from Ma
                            and
                                Your

Col. James Bordley, III., M.C. 0-396822

General Hospital 118

A.P.O. 72, c/o Postmaster

San Francisco, California, U.S.A.

Dr. James Bordley, Jr.

330 N. Charles St.,

Baltimore -1, Md.U.S.A.

April 3, 1945

Series IV., No. 40

Dear Boys,

A patient just dropped in and left me three packages of cigarettes. Did you ever think such a thing would bring joy to the heart? Well we are just that reduced in smokes. When people come to your home you let them smoke their own. Well that is not being niggerly, but only show a means of self preservation.

At three o'clock yesterday I went to the funeral of an old friend and patient, Morgan Marshall, Director of the Walters Gallery. A great loss to Baltimore. At four o'clock I went to the wedding and reception of Jim Foster and Miss Ruth. It was a very pretty affair and it was the entire living Brown Clan. It looked like an old home meeting at the reception. I have never seen the whole family together b fore and they represent every stage of civilization. Still we were all glad to see each other and ate, drank (lemon punch) and made merry. My, how old some of them looked! I don't know how they get that way.

It seems to me every boy we know in the services is in the Pacific and quite a few in the phillipines. I don't suppose you meet any of them, or, do you? If you ever do, write us so we can tell their families. So many fellows never write.

Our house is full of Anne's wedding. Mother is really having the time of her life planning and preparing. She has a shower next week with a slew of guests; Aunt Katherine comes in to try on her wedding gowns; Anne's wedding dress -- formerly Ellen's, has to be altered for length and ne fashion, Ma is the Director of the changes; Worthington is going to wear my cut-a-way and Ma had to pass on the fit and arrange to get the parts of the body in that stick out and over; my black shoes fitted exactly so that left Ma without a job. There is to be no reception because of the size of our homes. Anne is afraid of hurting someone's feelings without she invites a couple hundred, so it was decided to give up the idea.

Ma and I are coming out again, out for dinner three nights last week, all day Sunday at Ellen's (a wonderful Easter Day). This week we have slowed down to a cocktail party, a reception and one dinner out. I am afraid I will have to go away for a long rest.

More later.

Love from Mother and

Major John E. Bordley, M.C. O-403012

General Hospital 118,

A.P.O. 72, c/o Postmaster

San Francisco, California,U.S.A.

Dr. James Bordley,Jr.

230 N. Charles St.,

Baltimore -1, Md.,U.S.A.

April 9, 1945

Series IV.,No. 41

Dear Boys,

Well, I have been reduced in rank; I had to wash the windoes of the home. Not a soul have we been able to get since last September for such work and as the visibility was reduced to zero, I took a hand in the game and if I do say it, I did a pretty fair job. It as all done from the inside, as I was afraid tochance it from the outside. D made a mop and towel holder long enough to reach up and down. There is nothing now left domestically from cooking to mending that I have not tackled.

Bruno came in and spent the evening with us. We were going to give him a cocktail party and have the balnce of the Unit but he is so busy chasing around from New Haven to Asheville seeing relatives that we decided to wait until he is settled. He hopes to go to Walter reed where King is the chief of Medicine, if not there he will be with the 3rd Army command working out of Meade. This will enable him to get home often. He says all the other fellowswill be in this general neighborhood except those who live away from Baltimore who will get assignments in their respective areas. He was most interesting in the story of his travels and experiences, the most thrilling was his return by plane. I found him not so thrilled with the Chinese. He has not the exalted opinion with which our propagandists have filled us. His medical experience was in truth a sad story.

Mother is having a shower for Ann Bordley today. About twenty-five or thirty girls I think. That was all she could do in the way of entertainment. Ann really gets more and more pretty and has come out of most of her childlike simplicity.

We had akilling frost last night after three unprecedented weeks of summer weather. The fe flowers in our garden are all black as crows this morning and I hear the fruit loss in Western Maryland is tremendous and the same for the strawberries and early vegetables on the Eastern Shore. Of course, the Farmers' stories can be discounted but the loss must have been large.

Russia sort of dropped a bomb shell among our isolationists to defenders of the small nations against the overpowering strength of Russia "who was primarily out for Russia". They have tramped this country villifying Russia and now Russia's answer is overwhelming. They were confident -- or said so -- that Russia would have no part in the fight against Japan but would gobble things up in the Far East when we had defeated Japan. They are the same crew that is preparing next week to put up a great fight to prevent reductions in our tariff. They are also getting ready to try and break up the San Francisco Conference and split it wide open. They are a bunch of infected lice.

John Waters, Gen. Patton's son-in-law has been saved from one of the German prison colonies. We have not heard about his condition but hope for the best.

Love from Mother and

Your

Col. James Bordley,III., M.C. O-396822

General Hospital 118,

A.P.O. 72, c/o Postmaster

San Francisco, California, U.S.A.

Dr. James Bordley,Jr

330 N. Charles St.,

Baltimore -1, Md., U.S.A.
April 16, 1945

Series IV., No. 42

Dear Boys,   The King is dead, long live the King. It happened suddenly but for a lot of us not unexpectedly. He has had the pall over him for a good many months and showed it. Only his tremendous vitality kepy him going. It seems unfortunate that he did not give up before November so the American people could have followed their own inclination inelecting his successor. He knew it was coming and not so far away.

The new President was a county judge appointed by Prendergast but most men with whom I have talked think he is a level headed fellow. Great oaks from little acorns grow and maybe he will follow the pattern. I have great faith in the small town Judge, he is usually pretty well ac uainted with human nature and that is what we need right now. Personally, I have more faith in the possibility of a lasting peace now than before and I might add a less expensive one for this nation.

Roosevelt's objectives have always been excellent but he has been as devious in reaching for them as a heathen Chinee. As these objectives are the sole (and I might say soul) property of the American people I think theywill be as actively prosecuted as before and l hope with better balance. The country is truly hysterical over the sad news. I have s en two other Presidents die in office but not one tenth of the commotion caused by the present one. The radio, press, associations, churches have vied with each other in their adoration. Political parties are no more, etc. etc. His coffin was carried from the White House on an open railroad car to his home in New York and was lighted up so all the anxious crowd could see the last of their President. I never heard such eulogies from cabinet, preachers, judges, poets and from not only the great but the near great and even bower down the scale. The churches all held solemn services, all the orchestra played solemn music. No one ventured to play his favorite song -- "Pistol Packing Mamma". Why I don't know as Harry Hopkins had it played for him at the Cairo Conference and he thoroughly enjoyed it.

Well the King is dead, long live the new King and may he in his wisdom take of the good and discard the bad so that we as a nation may go the way of the righteous and prosecuting the war and the peace to a successful conclusion may make this a better world and a safer place for our children and their children. Took much credit cannot be bestowed on the past President for his great efforts to free the world from tyranny abroad and for such I shall ever be thankful.

Ann's wedding goes apace and on Saturday I have chosen to drive her to the church. My, I do a lot of odd jobs now-a-days! Her presents are really quite lovely and considering the times quite numerous and varied. I like her boy friend and am sure he will take good care of her.   It looks like we will not see Dudy and her kids before Summer in York Harbor. I hope if you get home this summer you willall by my guests (with your families) up at Rye Beach, of course.   I look forward to a family reunion with infinite pleasure. You have been away a long time and mother and I have grown no younger.

With love from Ma and

Your

Dr. James Bordley, Jr.

Major John E. Bordley, M.C. 0-403012   330 N. Charles St.,

General Hospital 118

A.P.O. 72, c/o Postmaster   Baltimore -1, Md.U.S.A.

San Francisco, California, U.S.A.   April 18, 1945
                                        Series IV., No. 43

Dear Boys,

    We have a new President and so far he has been impressive. He is to stick to the established military and foreign policy which is the wish of the country. As to his domestic policies he will take his time and make his own studies, which is hopeful. The cabinet is to remain the same for the present and according to the Commentators no change will be made until after the San Francisco Peace meeting, then the probabilities are large that Madam Perkins, Morgenthau and two or three others will be re-placed. He has made his first appointment: a Mr. Snyder, banker of St. Louis, to take the old finance job of Jesse Jones whom Jones says is the best qualified man in the nation.

    He also nominated General Patton for a full General -- a thing which Roosevelt's prejudice prevented before and which meets with the hearty approval of all. I liked his temperate speeches and for the first time in twelve years felt that I was listening to facts. No wise cracks, no mean suggestions, no bitterness. Most thoughtful people feel a sense of relief. We had a strike in one of the cracking plants, started yesterday morning and the President ordered it taken over by the Army by noon, the men go back to work this morning. What a difference!

    There is a rumor this morning of a junction between our Army and that of Russia. We have learned to await confirmation of rumors now. We have had too much jubilation over hot air coming in from Sweden, Switzerland, France and some of our imaginative commentators and newspapers. There is one thing sure if the junction has not taken place it is only a matter of hours before it will. Germany is so desperate she is shooting her own pilots. What a gang the Nazi crowds, not satisfied with destroying their neighbors, with nothing else to destroy they are destroying their own country. They are truly a land of madmen. We don't understand them because our education does not include lunatic asylums.

    We have had three days of nice rain which we were in need of. Our country wells have suffered so from the dry weather of the past two years they are in large measure still dry. The vegetation looks like mid-May and is today quite lovely. Our little garden patch is green, the lilacs have gone and the roses have buds.

    I have got to beat it to for the U.M.H. to operate, so more later.

          Love from Ma and
            Your

Col. J mes Bordley, III., M.C. O-396822

General Hospital 118

A.P.O. 1002, c/o Postmaster

San Francisco, California, U.S.A.

Dr. James Bordley, Jr.

330 N. Charles St.,

Baltimore -1, Md., U.S.A.
April 24, 1945
Series IV., No. 44

Dear Boys,   Well the wedding is over and except that Uncle Worthington got tight everything went off in good form.   She was married in the little church out on Charles St. by Baker. A lovely afternoon following a rainy morning made nature look bright and attractive and the girls in the wedding with their pretty faces and dresses added the finishing touch.   Carrol was flower girl and by far the most composed of the wedding party.   When the reception line formed at the church door and everyone was complimenting the girls no one said a word to Ca roll so she left the line and came over to me and said, "Pop, don't you think I look lovely?"   I told her she was the most lovely so she went back and got in line again.   She really was very cute. Anne, Brucie and Charlie were there and enjoyed the ceremony.   There was no formal reception as Anne's house is too small for the crowd she would have had to invite -- but the word was passed around among the families of the contracting parties and about fifty people went out for a sandwich and glass of champagne punch.   Dudy came down and would have brought Pat but it meant a too late return and she was afraid Pat would be exhausted.   We were all de- lighted o see her and Ann really appreciated the trouble she took.   Ann's presents were really lovely and while not so numeroud as I have seen, they made up in b auty and usefulness. Ma is resting after her labors.   There would have been no wedding without her, that is no pretty affair.   She arranged everything and while exhausted enjoyed ev ry minute.   She went down into the bowels of her 'ourteen trunks and found everything from wedding dress to dish clothes.

Well, the war is goin at a fast clip but 1 fear is still a long way from over.   Germany is getting hers good and plenty but you would be shocked at the sob sisters at home who are already devising ways and means to excuse the damn burglars and merderers for their atrocities. It may be unChristian to hang and shoot most Germans, but my, what a satisfaction to a lot of wearysouls who have been starved, maimedand had their children killed b fore their eyes.   May- be I am wrong but I am for cleaning Germany outonve and for all even if it means exterminat- ing every German.

The Baltimore base-ball club has st rted the season with big crowds and to date has lost but one game.   It is, as it was last year, made up of youngsters most of whom have either been rejected by the Army or are discharged casualities.   They have taken the Stadium for the season and all functions held there other than those of th team must come when they are away.   Every effort was made to brin the Naval Academt up here for all of their games but the authorities decided to put up a field of their own holding I think sixty thousand.

Everybody is watching with anxious hopes the San Francisco meeting.   If they fail to prepare for a long time peace, the whole world will go in mourning.   Already there are some disturbing indications but I hope common sense will have its days.

Love from Ma and

Your

Lt.Col. John E. Bordley,M.C. O-403012

General Hospital 118

A.P.O. 1002, c/o Postmaster

San Francisco, California,U.S.A.

Dr. James Bordley,Jr.

330 N. Charles St.,

Baltimore -1, Md.,U.S.A.
April 26, 1945

Seires IV., No. 45

Dear Boys,

The San Francisco meeting got under way last night. The President addressed it by radio. I think he made a perfect speech for the occasion, nothing but homely truths without any fireworks or back-biting. There are a lot of controversial issues but my guess is they will be compromised and settled. I am afraid the public is expecting more than it will get. The prevailing opinion is that it is a peace conference to settle the miiediate war and post war necessities of the various Allied Nations. This, of course, is not a fact as it is only to perfect a structure to which such difficulties can be later referred and after the establishment of peace. A glorified League of Nations with teeth and the United States participating.

The Army has uncovered the German atrocities just at the right time to impress both our country and our delegates. Of course we dimly knew of their existence but as our own men were not involved there was not the justified horror which s ould have followed their exposure, but, now our ox is gored and what a difference it makes. We have felt none of the real impacts of war, even our casualty lists are of scattered people of whoah the individual knows but one or less, that makes it hard for the average citizen to visualize the picture as a whole. In fact the great multitude visualizes little except that directly before them.

April 27, 1945

Last night Ma, Ellen Fisher, Katherine Bordley and Mary Foreman Brown were my guests at the Kennels for dinner. The world was out there with his wife. Howard Smith and his wife were celebrating their eleventh anniversary; Winford Smith and his wife their fortieth and a couple score others were out celebrating the eating of food without paying coupons.

What great news comes in over every radio and newspeper. Mussolini dead, Hitler dying (or dead). What could be more cheering to lovers of liberty. Even our great victories mean no more to civilization. And they shot Mussolini, trampled his body and spat in his face. Three cheers for the Italians who did their duty. What a vain thing is glory and how insignificant is false ambition.

The whole country was raised to its feet by the untimely story of the surrender of Germany. Some even started celebrating before the President denied the story. With eleven million boys in the Army the story sounded like sweet music to millions of families. I have been fooled before but not this time. I waited for official confirmation -- which never came.

Love from Ma and
Your

Dr. James Bordley, Jr.

Col. James Bordley, III., M.C. O-596822   330 N. Charles St

Gen ral Hospital 18

A.P.O. 1002, c/o ostmaster   Baltimore -1, Md., U.S.A.

San Francisco, alifornia, U.S...   May 2, 1945

Serie IV., No. 46

Dear Boys,   Things are exciting and moving so fast that it is a tax to keep abreast of events.
Mussolini hangs by his heels, Hitler dead (?), a new resident of the United States , a Commission trying to arrange an organization to insure perpetual peace, a U.S. Army marching at
will through the land of supermen, Russia an ally of western capitalism.   What an era in
which to live, what a potent force, if properly used for the safety and happiness of mankind.
No human mind can figure out all the implications.   President Wilson once said "I do not
want to be taken care of by Government.   Give me right and justice and I will undertake to
care for myself."   He did not succeed in his und rtaking to bring about the necessary right
and justice but his inspiration is the greatest factor in the present attempt.

        And what of eace? Can we ever get it on a substantial b sis?   Yes, I think we
can but not on the foundation now being erected.   There are two possibilities: a respect
for the rights of others -- a Christian foundation.   For this sacrifice of personal selfishness even this tragic war has not prepared us.   The other way is force -- in other words
not the love of the Lord but the fear of the devil.   It is a waste of time to try to consolidate the 1945 world, to bring every unit large and small into a uniform system of thought.
Their ideas and ideals, their economic and political ambitions can never be amalgamated into
a union for peace. The three great powers must first trust each other and then together
demand peace. I know this is contrary to the avowed purposes of the war but that does not
altar my ideas of human nature and man's ambitions.   I hope I am wrong because as I see it
Russia and the U.S. are not pulling as a team.   I don't know which is right but I do know
that right now with the war still going on, with the soldiers of the two armies fighting in
harmony and together there is a growing mistrust of Russia.   Whether right or wrong it is
building a road block against permanent peace.   It is the first call for sacrifice on both
sides, for faith and trust and if it fails there will be no peace, only an armistice until
man can create more infernal machines and more plausible excuses.   It takes a good sport
with Christian instincts not to get mad if your neighbor hangs his laundry in your back yard
but without that sporting Christian instinct who is to make and hold peace?

        If the world would think more in the terms of human lives and less in terms of
material independence, I honestly believe we could gain both.   The whole question now is
what are you willing to sacrifice for me, not what I am willing to sacrifice for you.   It
will take a strong hand to settle this question -- in fact three strong hands controlled by
unselfish motives.   I am glad the President has put the brakes on a national joy party on
V-day. He was wise and gained many friends among thoughtful people. What a travesty it
would have been with the war but half over and our sons still fighting and dying.

        The family is well and waiting with anxiety to hear the glad tidings of your return.

                    Love from Ma and
                          Your

296

Dr. James Bordley,Jr.,

Lt.Col.John E. Bordley,M.C. O-403012   330 N. Charles St.,

General Hospital 118   Baltimore -1,Md.,U.S.A.

A.P.O. 1002, c/o Postmaster   May 8, 1945

San Francisco, California, U.S.A.   Series IV., No. 47

Dear Boys,General von Runstedt says air power licked the Germans.   My what punishment the
bombs inflicted.   In Neurenberg the American prisoners say the bombers killed 300,000 people
in two days -- and these exclusive of the wandering Germans trying to get away from the
Russians.   What a travesty on civilization and out at San Francisco they are arguing over
national rights and boundaries.   The Germans may be dull and stupid but they have no patent
in the claim, we are all in the same boat.

Well we went all out to lick the Germans and that job is finished and now we are
going all out to lick the Japs and of course we will but I look for a lively scrap if the
island fighting as any criterion.   They have been tougher, I think, than the Germans.

We have just had a most damnable thing to happen.   The announcement of V.EL Day.
The stores closed, the streets were filled with celebrators throwing confetti and now it is
announced it is not official. This is the second time in two weeks.   Somebody should be put
in a German concentration camp -- that is the top of my imagination of horrors.   This upsets
everyone and interferes with the business of war besides being an unnecessary encouragement
to people with relatives in the German war.

There was an announcement over the loud speaker system which is established all over
the City.   I thought it was the President speaking but I guess I was mistaken because I am
sure he would never make such a mistake.

That was yesterday.   Today the President read his Proclamation telling of the
war's end in Europe.   Thank God it is over and thank also the fighting forces of the Allies.
Five years of horror to satisfy the insane ambitions of a gang og cut throats.   Maybe in the
long run the world will be better off but today it has too many mourners for me to be gay and
full of frivolity.   The President's speech you may have heard.   It was but the plain statement
of a fine citizen, no oratory, no voice display.   I believe we will thank God for him in the
trying times to come.

It will feel funny not to hear the news we have been listening to and reading for
three years.   It will be sort of anto climax, but we will hear more now from the area in
which we at home have been most interested in, Japan.   The news from there has been all too
scanty   The world and the people are funny.   As I walked up the street I heard one man say
to another, "Well the European war is over.   Now we will get more gasoline and food."   Not
a word about the dead soldiers and heart sick civilians.   You see we are not yet civilized
enough to put our neighbors' distress before our pleasures.   Maybe it is better but it galls
me no little.

This conglomerate letter is a sort of sign post along our hectic road.   The next
will be more connected.

                    Love from Ma and
                         Your

P.S.-- Is it so John is Lieut.Colonel?

297

Col. James Bordley,III.,M.C. O-396822   330 N. Charles St

General Hospital 118

A.P.O. 1002, c/o Postmaster   Baltimore -1, Md.
     May 16, 1945
San Francisco, California   Series IV., No. 48

Dear Boys,

    Well you cannot imagine the change that has taken place here since V E Day. It hasall the propagandists working overtime to the keep the public informed of the fact that war is not over.

    The Public is already to start and it is going to take strict regulations to hold it in check. You see when the war in Europe ended Lend-Lease automatically ended in the European field. This was the law. In order to start taking up the slack the Government started licensing plants no longer necessary, to do peacetime work. This was probably told in loud voices and everybody expected to get what they have been deprived of for many, many mnths, and they started shopping in a hurry. This is bad because few consumer goods have reached the stores. It must be checked or we will get more and more inflations, so the boys are out in force preaching war again.

    To add tothe confusion, the word of General Marshall that we may expect a protracted fight with the Japs has been largely discounted by more optimistic commentators. This is bad because it makes it moe difficult to keep war factories going at top production because the workers want permanent jobs in peacetime factories shops and offices.

    I have been too busy to write often but as we are all well and life goes on as usual there is little to write about.

        Love from Ma and
            Your

Lt. Col. John E. Bordley, M.C. 0-403012

General Hospital 118

A.P.O. 1002, c/o Postmaster

San Francisco, California

Dr. James Bordley, Jr

330 N. Charles St.,

Baltimore -1, Md.

May 26, 1945

Series IV., No. 49

Dear Boys,   This is the first time I have had a minute to sit down and write for several days.   Work, work, work and Pop is growing more and more tired of labor and resposibility but on July 9th I go to Rye Beach for a two months' stay, whichsounds good to me.

Paul Patterson's secretary called up to tell us that he # Paul - had been toyour Hospital and he was loud in his praises of Jim's ingenuity and having such a fine Hospital built under so many disadvantages. He said in an article in the morning Sun that your achievement made him proud of his Baltimore citizenship.   The afternoon Sun also carried a short story. I thought it very considerate that he should have had your mother called up.

If the Allies would go ahead and shoot a few of the German overlords it would be a great relief to the pent up feelings of a large portion of our population.   Why they delay the pleasure I can't figure.   There is a vast difference in the feelings in this country since the publication of the pictures of the concentration camps.   The Japs are rotten but their civilization is a mere assumption, but, the Germans have grown up with and formed part of civilization. They knew better than to turn beasts. It is really astounding to me and it seems to pervade their entire nation.   I have seen not the slightest indication that they even appreciate the horror of the whole rotten mess that have created and there are plenty of indications that if given another opportunity they will repeat.   God forbid the opportunity -- I hope so as I have lost faith in the get together of the Allies for post war security. Maybe I am getting old and impatient.

I have started this letter so often, I am tired of looking at it. The rush is endless and exhausting.

On every hand you hear praises of the President. It begins to look as if he intended to make this country a pleasant place in which to live and further intends to cut loose from a gang almost as rowdy as that of Germany. He believes every man should have a chance to make a living and that every man should take advantage of that chance and having worked he is entitled to save a little for hisold age and not be a ward of the Government.

Sen. Wagner has just introduced a bill to make the Social Security tax four percent. Such fellows forget the income tax the white collar people have to pay and the living expenses they have to meet. To make them pay four percent. is a tragedy. If the money were invested for their benefit it might help in their old age but when the Government puts it in the pool and then re-taxes them when their benefits are due it is pretty tough.   When employers begin to pay their part of the new 4% there will be fewer employees. The average old age pension is about thirty two dollars a month. This is a help but not a living and for it the taxes are pretty stiff.

The family stays well which is after all a great asset and for which we have much to be thankful.

Love from Ma and

Your

Col. James Bordley,,II. M.C. 0-396822   330 N. Charles St

General Hospital 118

A.P.O. 1002, c/o Postmaster   Baltimore -1, Md.,

San Francisco, California   June 2, 1945

Series IV. No. 50

Dear Boys,

The world still moves on a ziggy course, enough in fact to affect one's mind. Now France, that did not have the guts to defend its own country, is starting trouble in the Levant. They want to be classed as one of the great nations but they fail to show ny sign of greatness. With a Peace Conference going on they start a little private war. They are a decadent nation and the sooner the real powers come to that determination the better. It is tragic they always have to be rescued at the expense of world peace.

Food is getting hard to get. Ma spent from ten to six finding enough for two days. Sugar, chickens, meat and eggs are almost impossible to find. That has put such a strain on fish and vegetables that they too have nearly disappeared. Ellen Webb said it had been weeks since she had any beef or lamb for the children. If you want t go into the black market I hear you c n get most anything and if you live in a small town food is not scarce. There was quite an article by one of the childrens' doctors deploring the fact that insufficient meat was available for the kids.

The O.P.A. has made a foolish ruling on the sugar for Baltimore. As we have the largest refinery in the world we are not permitted to get off-shore sugar -- imported -- then the Government came along and commandeered all the refineries sugar. It left us with none. Now there is a hell of a mix up because our canneries, etc. which use sugar in large quantities cannot even fulfill their Government contracts and the householders are without sugar. Honestly, Washington can do more fool things. It is because there are forty agencies covering every job.

The President has taken a hand in the food situation and has appointed a very able Secretary of Agriculture and turned all the supply agencies over to him as of July 1st. This is one of the many sensible things the President has done to get away from the terrible confusion of the prior Administration. He has also appointed a live person for Secretary of Labor with authority to act. This isnone too soon either if a man is to own his business.

The point system the President says is to apply to officers as well as enlisted personnel and is to equally apply in the Atlantic and Pacific areas. This gives you both a better opportunity for getting home. I have been told that in response from the War Department, Longcope h s requested Jim's return -- a privilege extended to all medical schools.

I had a nice note from Dudy yesterday in reply to a message Firor asked me to deliver. Charlie Waters gave a cocktail party and came to see me to specially invite me. Miss Everist wrote the date on a card and gave to me to keep in my pocket and damned if I did not get the date confused and only knew it was over when Ellen asked me if I had a good time. I have been trying to analyze what happened and why. Whether it was my age or just plain damned stupidity.

Dudy says Pat had a great little tea party and had a wonderful time.
        Everybody is well.
                Love from Ma and
                        Your

LT.Col. John E. Bordley,M.C.0-405012

Gen ral Hospital 118

A.P.O. 1002, c/o Postmaster

San Francisco, California

Dr. James Bordley,Jr.

330 N. Charles St.,

Baltimore -1, Md.
June 5, 1945
Series IV., No. 51

Dear Boys,

This reminds me of the June before John's wedding. Every night blankets, every day cold. Not so good for maturing wheat or growing corn, but darned good for older people. Had a terrific storm down on the Eastern Shore which blew things to pieces. This followed a day of 85° temperature. The same day in Baltimore had a maximum temperature of 70° and in Vermont a snowfall of some eight or ten inches, while in Richmond it was in the nineties. The weather man says we have had ten such Junes in the past thirty years but I don't remember but one.

I went to a cocktail party at Firor's with Ma on Sunday. It was a joint affair given by Firor, Eaton and (the boy who married Miss Treide). Not a large crowd, mostly the wives of 118. It was very nice and the Firor's were delightful hosts. They told us much more than we knew before of your activities and your possibilities for returning. None of the trio have yet received assignments and have no idea what is in store for them. Firor says it will take a general court martial to send him back to the Pacific, he thinks for a married man three years abroad is ample. They were to report to the Surgeon General sometime this week. You know they have a rehabilitation center in Asheville where they sent the members of 18 for recuperation for two weeks. Bruno did not think he needed recuperating. He is located at Fort Myers and gets home twice a week and has two week ends a month. I am afraid the near home posts will be filled beforeyou all get back -- although the Surgeon General told Bruno that the policy was to keep the returning doctors near their homes.

Walter Buck is at Camp Meade and he gets home for Sundays. One or two others are in nearby Pennsylvania and they too get home frequently.

Invalided soldiers are being returned at the rate of thirty thousand a month and I imagine some of the returning doctors will get assignments in convalescent hospitals. They have a great shortage of nurses but I have heard no mention of doctors.

I had a long talk with Paul Patterson. He was highly pleased with what he designated as your "remarkable hospital". Said it was the best he had seen. He was a bit dubious about your return as the General told him your ultimate objective was Manila. I hope you get out before the move.

Have to run.

Love from Ma and

Your

301

Col. James Bordley,III., M.C. O-396822

General Hospital 118

A.P.O. 1002, c/o Postmaster   June 6, 1945

San Francisco, California   Series IV., No. 52

Dear Boys,

      We are about to enter a new field; To govern some eighty millions of people whose methods of life and political vision find no counterpart in our national life.   We are not to do it alone but in association with at least one nation which is ideologically as far apart from us as are the poles from one another.   We are starting with a military Government, but, not as in the war, free from political interference.   Preacher Niemohler says no Democracy yet discovered will fit the German people as they prefer to be governed, have always been governed and dislike the political requirements of Democracy.   Well there are such people all over the world but it seems strange that there can be a whole nation of people who prefer political regimentation.   This would seems to make our task more easy but I wonder whether they will like foreign leadership after being impressed for some twelve years with the idea that they are the master race.   How can we distinguish between the guilty and those who would never have taken part except through duress?   Who can we trust and we mus trust many.   It looks like a more difficult job than the fighting where the objective was clear and all were equally our enemies.

      It is currently believe the Russians are systematically purging out the undesirable but do our standars coincide with Russia's.   In their one purge at home it was indiscriminately the intelligencia, will they apply the same standard in Germany?

      Well,I have just had my principal technician -- Mrs. John Bordley -- sign a contract for five years.   You see I cannot dispense with her services and as she was a bit worried about her job after peace comes, I just killed two birds with one stone by signing her up.   She insisted on inserting certain conditions but we need not worry about them because cause my conditions are secure.   That is she wants time off for certain family affairs but I made the time when her services were not needed; then she does not want to work for certain persons in the organization, that was met by placing her services directly under me. You see I am really pretty slick, don't you think so?   This business of an independent income enjoyed by the women during the war is really going to raise a question for certain husbands who have been enjoying Army salaries.   I have met John's dilemma even before he gets home.   Pretty slick, don't you think so?

      With love from Ma and
            Your

Dr. James Bordley, Jr.

Lt.Col. John E. Bordley, M.C. O-403012   330 N. Charles St.,

General Hospital 118

A.P.O. 1002, c/o Postmaster   Baltimore -1, Md., U.S.A.
                                              June 11, 1945
San Francisco, California   Series IV. No. 53

Dear Boys,   I hate to write today because I am pretty low. No, no liquor! In fact I have had only one drink, and, that at Firor's, in weeks.   I find that age and liquor play he hell when mixed in one's system.

Ma and I took dinner at the Elkridge and the Club looks more like the Army and Navy Club in Washington than a sedate old civilian organization.   Every rank was represented from private to general.   Most of them were just home from Europe and had their families along and the whole atmosphere was charged with happiness.   A fe places were vacant at some of the tables which added a very serious note to the reunions.   Most of the smiles and laughter came from the young women whose husbands had been away a long time.   It was heart warming to hear and see them.   How long most of them will be here I guess is problematical. If you listen to the optimists you would think the Jap was about over.   It is a prevailing opinion the Japs will ask for peace.   I don't see one thing to make me think so.   Their island fighting is too serious and too deadly to make me believe they are looking toward surrender. I hope I am wrong.   Senator Tydings is home and the belief is he beat it out of the Phillipines to avoid their political struggle.   I don't see what was gained by his trip either for the Philippines or the U.S.

Most of the critics think the San Francisco meeting has all in all gine a long way toward peace. They have ironed out their difficult problems and left the big five in control of the machinery.   Maybe this is good -- I think so in spite of the many failures to preserve peace through power.   I am not much of a believer in international Christianity. Gen. Isenhower says the Army is determined to preserve peace even if they have to fight for it.   That I think will be the only way.

General Patton addressing the Sunday School children of his old school, said: "This war is about half over but there will be others as there have always been wars since the world was settled".   Well, he has a knack for making the old crows caw and if that settlement fails him I will be surprised.   Even the suggestion -- made in California -- may result in his condemnation if not in his demotion.   The country is thinking peace -- or dreaming it -- and does not want to be disturbed by contrary suggestions.

Dudy is down for her dentist -- but I guess I will not see her.   She is taking lunch with Ma and dinner with some of her young friends and goes back tonight.   She says she and the kids are very well.

                    Love from Ma and
                         Your

303

Col. James Bordley,III.,M.C. O-396822   330 N. Charles St

General Hospital 118

A.P.O. 1002, c/o Postmaster   Baltimore, Md.
    June 14, 1945

San Francisco, California   Series IV., No. 54

Dear Boys,

    Bumped right into the middle of summer after the most wonderful two June weeks I recall. This is our first experience in the little house with heat. I am delighted to find it as cool as 4 Charlcote. You see we have done everything to make it warm in winter and cool in summer and it has paid in dividends of comfort.

    I heard a very interesting story by a man who was told by one of the Peace envoys at San Francisco why the Russians hold up the show and then in the end give in. He said it was the dual meaning of our words when translated into Russian. Sometimes the historical significance of the word is clearly lost in Russian. Most of the Russian translators are not highly educated and they confuse our meaning. This is very interesting especially when coupled with the gentleman's idea that the Russians want to be perfectly fair and are interested only in perfecting a permanent peace. He believes that with Japan a stumbling block to character of peac desired by the Russians they are certain to join us in the fight provided we want them? I think we do!

    You never heard of as many receptions and we get invited to all of them and I have a devil of a time getting out of some of them. Yesterday, Dr. Winford Smith's office called up and said Sir and Lady (somebody) were in town and that you had requested they be entertained. The Hopkins gives them a tea in a few days. I thought it would be nice to give them a cocktail party out at the Kennels and invite among others the returned 118s. We would give them a dinner but house is small and the supply of food is even more restricted. If they ere nice to you we will certainly be nice to them. So many people have gone away and the balance have so little gasoline you have to give them about two weeks' notice so they can save up. The returnees are getting some attention in the way of arties but not half as many as they would if coupons and ration tickets were not so scarce. You cannot buy any good liquor, gin or vermouth. I would give a war party but this country has never learned how to take it. They say in England a lemonade party was the rare affair. We have no lemons.

    Your friend Elliott Roosevelt is in the dog house again. "Borrowed" two hundred thousand from the head of a large corporation and at the request of the "Roosevelt family" the debt was settled for four thousand. A Congressional investigation impends but will probably not come off as it might embarrass the Democratic Party. I must say for that family they never lost an opportunity to profit by Papa's job and they did it in large figures.

              Love from Ma and
                Your

P.S.--I had about an hour with Dudy. She looks better than ever. Says the children are fine and Jim brags about his morals. We will see them up North before long.

June 15, 1945.

Dear John,

Last evening I went to a play -- the
enclosed program explains. It was very cute and
I can tell you that your daughter, Anne, has a very
attractive singing voice and your daughter, Brucie
can play a mean flute and has much poise -- inter-
spersed a little with twelve year consciousness.
After the play the audience was treated to a nice
cold beer and a very enjoyable time.   Playhouse --
the old Fisher mansion; head host, old Doc Fisher.

The Hopkins is entertaining the Lord and
Lady and their fellow travelers.   If they can
spare the time I am going to give them a dinner
at theClub, having as our other guests the returned
members of 118 and their wives and the wives of
some of the other members. To do this I will have
to petition the Board of Governors as they have
passed a rule stopping all dinners except family
affairs and out of town guests of the families.
There is no variety of food or drinks and we will
have to take what is served on the day of the dinner.
We could not possibly entertain them at home
because we have only a second rate cook, can secure
no additional help and have not the necessary
food coupons.
Ellen says you wrote not to spare money.
Wait until you get home and find out how little
there is to spare and how much it costs to meet
inflated values.   Boy, there is no extra cash
even for the rich.   Our property is all re-assessed
upwards, City tax rate the highest ever, State
income tax, personal property tax and a crushing
Federal tax on everything.   With a large practice
I have had to dip into my savings for several
thousand needed dollars.   I only want you to get an

305

idea what is coming your way when you get home.
We, too, are fighting a war -- the war against want.
So far we have had enough to eat but that is taking
a turn for the worse. Ask any woman who does the
marketing. There are a few favored customers but
the rank and file to which we belong is having a
tough time.

Love from Ma and
Your

Lt. Col. John E. Bordley, M.C. O-403012   330 N. Charles St

General Hospital 118

A.P.O. 1002, c/o Postmaster   Baltimore -1, Md.
                                           June 22, 1945
San Francisco, California   Series IV., No. 55

Dear Boys,

Well the Gov. General and his lady plus the daughter and Peter arrived yesterday. Ma and I had them for luncheon with eighteen others at the Kennels. If I do say it myself it was a bang up affair. It was on the porch. In the background were placed a British and U. S. flag. The place cards were on a little basket at each place. With the place cards were U.S. miniature flags on staffs except at the Governor General's place where the flag was that of Australia and at his Lady's place where it was the British flag. The table decorations were beautiful, in fact the most beautiful I ever saw. The predominant flower was the pink water lily. In the center the flowers were in an oblong dish about two feet long and at the ends of the table in round dishes where they were mixed with white and yellow field flowers. Instead of cocktails we served mint juleps made of fine old Maryland rye. They were served on the lawn with chairs placed in a circle around a round table filled with large pretzels and potato chips. This function took about half an hour.

The first course was melon, them imperial crab served in the shell like devilled crabs. With it were served broiled tomatoes (which greatly pleased the Gov. and Lady). Then a salad of Avocado pears followed by an ice.

The Governors of the Club turned everything over to us. The other guests besides those of honor were the returned Doctors and their wives and the wives of the un-returned, Dr. and Mrs. Winford Smith, Ellen and Charlie. The Governor's party went to the Hopkins on an inspection trip at three o'clock, they were given a large reception after which the Governor showed in the Hurd Amphitheatre two long rolls of New South Wales and New Guinea.

The Jones of Australia arrived yesterday too late for the functions and were given a supper at Dr. Johnson's sister's home. Ma and I were invited but we were too tired to go so we missed that function.

The Governor and his wife made a fine impression and I think they really had a very good time. They leave for Canada today but will return before going to England but not until we leave for Rye Beach.

I thought you would like to know so I write at once.

        Love from Ma and

            Your

307

Col. James Bordley,III.,M.C. O-396822   330 N. Charles St

General Hospital 118

A.P.O. 1002, c/o Postmaster   Baltimore -1, Md.
                                                    Series IV., No.56
San Francisco, California   July 2, 1945

Dear Boys,

Good old summertime?   Well with the outside temperature at 100° and the inside temperature at 98°, figure out why the good old summertime. I know you have had much of the same, I hope with less humidity.

The Navy has decided to take over St. John's College. It is the old story, give a government power and it runs roughshod over the people. There is not the slightest reason to destroy the old college, the Navy could move its golf course back a mile and give the Academy twice as much land as they get at St. John's. The Academy holds over the head of Maryland that if they don't get what it wants it will fold its tent and go to the Pacific. This is a bluff, they have too large an investment and have the place at Annapolis surrounded with too many traditions to think of moving. They not only want St. John's but as well a group of the fine old Georgian houses which they intend to destroy.

Just before the war bus lines north and south were carrying to Annapolis a half million persons a year and they told me that the people went to see Annapolis and incidentally only the Naval Academy.

We leave next week for Rye Beach to be gone until after Labor Day. My, how ready I am to go and how much I need the rest. We expect to see more of Dudy and the children this summer as Dudy will have a car. I hope it worksout all right. We can't take a car because I will not use my gasoline given for professional use and my tickets on my "A" card give me too little gas even if I ship my car which I would not because the freight space is needed for Army purposes. Barring the heat, the family is well.

                    Love from Ma and
                              Your

Dr. James Bordley,Jr

Lt.Col. John E. Bordley,M.C. 0-403012

General Hospital 118

A.P.O. 1002, c/o Postmaster

San Francisco, California

330 N. Charles St

Baltimore, Md. -1

July 5, 1945

Series IV., No. 57

Dear Boys,

Well the heat wave broke with multiple storms and for two daysthe weather was wonderful. It seems to be working up to another sweat now. What do I care? On Monday, the 9th, mother and I set sail for Rye Beach and I hope cool winds and a good long rest. I am really ready to call it a day. Where all the patients have come from in th past three years I don't know, but, come they have and Pop has tried to serve them well. It grows increasingly hard as the years roll by but I believe without them I would go crazy.

I saw Dick Follie, Sr. the other day/ He is broken, record of idleness, white bent and haltering. None of that doe me. I play golf, he has a hard time walking. I am still comparatively alert, he has to think hard and forgets much. I am his senioir by a couple of years. Some day I will die, but I bet I will have my boots on.

I went out to see the movie of Anne's wedding. It was beautifully done and the pictures were wonderful. The trick was arranged by Mr. Lycett, her new uncle. He has a lovely home beyond the Garrison Church, with a wonderful collection of trees. I operated on his two sisters some thirty-five years ago.

We hear a great deal about your coming home. All rumors, the origin of which leads exactly nowhere. We heard yesterday that George Shriver is on his way home. I thought that might mean an early return for others. I really think three years plus is long enough to be in a tropical and sub-tropical climate. We heard that MacArthur snubbed General Kirk and has taken full authority and that cooperation between the two is at a low ebb. Probably another rumor and certainly should not influence your return. Someone, or, maybe a coalition have tried to smear MacArthur for months. Knowing the Army pretty well I have some ideas why. It was clear from many of the comments that certain elements were working to have Eisenhower sent out to take charge. I think it will be hard to get such a scheme by the President. He does his own thinking and frequently talks out of turn on basic matters. He has no masters.

Ellen and her family are going to Atlantic City. I can never tell you how much Ellen has helped me. She is a real asset to the office and a mighty sweet one.

Love from Ma and
Your

P.S.--If you ever run across Pfc Earl J. Adams, say a kind word to him. His father is a patient and Secretary to Bill Hubner.

309

ABOUT THE AUTHOR

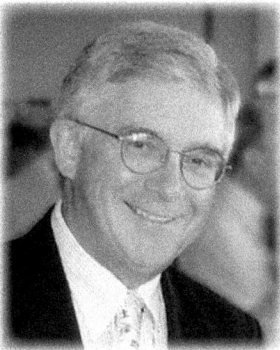

Charlie Webb was born in Baltimore, graduated from Gilman School, Trinity College and Columbia University medical school. He completed an orthopedic surgery residency at Johns Hopkins and served in the army medical corps in Viet Nam. Upon return he joined a private practice on the Eastern Shore. He has an interest in colonial history, served on the board of the Hammond Harwood House in Annapolis, and published an article in the Maryland Historical Magazine on an attempted historic restoration of Annapolis.

9 798822 928237